KEY ISSUES IN METHADONE MAINTENANCE TREATMENT

First published in Australia 1992

Available in North America through
International Specialized Book Services
5602 N.E. Hassalo Street
Portland Oregon 97213-3640
United States of America
Tel: (503) 287 3093
Fax: (503) 284 885

KEY ISSUES IN METHADONE MAINTENANCE TREATMENT

JEFF WARD
RICHARD P. MATTICK
AND WAYNE HALL

National Drug and Alcohol Research Centre
University of New South Wales

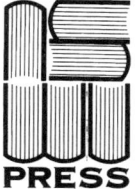

PRESS

This project was funded by the Drug and Alcohol Directorate of the New South Wales Department of Health

JW: For Kirstin and Isabel

RPM: For Susan

WH: For Pat, Tess and David

Published by
NEW SOUTH WALES UNIVERSITY PRESS LTD.
PO Box 1 Kensington NSW Australia 2033
Phone (02) 398 8900 Fax (02) 398 3408

Ward, Jeff.
    Key issues in methadone maintenance treatment

    Bibliography.
    Includes index.
    ISBN 0 86840 069 6.

    1. Methadone maintenance. 2. Narcotic addicts — Rehabilitation.
    I. Mattick, Richard P. (Richard Phillip). II. Hall, W. (Wayne).
    III. Title.

362.2937

Typeset by Character and Caps, North Sydney.

CONTENTS

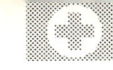

A NOTE FROM THE NSW DRUG AND ALCOHOL DIRECTORATE

ealth policies are intended to influence decisions about the design and delivery of services and the resources allocated to them. To achieve this health policies should be clear and authoritative; they should give confidence to service planners and providers in establishing or modifying health services. This confidence, in turn, is influenced by the extent to which the policy is perceived as relevant to the health problem in question and this is most successfully achieved where policies are founded on the best available information in the subject area. The key sources of this information are the scientific or research literature and expert opinion.

There is no shortage of opinions about most aspects of methadone maintenance treatment. Methadone treatment continues to be discussed as an ethical and even moral question, as a social issue, and still too frequently as a political phenomenon subject to a contest of wills and reputations.

Policymakers have a responsibility not to ignore the broad range of interest groups and issues which influence opinions about methadone treatment; however, they must at the same time avoid allowing particular groups or issues unreasonably dominate the content or direction of health policies. Opinions and practices about methadone treatment which are unproven, or which at best have ambiguous support from the literature, may become accepted as authentic over time if not called to account for themselves. If opinions and practices of this kind become enshrined in policy they are given authority and may therefore be subject to less scrutiny than necessary and contribute to suboptimal treatment.

Key Issues in Methadone Maintenance Treatment is the product of a project which had the aim of ensuring that health policies concerned with methadone maintenance treatment were based on the best available information. The core element of this information was the scientific literature and this was augmented by comments about the literature and clinical practice from experts in methadone treatment throughout Australia.

The New South Wales Drug and Alcohol Directorate, the State policymaking organisation for methadone treatment, commissioned the National Drug and Alcohol Research Centre (NDARC) to undertake a major review of the methadone literature. NDARC was chosen because of its suitability, competence and independence.

Nine key clinical issues were identified as requiring particular attention in policy review. These were:

- an assessment of the overall effectiveness of methadone treatment;
- methadone maintenance and infectious diseases, especially HIV/AIDS;
- the duration of methadone treatment;
- methadone dosage;
- assessment for treatment;
- the use of urinalysis;
- the role of counselling in methadone treatment;
- pregnancy as a special issue; and
- withdrawal regimens at the end of treatment.

This book is an essential resource for developing relevant and effective policy concerning methadone treatment and is also a useful guide to those involved in planning, delivering, evaluating and researching methadone maintenance services. It is indeed a solid basis for policy development, confident clinical practice and general progress in this field.

Danny O'Connor

Manager, Treatment Policy
New South Wales Drug and Alcohol Directorate.

The world seems split into three camps — those who know methadone maintenance to be good and efficacious, those who know it to be bad and ineffective, and a minority who are still receptive to new data and analyses of benefit and cost. At first glance it would seem that this latter group is the most obvious target population for this book. But more of this later.

There can be no doubt that a thorough and independent review of the literature is required. Despite the plethora of descriptive studies of methadone programs, and despite vociferous criticisms of the alleged legitimisation of private sin, it is extraordinary to discover that there has been such a dearth of disciplined study of methadone maintenance. If clinical research was an animal, then its backbone would presumably be the randomised controlled trial (RCT), with other forms of study perhaps being the attached muscle, flesh or flab. With methadone maintenance, what does the animal look like? There is certainly no shortage of muscle and flesh, but it must surely be concluded that the backbone is sadly lacking. Indeed the weight of other studies being carried by the feeble backbone can perhaps only be sustained by the uncritical faith of many of methadone's supporters. For the reader who is offended by this analogy and implicit criticism of the research community and their efforts in this area, consider the brevity of Chapter 2. Jeff Ward, Richard Mattick and Wayne Hall have looked extensively for properly controlled RCTs, and have been able to find only five studies. Extraordinary when one considers that methadone has been available for nearly half a century, and has been extensively used in methadone maintenance programs for a quarter of a century.

But does it really matter? After all, there are other areas of medicine in which treatments have become firmly established without the need for the scientific rigour of an RCT. But the reality of the situation is that methadone maintenance is not universally or uncritically accepted. For example, although methadone maintenance programmes might be widely accepted in many cities in the USA, Canada, the Netherlands and Australia, there are nevertheless countries in which methadone does not even exist as a tool within the armentarium. Until there is consensus about the observed benefit of methadone maintenance, it is beholden upon the policy maker, practitioner and researcher to pay particular attention to the findings of research studies. These people will derive considerable benefit from this book, enabling them to become more aware of the possible short-comings in their own present policy, practice or research activities.

Item by item, the authors lead the reader through consideration of the influence of different dose schedules, duration of prescribing, the role of urine analysis, the associated counselling and psycho-therapy and withdrawal at the end of maintenance. The reader is enabled to build up a composite picture of methadone maintenance treatment, with an awareness of both the place and the significance of different component parts.

At the opening of this Foreword, I suggested that the book may be most appropriately directed at the minority group who are still receptive to new data and analyses. On reflection, however, it may be that the more important audiences are the other two groups (those who know maintenance to be good and efficacious, and those who know it to be bad and ineffective) for it may be in these two groups that the critical perspective of the authors may confer the greatest benefit.

JOHN STRANG
Maudsley and Bethlem Royal Hospital, Kent, UK
May 1992

PREFACE

his book is the outcome of a project which was funded by the Drug and Alcohol Directorate of the New South Wales Department of Health in the form a grant awarded to Dr Richard Mattick. For the idea of a review of the research literature on methadone maintenance treatment and the turning of that idea into a project, credit should go to Danny O'Connor, Mel Miller and John Leary. The project was overseen by a joint National Drug and Alcohol Research Centre and New South Wales Drug and Alcohol Directorate steering committee which consisted of John Leary, Danny O'Connor, Pat Ward, and the authors. We would like to thank the members of the committee from the Directorate for their important involvement, and especially Danny O'Connor who made the completion of the project and this book possible. The National Drug and Alcohol Research Centre is funded by the National Campaign Against Drug Abuse which is an initiative of Federal, State and Territory governments of Australia.

As part of the project a number of reviewers expert in methadone maintenance treatment read and commented on the draft literature reviews on which this book is based. We would like to thank the following people for their time and for making this book much better than it otherwise would have been: Dr Robert Ali, Drug and Alcohol Services Council, South Australia; Dr James Bell, Prince of Wales Hospital, Sydney; Dr Edith Collins, Drugs in Pregnancy Service King George V Hospital, Sydney; Dr Paul Holman, Larunde Hospital, Bundoora, Victoria; Ms Jennifer Holmes, Drugs in Pregnancy Service, King George V Hospital, Sydney; Dr Keith Powell, The Royal Canberra Hospital South, Canberra; Dr Allan Quigley, Western Australian Alcohol and Drug Authority, Perth; Dr Adrian Reynolds, Alcohol and Drug Dependence Services, Queensland Department of Health, Brisbane; Dr Gary Swift, Eastern Area Health Service, Sydney; Ms Grace P. Thomas, Westmead Hospital, Sydney; and Dr Alex Wodak, St Vincent's Hospital, Sydney. However, they bear no responsibility for any errors that remain, and it should not be assumed that they necessarily agree with everything we have written.

We would also like to acknowledge the following people and organisations who contributed in various ways to the completion of the book. James Bell and Bruce Flaherty read and commented on the penultimate draft. Julie Hando was a co-author of an earlier paper on which the chapters on the effectiveness of methadone treatment were based. Andrew Baillie gave his time and expertise to producing the graphs. The library of the Australian Council on Alcohol and Other Drug Associations and Andrew Baillie and Pam Webster provided us with extensive bibliographies of their listings on methadone treatment at the beginning of the project. The librarian of the National Drug and Alcohol Research Centre, Eva Congreve, assisted throughout the project in ordering material and alerting us to new publications. The secretarial staff of the National Drug and Alcohol Research Centre — Libby Barron, Margaret Eagers and Gail Merlin — helped in a variety of ways towards the successful completion of the project. Allan Quigley's colleagues Simon Lenton, Richard Saker and Greg Swensen provided comments on some of the draft reviews. Finally, we would like to thank Amanda Baker, John Caplehorn, Shane Darke, Robert Newman and Wendy Swift who read early drafts of some of the chapters and provided valuable commentary, although again the authors bear the full responsibility for any remaining errors and it should not be assumed that they agree with everything that we have written.

JEFF WARD
RICHARD P. MATTICK
WAYNE HALL
National Drug and Alcohol Research Centre
University of New South Wales

INTRODUCTION

THE ORIGINS, RATIONALE AND OBJECTIVES OF METHADONE MAINTENANCE

n the early 1960s, Dole and Nyswander introduced orally administered maintenance doses of the synthetic opioid drug methadone as a drug-substitution treatment for opioid dependence. According to Dole and Nyswander, opioid dependence was 'a physiological disease characterised by a permanent metabolic deficiency' which was best managed by administering to the opioid-dependent patient 'a sufficient amount of drug to stabilise the metabolic deficiency' (Dole & Nyswander, 1965). The use of methadone as a substitute opioid provided a legal and controlled supply of an orally administered opioid drug which had to be taken only once a day because its long duration of action eliminated opiate withdrawal symptoms for 24 to 36 hours. It was claimed that high or 'blockade' daily doses of oral methadone removed the craving for heroin and blocked its euphoric effects, thereby providing an opportunity for the individual to improve his or her social functioning by taking advantage of the psychotherapeutic and rehabilitative services that were an integral part of the program (Dole & Nyswander, 1967).

Once methadone maintenance treatment had been shown to reduce heroin use and criminal activity (Dole & Nyswander, 1976) it quickly became the most common form of drug replacement therapy for opioid dependence. In the process of this popularisation in the USA, methadone maintenance underwent a number of important changes in treatment goal, dosage, and the extent of ancillary services that were provided in addition to the provision of methadone (Gerstein & Harwood, 1990). The treatment goal of many programs shifted from long-term maintenance towards achieving abstinence from all opioid drugs, including methadone, within a period of a few years. The average dose of methadone also declined from the high blockade doses favoured by Dole and Nyswander to the much lower doses that were required to avert withdrawal symptoms, and in some recent programs to doses that failed to avert withdrawal symptoms. Furthermore, under the exigencies of Federal funding cuts for methadone maintenance programs, the extent of ancillary services declined.

The proliferation of variations on the basic Dole and Nyswander model of methadone maintenance makes it difficult to draw strong conclusions about the effectiveness of methadone maintenance treatment from the research and clinical literature. As will become apparent, because these program variations differ in effectiveness, conclusions can only be drawn about the 'average' effectiveness of methadone maintenance. The variability in the outcome of methadone maintenance treatment has been addressed by discussing the characteristics of programs that appear to affect treatment outcome, namely, methadone dose, duration of treatment, and ancillary services.

An additional complication in drawing conclusions about the effectiveness of methadone maintenance is the variety of goals that it may serve, the relative importance of which may depend upon which perspective is used — that of the individuals in treatment, or of the community that funds many of the programs. From the perspective of the community, the major treatment goals are reducing illicit drug use and the predatory criminal activity by which many users finance their drug use (Dobinson & Ward, 1985, 1987), and preventing the transmission of HIV and hepatitis by needle sharing. The community also has an interest in improving the users' health, employment status and personal relationships, and minimising the spread of drug addiction by reducing the recruitment of new users from the social networks of existing addicts who finance their own drug use by selling drugs to others. Opioid-dependent drug users may share some of the community's treatment goals but give them very different priorities. The prevention of HIV and improvement of health and social well-being, for example, may be given a higher priority by dependent opioid users than reducing drug use and criminal activity.

The focus of this book is unavoidably on the impact of methadone maintenance on illicit drug use and criminal acts. Since the reduction of these activities was the main aim of methadone treatment, and the major reason why it continues to be publicly supported, the outcome in these areas is what has been most consistently assessed in studies of methadone maintenance treatment. The important role of methadone maintenance treatment in the containment of HIV transmission, which has been much less extensively investigated, will also be discussed. The focus on the goals of reducing injecting drug use and criminal activity does not mean that the patients' perspective on treatment should be ignored. Indeed, as we argue throughout the book, methadone maintenance should become more patient-centred. If this is to happen, future research on methadone maintenance will need to evaluate not only its effectiveness in reducing opioid drug use and involvement in criminal acts but also the extent to which it improves patients' personal health and social well-being. The recent development of multidimensional assessment instruments such as the Opiate Treatment Index (Darke et al., 1992) should make this task easier to achieve.

HOW THIS BOOK CAME ABOUT

n 1990 the National Drug and Alcohol Research Centre was approached by the New South Wales Drug and Alcohol Directorate to undertake a review of the research literature on methadone maintenance. The results of this review were to be used to revise methadone maintenance treatment guidelines. Nine key areas were identified:
- the effectiveness of methadone maintenance;
- methadone maintenance and HIV/AIDS;
- the duration of methadone maintenance;
- methadone dosage;
- assessment for methadone maintenance;
- the role of urinalysis;
- the role of counselling;
- methadone maintenance during pregnancy; and
- withdrawal regimens at the conclusion of treatment.

A full-time member of staff was employed for the following year to review the research literature. The method used to review the literature was a modification of the procedure used in the quality assurance project (Mattick & Grenyer, 1990) which in turn was based upon a similar project in psychiatry (Andrews et al., 1982). The review process for each of the nine topics went through three stages. First, the relevant literature was identified from a variety of sources: commercial computer data bases (Psychlit, Medline); a bibliography compiled by the library of the Australian Council on Alcohol and Other Drug Associations; bibliographies in papers collected from the literature; and in a few cases from papers provided by people working in the field. The literature so retrieved was critically read and a review drafted for each of the nine topic areas.

Secondly, the draft reviews were forwarded to an Australia-wide panel of commentators who had been selected for their clinical expertise in methadone maintenance treatment. These commentators not only represented a range of views on the practice and philosophy of methadone maintenance treatment, but many of them also had an active research interest in the field. They were asked to comment on three things: any important studies that were not included in the review; any errors in the interpretation of the research literature; and the extent to which the findings of the reviews conformed with their clinical experience. Thirdly, the draft reviews were revised to take account of the comments of the clinical experts although no attempt was made to arrive at a consensus of expert opinion in the process of revision.

OUR APPROACH

This book provides a perspective on key issues in methadone maintenance treatment for opioid dependence which is research-based where possible. The key issues addressed were the following:

- Is methadone maintenance treatment effective in reducing drug use, criminality and rates of HIV transmission?
- If so, what is the best way to deliver the treatment?
- What sorts of persons are most appropriate for methadone maintenance?
- How should patients' suitability for methadone be assessed?
- What dose range of methadone should be used?
- How long should treatment last?

- Should urinalysis play a role in methadone maintenance programs?
- If so, how should the results of urinalyses be used?
- How should programs respond to continued drug use?
- What role should counselling play?
- How should special groups of patients, such as pregnant women, HIV positive people, and people with psychiatric co-morbidity, be managed within methadone maintenance programs?

A research perspective has been adopted in which conclusions are based on the best available research evidence. As with any therapeutic approach, there are issues which have not been adequately researched. When there is little or no research evidence, we have relied upon the plausibility and logic of the practitioners' views as expressed in the professional literature. What is meant by the 'best available research evidence' is outlined in Chapters 2 and 3.

Not all the controversies surrounding methadone maintenance treatment can be empirically resolved. There are critics, for example, who have strong moral reservations about methadone maintenance treatment. The underlying basis for these moral reservations, and the bearing of research evidence and clinical opinion on them, needs to be briefly discussed. While we accept Hume's (1739) argument that statements about what one ought to do cannot be inferred from statements about what is the case, we nonetheless believe that empirical evidence has a bearing upon the evaluation of moral principles, as do many modern ethicists (for example, Rachels, 1986). This is clearest in the case of the moral justification offered for methadone maintenance by its proponents who argue on utilitarian moral grounds that the benefits of the treatment to both the patients and the community outweigh its costs. They accordingly have an obligation to demonstrate that it achieves its aims of reducing injecting heroin use and crime, while improving the health and well-being of a substantial proportion of its patients, and without incurring greater social harms. Some opponents of methadone maintenance argue that it fails to achieve these goals in that substantial numbers of methadone patients continue to inject illicit drugs and engage in criminal activity. Research evidence on the outcome of methadone maintenance is clearly relevant to an evaluation of these competing claims.

A utilitarian appraisal of costs and benefits does not address all the moral objections to methadone maintenance. Some of its opponents, for example, argue that methadone maintenance is unacceptable because it simply 'replaces one drug of dependence with another'. These critics often insist that all opioid addicts should become abstinent from all opioid drugs, including methadone.

Empirical evidence is relevant to the evaluation of this moral objection to methadone maintenance treatment for the reason outlined by Kant in the late eighteenth century — namely, showing that a moral obligation is empirically impossible, or at least extremely difficult to meet, provides a good reason for rejecting or modifying it. An appraisal of this moral objection to methadone maintenance is made difficult by the fact that the reasons why such critics find drug substitution so morally objectionable are rarely spelt out. Its appraisal requires a brief consideration of the possible underlying reasons for this moral objection.

The opposition to methadone maintenance is rarely based upon an objection in principle to the therapeutic use of opioid drugs (although one of the side effects of the hostility to opioid drugs has been an aversion to their legitimate medical use on the part of both doctors and patients). If the objection to methadone maintenance was simply one consequence of a general opposition to the medical use of opioid drugs, then the use of opioid drugs to produce analgesia for childbirth and post-operative pain would also be morally objectionable.

If methadone maintenance is objectionable because long-term opioid use may produce, or maintain, opioid dependence then similar objections would have to be made to the use of opioid drugs for analgesia in palliative care, and the management of chronic intractable pain of non-malignant origin. In cases of life-threatening illnesses and chronic painful conditions, patients may be maintained for months, and sometimes years, on substantial daily doses of opioid drugs, with many of them developing signs and symptoms of opioid dependence.

If the long-term medical use of opioid drugs is condoned, it is difficult to understand the basis for the moral objection to methadone maintenance. Is it because heroin addicts were not 'ill' when they began to use opioid drugs for their euphoric effects? Is it because they are in some sense 'responsible' for becoming dependent upon non-medically prescribed opioid drugs? A focus on the original 'blameworthy' reasons why people become dependent, such as the pursuit of euphoria, ignores the real distress and adverse effects of opioid dependence on the user's health. It is also a moral appraisal that is rarely applied consistently. Our community, for example, provides expensive medical treatment to deal with the consequences of behaviour that was in some limited sense 'voluntarily' entered into. These consequences include conditions as varied as: alcoholic liver disease, AIDS, lung cancer, heart disease, obesity, and sexually transmitted diseases. If treatment for these conditions is regarded as morally acceptable while methadone maintenance is not, the suspicion is aroused that the objection to methadone maintenance is based upon the prejudice that opioid drug users are 'undeserving' of treatment.

Whatever the underlying rationale for the objection to methadone, research evidence is relevant to an evaluation of the moral claim that abstinence is the only acceptable treatment goal for opioid-dependent people. An insistence on abstinence from all opioids presupposes that abstinence is relatively easily achieved and sustained by those who have become dependent upon opioids. This assumption is contradicted by the research evidence on the results of opioid detoxification and drug-free treatment, and the small number of studies of the 'natural history' of opioid dependence (Gerstein & Harwood, 1990, Chapter 4; Stimson & Oppenheimer, 1982; Thorley, 1980; Vaillant, 1966; 1973).

The evidence indicates that the majority of opioid addicts relapse to heroin use shortly after detoxification. Drug-free treatments attract fewer patients than methadone maintenance, have lower rates of retention in treatment, and lower rates of successful graduation to a sustained drug-free lifestyle, although they do reduce the frequency of injecting drug use and benefit their patients in other ways (Gerstein & Harwood, 1990). The evidence on the natural history of opioid dependence shows that the proportion of people who become and remain abstinent is of the order of 10% within the first year after treatment, and that about 2% per annum achieve abstinence thereafter (Wodak, 1985). While people remain opioid dependent, their annual chances of becoming abstinent are not much higher than their risk of dying prematurely from an opioid overdose or other opioid-related cause.

The difficulty of achieving abstinence does not preclude abstinence as one of the treatment goals offered to opioid-dependent people. Drug-free treatments which aim to achieve abstinence clearly have a place in the treatment response for those opioid-dependent people who want to become abstinent and some drug-dependent people also choose to enter drug-free treatment programs after a trial of methadone maintenance. But it is clear from the high failure rate of abstinence oriented programs that there is no compelling moral reason for insisting that abstinence is the only acceptable treatment goal for those who are opioid dependent.

THE PLAN OF THE BOOK

Section I of this book provides an evaluation of the effectiveness of methadone maintenance as a treatment for opioid dependence. It addresses the fundamental question: Do opioid-dependent people have a reasonable chance of benefiting from methadone maintenance in that their heroin use and criminal activity will decrease? If the answer to this question is 'no' then there is little point in considering how methadone maintenance is best provided.

Chapter 2 reviews the results of the small number of randomised controlled trials of methadone maintenance which have been conducted. In Chapter 3 the best available observational research evidence on the effectiveness of methadone maintenance treatment is reviewed. In Chapter 4 the small research literature which has evaluated the impact of methadone maintenance treatment on the transmission of HIV/AIDS among injecting drug users is considered. With the advent of HIV in the early 1980s and the rapid increase in its prevalence among injecting drug users in Europe and parts of North America, its containment has become a relevant outcome on which to assess the effectiveness of methadone maintenance.

Section II reviews evidence on the components of methadone maintenance treatment. Chapter 5 reviews the research evidence on the assessment of patients for methadone maintenance treatment. In Chapter 6 the effect of methadone dose on retention in treatment and heroin use is examined. Chapter 7 deals with the contentious issue of monitoring illicit drug use in treatment. This includes the role that urinalysis should play in monitoring patients' drug use, and the appropriate response to continued illicit drug use. Chapter 8 considers the evidence on the contribution that counselling makes to the outcome of methadone maintenance treatment. Chapter 9 considers the contentious but under-researched issue of the optimal duration of treatment. It reveals the fundamental division between two influential opposing philosophies of methadone maintenance treatment: the model of potentially indefinite maintenance on methadone originally espoused by Dole and Nyswander, and the more recent model of methadone as a step towards achieving abstinence from all opioid drugs, within a limited period of approximately two years. Chapter 10 deals with the question of how best to withdraw a patient from methadone when they have succeeded in stabilising their lives after some years of maintenance treatment, or when they decide to leave the program against staff advice.

Section III deals with a number of special issues. The novel issues raised for the goals and practices of methadone maintenance treatment by the advent of HIV/AIDS are discussed in Chapter 11. In Chapter 12 the research and clinical evidence on the role of methadone maintenance in managing the pregnancies of opioid-dependent women is reviewed. In Chapter 13 the special issues raised by the high prevalence of psychiatric co-morbidity among methadone patients are discussed.

In Section IV the evidence presented in the earlier chapters is integrated. Since the best evidence is largely American, in Chapter 14 we begin by discussing the degree to which this and other international evidence can be applied to Australian methadone maintenance programs. Chapter 15 provides an overall appraisal of methadone maintenance treatment by summarising the average effectiveness of methadone maintenance and the characteristics of effective forms of methadone maintenance treatment. It concludes with a brief discussion of the high priority issues for research on methadone maintenance treatment.

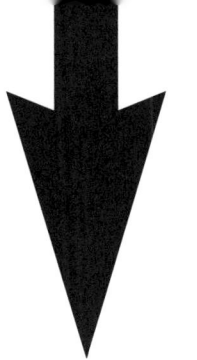

SECTION I

OUTCOME

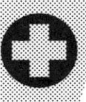

TREATMENT EFFECTIVENESS I: RANDOMISED CONTROLLED TRIALS

THE RANDOMISED CONTROLLED TRIAL

The gold standard for establishing the effectiveness of any treatment in modern medicine is a *reproducible* demonstration in a *randomised controlled trial* that the treatment produces a superior outcome to a relevant comparison treatment, such as no treatment or minimal treatment. The simplest type of randomised controlled trial is one in which people with a condition (e.g. opioid dependence) are randomly assigned to receive either the *active* treatment (e.g. methadone maintenance) or a comparison treatment (e.g. drug-free counselling). The evaluation of treatment effectiveness presupposes a comparison treatment so that one can discover what would have happened if the patient had received a different treatment, including no treatment at all. The aim of randomisation is to ensure that the subjects who are allocated to the treatment and the comparison conditions are equivalent *in the long run*, that is, over a large number of trials in which subjects have been randomly assigned to the treatment and comparison conditions. Only when the two groups have been assigned in this way can one be confident that a difference in treatment outcome is more likely to reflect the effects of the treatment than the pre-existing characteristics of the subjects who were assigned to the different treatments.

In order to minimise bias in assessment, both the administration of treatment and the assessment of treatment outcome should be conducted in such a way that neither the person receiving the treatment nor the person assessing its effects are aware of which treatment the patient has received. When this is not possible, at least the assessment of treatment outcome should be conducted by an assessor who is unaware of which treatment the subject has received. The measurement of outcome should also be of demonstrated validity, and a statistical test should be used to decide if any difference in treatment outcome observed between the treatment and control is too large to have arisen by chance.

The demonstration in a single study that a treatment produces a better outcome than a control condition is rarely decisive in evaluating therapeutic effectiveness. It is the ability to reliably reproduce or replicate such findings that establishes therapeutic effectiveness. The importance of successful *replication* of both positive or negative results derives from the possibility of making errors in the statistical comparison of the outcomes of the treatments being compared. We will falsely conclude that treatment is superior to the comparison in 5% of tests, and on occasions we will also incorrectly conclude that treatment is no different from the comparison condition. The percentage of occasions in which the latter happens depends upon the size of the difference we are seeking to detect and the sample size we use in our attempts to detect it. The more reliably a result is reproduced, the greater our confidence in it, because the chance of a run of consistent decision errors decreases dramatically as the number of replications increases. So, for example, if we always demand that the chance of our falsely rejecting the null hypothesis is no greater than 0.05 then the chances of obtaining five false positive results is $(0.05)^5 =$ 0.00000003125.

RANDOMISED CONTROLLED TRIALS OF METHADONE MAINTENANCE

There have been few randomised controlled trials that compared the effectiveness of methadone maintenance with an appropriate control condition. When methadone maintenance was introduced (Dole & Nyswander, 1965), the randomised controlled trial was not part of the culture of treatment evaluation to the same degree it is today. This meant that the opportunity to randomly assign patients to methadone and minimal treatment was only rarely exercised before methadone became a widely available form of treatment. By the time that methadone maintenance had become an important part of the publicly-funded treatment system for opioid dependence in the early 1970s, it was no longer politically acceptable to deny the treatment to people who might have benefited from it. Although it was still ethically acceptable to randomly assign opioid addicts to methadone and other competing forms of treatment, in practice it became difficult to do so because patients who were randomly assigned to treatments of which they did not approve, could obtain their preferred treatment elsewhere (for example, Bale et al., 1980; Bell et al., 1992).

Only three randomised controlled trials have been performed in which comprehensive methadone maintenance has been compared with a control condition over a substantial period of time (Dole et al., 1969; Newman & Whitehill, 1979; Gunne & Grönbladh, 1981). All three studies were undertaken in a context in which methadone maintenance program places were strictly rationed — a fact that made it ethically acceptable to randomly assign patients to either methadone or a control condition. More recently, two randomised controlled trials have compared some form of methadone maintenance with an alternative treatment over short periods of time (45 days or less). These two trials will also be reviewed. Randomised controlled trials have also compared variations of methadone maintenance treatment with one another (e.g. high and low dose methadone maintenance), or methadone with other forms of maintenance using synthetic opioids such as LAAM. However, these studies do not bear as directly on the effectiveness of methadone as do the studies that have been included in this chapter. They are reviewed where relevant in subsequent chapters (for example, on methadone dose).

Dole, Robinson, Oracca, Towns, Searcy and Caine (1969)

These investigators conducted the first randomised controlled trial of methadone maintenance in New York using imprisoned, recidivist opioid addicts who had at least a four-year history of opioid use. Thirty-four men who became eligible for release over a four month period were invited to participate in the trial, of whom 32 accepted. Half of these (16) were randomly assigned to methadone maintenance (of whom 12 entered treatment), and the other 16 were assigned to a no treatment waiting list. Methadone maintenance was commenced before they left prison and continued after their release.

Both groups were followed up at 12 months post-release, and only one subject in each group was lost to follow-up. There were dramatic differences in favour of methadone maintenance when outcome was assessed by rates of imprisonment and return to daily heroin use. Six of the 12 men who entered methadone maintenance were employed or in school, and three had been gaoled, whereas all 16 of those in the control condition had returned to gaol. Similarly, while all 16 men in the control condition had returned to daily heroin use, none of the men in methadone maintenance had done so, even though 10 out of 12 had used heroin since their release, and three continued to use intermittently.

Even a conservative analysis on the basis of 'intention to treat' favours methadone maintenance — that is, an analysis in which all 16 men who were originally assigned to methadone maintenance were included (rather than the 12 who entered treatment), and all subjects who were lost to follow-up were counted as treatment failures. The outcomes from an analysis by intention to treat are shown in Table 1 expressed in terms of odds ratios with their accompanying 95% confidence intervals. The odds ratios express the ratio of the odds of the control and methadone maintenance conditions returning to daily heroin use or being imprisoned in the year after treatment. The 95% confidence intervals indicate the smallest and largest values of the odds ratio that are consistent with the sample results.

Table 1 shows that the odds of being imprisoned were 53 times higher, while the odds of returning to daily heroin use were 92 times higher, among those in the control condition than those in methadone maintenance. The number of cases in each group are

Table 1: The one year outcome of the Dole et al. (1969) randomised controlled trial from an analysis by 'intention to treat'.

| | Reincarcerated | | Daily Heroin Use? | |
	Yes	No	Yes	No
Methadone	6	10	4	12
Control	16	0	16	0
Odds Ratio*	53.31		91.67	
95% confidence interval	2.71 to 1048.20		4.51 to 1864.92	

*Odds of control versus methadone, calculated by adding 0.5 to each cell frequency.

small which makes the estimates of the odds ratios uncertain, as is reflected in the width of the 95% confidence intervals around each odds ratio. In the case of daily heroin use, for example, the confidence interval ranges between a lower limit of 2.7 and an upper limit of 1048. Contrary to popular prejudice, the fact that such differences are statistically significant with such small samples makes the size of the differences in favour of methadone all the more impressive.

Newman and Whitehill (1979)

These investigators conducted a randomised controlled trial of methadone versus placebo maintenance among heroin addicts in Hong Kong. The trial was made possible by the late introduction of methadone maintenance treatment to the colony, which meant that people who were randomly assigned to the control condition were unable to obtain it elsewhere. The patients included in the trial were the first 100 male addicts who met the same criteria that had been used in the Dole et al. (1969) study, namely, they had at least a four-year history of opioid addiction, at least one failed attempt at rehabilitation by other means, and evidence on urinalysis of daily opioid use.

All those who consented to participate in the trial were first admitted to the treatment unit for two weeks and stabilised on 60 mg of methadone. They were then randomly assigned to be placed on methadone maintenance or placebo maintenance after discharge. Both groups were offered extensive follow-up counselling and treatment. The methadone group received a high dose of methadone determined by the patient (average 97 mg per day) while those in the placebo condition were withdrawn from methadone under double blind conditions. In the methadone condition, patients who continued to use heroin as monitored by urinalysis (more than six positive urines), and those who failed to comply with the requirement for daily dosing (by missing six consecutive doses) were discharged from the program.

Both groups were followed for three years and outcome was assessed in terms of the numbers retained in treatment. The differences in treatment retention were dramatic (Table 2). By the end of 32 weeks five of the 50 placebo controls and 38 of the 50 methadone treated group were still in treatment. By the end of three years the numbers still in treatment were one and 28 respectively (OR = 62.4, 95% CI: 8.0, 487.9). The reasons for discontinuing treatment also favoured the methadone group: 31 of the 49 patients from the placebo group were discharged for continued heroin use compared with only eight of the 22 patients in the methadone group. There were three deaths in the study, all in the methadone group. In only one case was there any suspicion of an overdose. The other two deaths were from causes not related to continued heroin use (although both deaths were probably attributable in part to the adverse health effects of prior opioid use).

Table 2: Results of the Newman and Whitehill (1976) randomised controlled trial at three-year follow-up.

	Retained in Treatment?		Discharged for Heroin Use?	
	Yes	No	Yes	No
Methadone	28	22	8	14
Control	1	49	31	18
Odds Ratio	62.36		0.33	
95% confidence interval	7.97 to 487.90		0.12 to 0.94	

Gunne and Grönbladh (1981)

These authors conducted a randomised controlled trial of the Swedish methadone maintenance program that was closely modelled on the original Dole and Nyswander (1965) approach. As with the Newman and Whitehill (1979) study, it was possible to undertake such a study because methadone maintenance was only introduced into Sweden in the early 1970s, and the number of places in the program was strictly rationed because of political opposition to methadone maintenance as a form of treatment (Grönbladh & Gunne, 1989).

The criteria used to select persons who were eligible for inclusion in the study were substantially the same as those of Dole et al. (1969), and Newman and Whitehill (1979), namely, at least a four-year history of opioid addiction, a previous failed attempt at rehabilitation, and evidence from urinalysis of daily opioid use. Those who were under the age of 20 were excluded, as were those who used other drugs, or who were facing criminal charges. The methadone maintenance program in this case involved substantial vocational rehabilitation during an inpatient admission of up to six months. All subjects who were assigned to the control condition refused drug-free treatment. The two conditions under comparison, then, were methadone maintenance in a setting of intensive vocational rehabilitation and no treatment.

This study differed from the other two in that it used a sequential design. Instead of assigning a predetermined number of subjects to methadone or a control condition, the trial continued until a statistically significant difference emerged in favour of either condition. This occurred after 36 subjects had been recruited, 17 of whom were assigned to methadone, and 19 to the comparison treatment (with two subsequently being excluded because they enrolled in methadone elsewhere).

The outcomes were initially assessed at the end of two years — the point at which those initially assigned to the control condition became eligible for entry to methadone. Twelve of the 17 in the treatment condition were no longer regularly using opiates or other drugs, and were either employed (10) or undertaking further education (2). The remaining five treatment subjects continued to abuse opioids or hypnotics, and had been discharged from the program. Only one of the 17 subjects in the control condition had ceased drug abuse; 12 continued to abuse opioid drugs; two had died and two were in prison (OR = 38.4, 95% CI: 4.0, 373.1). That is, at the end of the two-year follow-up, among subjects who entered methadone treatment the odds of discontinuing regular illicit drug use were 38 times the odds of doing so among the subjects who were initially offered drug-free treatment. The results reported by Gunne and Grönbladh among the treatment patients in their study were the same as those obtained among another 174 patients who were admitted to the methadone maintenance program over a 20-year period (Grönbladh & Gunne, 1989).

Vanichseni, Wongsuwan, Staff of BMA Narcotics Clinic No. 6, Choopanya and Wongpanich (1991)

Vanichseni et al. conducted a randomised controlled trial comparing 45-day methadone detoxification with 45 days of methadone maintenance. The subjects of the trial were 240 heroin injectors in Bangkok, Thailand who applied for detoxification and who had at least six prior detoxifications. They were randomly assigned to methadone assisted withdrawal over 45 days (the standard detoxification regime in Thailand), or to methadone maintenance for the equivalent period (average dose 74 mg per day). Outcome was assessed by continued illicit heroin use, as indicated by morphine positive urines during twice-weekly urinalysis, and retention in treatment. There was no further description of the treatment program.

Predictably there were major differences between the withdrawal and maintenance groups on both outcome measures. The drop-out rates by the end of the 45-day period were 66% and 24% respectively (OR = 6.05, 95% CI: 3.44, 10.62), with the withdrawal group showing dropping-out of treatment earlier than the maintenance group. That is, the odds of dropping-out of treatment were six times higher among those on the withdrawal program than those on the maintenance regimes. The percentages of morphine positive urines were 53% and 28% in the withdrawal and maintenance groups respectively (OR = 10.33, 95% CI: 3.40, 31.35). That is, the odds of providing a morphine positive urine were more than 10 times higher for those on the withdrawal program than among those on the maintenance regime.

The practical significance of the findings for the effectiveness of methadone maintenance is uncertain. It is reassuring, if unsurprising, that Thai heroin addicts who enter methadone maintenance are more likely to remain in treatment, and less likely to continue to inject heroin while in treatment, than are those who are placed on the standard withdrawal regime. But this is hardly a rigorous test of the effectiveness of methadone maintenance in retaining patients in treatment and minimising their injection of heroin in the longer term, which is measured in years rather than days.

Yancovitz, Des Jarlais, Peyser, Drew, Friedmann, Trigg and Robinson (1991)

These authors reported a randomised controlled trial of 'interim' methadone versus limited contact while on a waiting list to enter a comprehensive methadone maintenance treatment program. 'Interim' methadone involved the 'provision of limited services to patients awaiting treatment positions in comprehensive methadone programs'. It consisted of an initial medical examination, education about AIDS, and the daily dispensation of oral methadone medication 'to prevent narcotic withdrawal symptoms and to block the euphoric effects of heroin' (p. 1185). No vocational or other social rehabilitation or counselling was provided.

The subjects for the study were 301 heroin addicts recruited from the waiting lists of 23 methadone maintenance treatment programs in New York. Initially, patients were randomly assigned to one of three conditions: interim methadone; waiting list with frequent contact and urinalysis; and waiting list without contact. Once a treatment place became available they entered comprehensive treatment and left the study. Initially, recruitment into the trial was good but this soon slowed dramatically when potential participants perceived the one in three chance of receiving methadone as too low. The protocol was subsequently simplified to a two-group design (interim methadone versus frequent contact) and the duration of both conditions was limited to one month, after which all entered comprehensive treatment.

By comparison with the results of urinalysis, the self-reports under-reported drug use; therefore, only the urinalysis results were reported. These showed that the proportion of patients in interim methadone who had used heroin declined from 63% to 29% while the proportion remained stationary in the frequent contact control group (62% and 60%) (OR = 3.55, 95% CI: 1.86, 6.77). That is, the odds of using heroin during the one month trial were over three times higher among the frequent contact control than among the interim methadone maintenance group. There was no change in cocaine use in either group.

The difference in favour of interim methadone persisted when the partial results of the patients with incomplete data were examined (by using the urinalysis result closest to the conclusion of the trial). In this case the proportions of patients with urines positive for morphine were 36% in the interim methadone group and 60% in the frequent contact control group. Sixteen months after the trial the proportion of patients who had subsequently enrolled in comprehensive methadone maintenance treatment were 72% in the interim methadone condition and 56% in the frequent contact condition. Thus, the odds of subsequently enrolling in comprehensive methadone maintenance were two times higher in the interim methadone group than in the frequent contact control group (OR = 2.01, 95% CI: 1.24, 3.24).

This study illustrates the difficulties of conducting randomised controlled trials of methadone maintenance treatment. The need to entice participants into the trial, and to keep them in treatment, limited the duration of the trial, and hence limited the inferences that could be drawn about the effectiveness of interim methadone. As was the case with the trial of Vanchseni et al., the reduction in heroin use was reassuring but hardly compelling proof of the effectiveness of interim methadone. The increase in the number of persons who subsequently entered comprehensive treatment was perhaps of greater clinical significance.

SUMMARY

The three controlled trials of comprehensive methadone maintenance produced similar results: all showed that methadone maintenance was more effective than either placebo or no treatment in retaining people in treatment, in reducing opioid use, and in reducing the rate of incarceration. This is an impressive result for studies that have included small sample sizes, and have been conducted in three different countries over a period of about 15 years.

The two more recent controlled studies of time-limited methadone maintenance programs with a minimum of support services provide evidence of the short-term effectiveness of methadone maintenance in retaining patients in treatment and reducing their heroin use while they remain in treatment. Although the results of the randomised controlled trials are strongly supportive of the effectiveness of methadone, there are arguably too few replications to enable definitive conclusions to be drawn about the effectiveness of methadone. Our confidence in the results of the randomised controlled trials will be enhanced to the degree that similar results have been reported in larger observational studies of effectiveness.

3

TREATMENT EFFECTIVENESS II: OBSERVATIONAL STUDIES

OBSERVATIONAL STUDIES OF TREATMENT EFFECTIVENESS

In the absence of a sufficient number of randomised controlled trials to draw strong inferences about treatment effectiveness, the assessment of the effectiveness of methadone maintenance depends upon the results of observational studies of patient outcome. In such studies the outcomes of treatment are observed among patients who have assigned themselves to different forms of treatment rather than being randomly assigned by a treatment researcher. Observational studies of treatment effectiveness comprise two major types. First, there are comparative studies in which the outcomes are compared in persons who selected themselves into different treatments (for example, methadone maintenance, therapeutic communities, and drug-free counselling). Secondly, there are pre-post evaluations of treatment in which a group of people entering a single type of treatment are assessed at intake and at some time after treatment, with the effect of treatment being assessed by changes in outcomes such as drug use between pre-treatment and post-treatment.

CONTROLLED COMPARATIVE STUDIES

The major problem with all observational studies is whether the people receiving different forms of treatment were comparable prior to treatment. As a consequence, it is difficult to rule out the possibility that apparent differences in treatment outcome arise because of differences in patient prognosis prior to treatment. The strategy of quasi-experimentation (Cook & Campbell, 1979) provides a way of making cautious inferences about treatment effectiveness from observational studies. This involves three processes. First, plausible rival hypotheses are generated which may explain any differences between treatments in outcome. Of these the most plausible is that the treatments differed in the number of patients who had a good or a poor prognosis regardless of treatment. Secondly, patients are measured on variables that may predict a better or worse outcome, such as prior history of drug use, degree of criminal involvement, and severity of drug dependence. Thirdly, statistical methods of control (e.g. stratification and covariate adjustment) are used to decide whether these rival hypotheses explain the differences in outcomes between treatments. That is, do the differences in treatment outcome persist when account is taken of pre-existing patient differences? If the differences in outcome persist after statistical adjustment, one can be more confident that there is a treatment effect.

The inclusion of evidence from the quasi-experimental studies in a review of the effectiveness of any form of treatment is unavoidable, even when there is abundant evidence of effectiveness from randomised controlled trials. In order to conclude from the evidence of the randomised controlled trials that the treatment under investigation is effective, a quasi-experimental comparison is required to justify the inference that the people who have been included in the randomised controlled trials are comparable in all relevant respects to the patients who receive such treatments in clinical practice. Moreover, a refusal to accept anything other than the evidence from randomised controlled trials (e.g. McMaster Department of Clinical Epidemiology, 1981) would have the unintended effect of endorsing minimally evaluated treatments for opioid dependence. Given the serious individual and societal consequences of opioid drug dependence, the community will insist upon offering some form of treatment, and in the absence of evaluation by randomised controlled trials, the proponents of all therapeutic approaches have an equal claim for public support.

COMPARATIVE STUDIES OF METHADONE MAINTENANCE TREATMENT

Bale, Van Stone, Kuldau, Engelsing, Elashoff and Zarcone (1980)

Bale and his colleagues (1980) planned to conduct a randomised controlled trial in which the outcomes of methadone maintenance and therapeutic communities would be compared with detoxification; however, ethical and practical problems prevented random assignment of subjects to treatment. The result was a study that compared the outcomes of patients who selected methadone maintenance treatment, therapeutic communities and detoxification at 12 months post-treatment.

There were several distinctive features of this study. First, subjects who entered methadone and therapeutic communities were very nearly comparable, as indicated by a comprehensive pre-treatment assessment. The main reasons for this were that subjects were recruited from a common pool of potential patients (opioid-addicted veterans in the Veterans' Administration treatment system), and that staff from each of the treatment programs competed for the patients on conditions of near equality. All program staff had access to the potential subjects while they were in hospital, and subjects were encouraged to spend three weeks in the program to which they were assigned before they changed to the program of their choice.

Secondly, a number of different programs were represented within each treatment modality. There were three therapeutic communities with a variety of orientations, and two low-dose methadone maintenance programs that were compared with detoxification only, which was provided in the main treatment centre from which all subjects for the study were recruited. Thirdly, 93% of patients were followed up at six and 12 months. The results of treatment were therefore available for almost all who entered treatment, regardless of how long they stayed, and not just for the treatment successes. Fourthly, the 12-month outcome was assessed by an independent interviewer who was unaware of which treatment the subject had received, and efforts were made to validate self-reports of drug use and criminal activity.

The major results of relevance to this review are those that compared the outcomes of methadone maintenance with those of simple detoxification. The comparison between methadone maintenance treatment and therapeutic communities — which failed to find any difference between the two in average effectiveness — will not be discussed. The results indicated that the two methadone maintenance programs produced better outcomes than did detoxification when measured by reductions in opioid drug use during the past month, and the number of convictions recorded during the past year. Moreover, the differences in outcome between methadone maintenance and detoxification persisted after adjustment for 10 patient characteristics that had been shown to predict outcome.

A number of issues need to be considered in interpreting this study. First, the methadone maintenance programs provided in this study differed from that recommended by Dole and Nyswander. Both programs prescribed low doses of methadone and encouraged their patients to become abstinent from all opioids, including methadone. Secondly, the combination of a small sample size for methadone and the use of crude dichotomous measures of outcome reduced statistical power, and hence the sensitivity of the study to detect differences in outcome between treatment modalities. Thirdly, those who received detoxification only were entirely self-selected in that they consisted of people who had declined any other form of treatment.

Even allowing for these qualifications, the Bale et al. study provided evidence for the effectiveness of methadone maintenance which supported the results obtained in the three randomised controlled trials. The methadone maintenance programs produced better outcomes in terms of drug use and criminality than detoxification, and this difference in treatment outcome was not explained by the covariates that Bale et al. measured. In terms of the quasi-experimental strategy outlined above, this study provides qualified support for the conclusion that the differences in outcome between methadone maintenance and detoxification were caused by the difference in treatment.

Anglin and Associates

Anglin and his colleagues conducted a series of studies in California to evaluate the impact of treatment on the behaviour of patients in a number of methadone clinics (Anglin & McGlothlin, 1984). In each study, retrospective data were collected using a time line technique in which the interviewer went over a detailed chart marked with the subject's criminal and treatment history. After establishing the date of first opioid use and the date of first dependence, the interviewer and subject filled in details of opioid use, criminal activity, and other relevant outcome measures up until the time of interview.

The authors claim that this technique yielded reasonably accurate, retrospective information.

METHADONE VERSUS NO METHADONE TREATMENT

The authors originally set out to study a group of opioid-dependent people who were committed for seven years to compulsory inpatient treatment as an alternative to imprisonment during 1962–64 as part of the California Civil Addict Program (CAP) (Anglin & McGlothin, 1984). Of the 439 subjects in this early study, 118 later entered methadone maintenance treatment when it was commenced in California in the early 1970s. By this time nearly all of the subjects in the CAP had finished their first commitment period (Anglin, 1988). Among the subjects who did not enter methadone maintenance treatment, two groups were defined on the basis of their opioid use post-CAP: a group of inactive recovered heroin users who gave up their addiction during CAP treatment; and a group of active users who relapsed to daily heroin use. For the purposes of evaluating the effectiveness of methadone maintenance treatment, the comparison group for the methadone patients was the active heroin-using group.

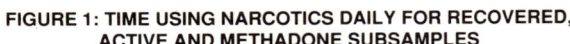

FIGURE 1: TIME USING NARCOTICS DAILY FOR RECOVERED, ACTIVE AND METHADONE SUBSAMPLES

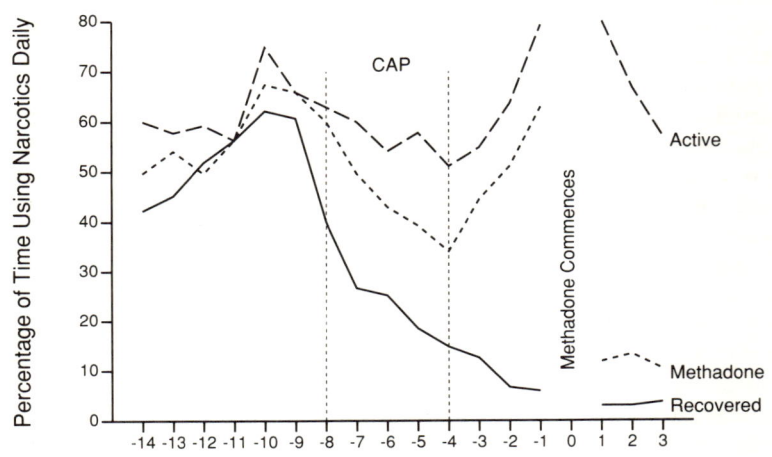

Years Before and After Use of Methadone

(Adapted from Anglin & McGlothlin, 1984)

Figure 1 is a graph of retrospective time series data that shows the percentage of non-incarcerated time that subjects in each of the three groups (recovered, active heroin users and methadone patients) were involved in daily heroin use. The two dotted vertical lines at 4 years and 8 years mark out the time spent in the CAP. The year 0 on the abscissa represents the time of admission to methadone maintenance treatment for the methadone group. For the recovered and active groups, the median admission date for the methadone group was used to establish the comparative reference point (Anglin, 1988).

The effect of entry to methadone maintenance treatment for the methadone group is apparent when compared with the active group. An increase in heroin use is shown for both groups just prior to admission, which was probably due to a dramatic increase in the supply of heroin in the USA at that time. Entry into methadone maintenance brought about a marked reduction in heroin use which endured throughout the three-year follow-up period. Although not represented here, a similar pattern of results was found for criminal activity (Anglin & McGlothlin, 1984).

INVOLUNTARY TERMINATION OF METHADONE TREATMENT VERSUS METHADONE MAINTENANCE

In 1976 the only methadone program operating in Bakersfield, California was closed. The nearest clinic was 70 miles away in Tulare. The closing of the Bakersfield program provided McGlothlin and Anglin (1981b) with the conditions for a natural experiment in which the Bakersfield patients could be compared to a group from nearby Tulare who were not involuntarily discharged from treatment. Follow-up interviews were conducted two years after the closure of the Bakersfield clinic. Overall, the Tulare group spent 73% of non-incarcerated time during the follow-up period in methadone maintenance compared with 8% for the Bakersfield group.

There were substantial improvements in heroin use and criminal activity reported by both groups when the pre-treatment and treatment periods were compared. In terms of the effect of the closure of the Bakersfield program, 60% of the men and 56% of the women became dependent again, excluding the eight patients who managed to transfer to another clinic. At the time of interview, an unexpected urine sample was taken, and the rate of morphine-positive urines was higher for the Bakersfield group. Of the 14 subjects who tested positive in the Tulare group only two were still on methadone. The Bakersfield group also had about twice the percentage of individuals arrested during the follow-up period when compared with the Tulare group. The overall outcome for the Bakersfield group was poor: 54% became dependent on opioids again, 73% were arrested, 61% were imprisoned for more than 30 days, and two died from drug overdoses.

Anglin, Speckart, Booth and Ryan (1989) conducted a similar study after the closure of the San Diego public methadone program, using a similar comparison group. However, the study found few differences between people in the involuntarily terminated and continuing methadone maintenance programs, largely because a substantial proportion of the San Diego group transferred to private methadone programs. Even so, it should be noted that the patients who did not transfer had poorer outcomes than those who did.

Overall, the studies reviewed here by Anglin and his colleagues include two reasonably powerful tests of methadone maintenance treatment: a comparison of the effects of the introduction of methadone maintenance treatment to a group of opioid-dependent patients with a no-treatment comparison group; and a unique study of the effects of involuntary cessation of methadone maintenance treatment with a comparison group of patients who remained in methadone maintenance treatment. Although the results of both studies showed the expected effects of the introduction and removal of treatment, our confidence that these results were due solely to the effect of treatment is somewhat reduced by the reliance on long-term retrospective self-reported drug use.

The Drug Abuse Reporting Program

The Drug Abuse Reporting Program (DARP) was a large-scale treatment outcome study that collected data on approximately 44 000 clients who applied for treatment at 52 drug treatment agencies in the USA and Puerto Rico during 1969 to 1973 (Simpson & Sells, 1982). The treatment modalities represented by the participating agencies were methadone maintenance, residential therapeutic communities, outpatient drug-free treatment, and short-term detoxification programs. Another category was created to include those people who applied for, but never began treatment. Bi-monthly status reports were received over a year for those clients who entered treatment.

Follow-up interviews took place five to seven years after initial assessment for treatment. A total of 4627 subjects were interviewed from each of three annual cohorts for the years 1969–71, 1971–72, and 1972–73. Treatment outcome was assessed retrospectively by interviews in which subjects were asked about their behaviour during each month between the end of treatment and the time of the interview. The outcomes assessed in these interviews were: drug use, crime, employment status, alcohol consumption, living situation, and further treatment episodes.

The findings from the DARP have been reported in a series of papers (e.g. Bracy & Simpson, 1982–83; Simpson, 1981; Simpson et al., 1982; Simpson & Sells, 1982). In terms of comparisons between treatments, patients in methadone maintenance, therapeutic communities and outpatient drug-free programs had better outcomes than those who went through detoxification programs or had no treatment at all (Simpson & Sells, 1982). This finding was apparent in the year immediately following treatment, and was still evident, although the differences had diminished, at the five-year follow-up (Bracy & Simpson, 1982–83). One DARP study, however, found that these differences in treatment outcome did not persist for such long periods (Simpson et al., 1982).

The finding of the DARP research that is most often quoted is the positive relationship between time spent in treatment and the post-treatment performance (see Chapter 9 for an extensive discussion of this issue). The length of time spent in treatment was predictive of improved treatment outcome for treatment periods of at least one year for methadone maintenance. In general, there was a linear relationship between improvement and treatment duration between three months and two years, the longest treatment period given the duration of the project (Simpson, 1981). The only other variable that predicted post-treatment performance was the pre-treatment criminal history of the person, in which case higher levels of criminal activity predicted poorer outcome in terms of opioid use, employment and crime (Simpson & Sells, 1982).

There are a number of problems with the DARP studies as evaluations of the effectiveness of methadone. The major problem was that the follow-up data on post-treatment outcome was collected retrospectively for the four years preceding follow-up. The credibility of month by month recollections of drug use over such a period is doubtful. Behaviour during periods closer to the follow-up period would be more reliable, but could be confounded by a number of unknown variables that may have nothing to do with treatment, as the authors acknowledge.

The Treatment Outcome Prospective Study

The Treatment Outcome Prospective Study (TOPS) (Hubbard et al., 1984; Hubbard et al., 1989) was a prospective study of over 11 000 illicit drug users who applied for treatment in 41 programs in the USA. The major drug treatment modalities represented by the participating programs were methadone maintenance treatment, residential therapeutic communities, and outpatient drug-free treatment. All the applicants for treatment in the participating treatment programs for the years 1979, 1980, and 1981 were interviewed about their drug use, criminality and other behaviour before treatment, and were then followed up during treatment.

The purposes of the study were to assess the effect of treatment on clients' behaviour, and to identify client and treatment factors that predicted different treatment outcomes. The key outcomes measured were illicit drug use, criminal activity, employment, depression and suicide. All outcomes were assessed by subjects' self-reports which were validated by a variety of procedures. An important feature of the TOPS study was the use of statistical techniques to control for the influence on outcomes of potential confounding variables such as sex, marital status, education level, age, race/ethnicity and number of prior admissions.

The study can be divided into two phases. In the first in-treatment phase all applicants for treatment were interviewed and followed up every three months while they remained in treatment. In the second phase, selected cohort subgroups for each admission year were followed up at three months, one year, two years and at three to five years after treatment (the length of the latter follow-up depending on their year of admission).

The results of the TOPS study confirmed those of previous studies in that all three treatment modalities were associated with a reduction in illicit drug use. TOPS also confirmed the observation that length of time in treatment was an important predictor of post-treatment behaviour for some of the outcomes measured (see Chapter 9).

Methadone treatment had the best retention rates of the three treatment modalities in TOPS. Patients in methadone maintenance treatment were less likely to drop out of treatment than those in drug-free outpatient and therapeutic communities: after three months, 65% of methadone patients remained in treatment, whereas less than 40% of the outpatient drug-free clients and 44% of the residents in therapeutic communities remained in treatment more than three months. At the end of six months 50% of patients were still in methadone maintenance treatment.

Patients in methadone maintenance substantially reduced their heroin use while in treatment, with less than 10% regularly using heroin (weekly or daily) after three months. Table 3 summarises the results of a logistic regression analysis which examined the likelihood of regular heroin and predatory criminal activity in the year after leaving treatment (or the past year in the case of patients who remained in long-term methadone maintenance) on the part of patients grouped by time in treatment. The comparison group consists of those patients who remained in methadone maintenance for less than one week. The numbers in the table are odds ratios which can be interpreted as follows. In contrast to the comparison group, odds ratios of less than one for each of the groups who spent more than one week in methadone maintenance represent a reduction in the likelihood of the outcome (for example, heroin use) and odds ratios greater than one indicate that the outcome is more likely. When the decreases or increases in the likelihood of the behaviour become statistically significant this has been indicated. The logistic regression analyses controlled for a variety of potential confounding variables and its results can be understood, in simple terms, as representing the patients' outcomes when all other important variables have been controlled for.

Table 3: Summary of TOPS findings on the relationship between time in methadone maintenance and outcome during first year after treatment expressed as odds ratios.

	Time in Methadone Maintenance				
	<1 week#	1-13 weeks	14-52 weeks	>52 weeks	Long-term maintenance
Outcome	n=86	n=161	n=268	n=137	n=183
Regular heroin use	1.00	1.16	0.83	0.47*	0.23*
Predatory crime	1.00	0.81	0.81	0.59	0.36*

(*Source*: Hubbard et al., 1989)
comparison group for calculation of odds ratios.
* p<.05

As can be seen from Table 3, a significant reduction in regular heroin use was observed among patients who spent more than a year in methadone maintenance but who had subsequently left at some time before follow-up interviews took place. Patients who left treatment within one week of entry were twice as likely to be regular heroin users as were those who stayed for a year or more. Similarly, compared with those patients who remained in methadone maintenance throughout the period to follow up, the group that stayed less than a week were four times more likely to be regularly using heroin.

Criminal activity was assessed by self-reported predatory crimes such as breaking and entering and robbery. Among patients in methadone maintenance, one-third reported committing a predatory crime in the year before treatment. This dropped to 10% during the first month of treatment. As Table 3 suggests, significant reductions in self-reported predatory crime were only observed while patients remained in methadone maintenance. Post-treatment criminal activity was predicted by level of pre-treatment involvement in crime but was unrelated to aspects of treatment. Methadone treatment, therefore, was associated with a reduction in criminal activity during treatment but did not permanently change the behaviour of the more criminally involved patients in the post-treatment period.

TOFS is the largest controlled prospective study of drug treatment to be conducted in recent times. It provides information on the behaviour of a large number of subjects before, during and after treatment in methadone maintenance, therapeutic communities, and outpatient drug-free programs. The use of statistical procedures to control for the influence of variables like client characteristics on treatment outcome lends more weight to the findings. The results of the study suggest that participating in methadone maintenance treatment is associated with marked and enduring reductions in heroin use and criminal activity.

PRE-POST-STUDIES OF TREATMENT EFFECTIVENESS

The interpretation of pre-post-observational treatment studies is even more problematic than the interpretation of comparative observational studies because of the absence of a comparison treatment condition. Inferences about treatment effectiveness from pre-post-studies are often made either by comparing the outcomes of people who dropped out of treatment with the outcomes of people who remained in treatment, or by examining the relationship between length of time in treatment and outcome. Such inferences are of uncertain value because of the existence of a plausible rival explanation of a positive relationship between length of time in treatment and patient outcome — namely, that those with the best outcome (e.g. who were the least dependent on opioids, and the most motivated to discontinue drug use) were more likely to be retained in treatment. This is a form of 'selection' bias.

The quasi-experimental strategy can provide a limited evaluation of such alternative explanations. First, the hypothesis that patients with a good outcome were more likely to be retained in treatment can be tested by measuring the relevant characteristics (e.g. degree of dependence, previous treatment history, and motivation to change) of those who do and do not remain in treatment. Secondly, if selection bias is operating, statistical methods (e.g. covariate adjustment) can be used to discover whether the relationship between treatment duration and patient outcome persists when differences in patient characteristics are taken into account.

Gearing and Schweitzer (1974)

Gearing and Schweitzer (1974) provided an independent evaluation of 17 500 patients admitted to Dole and Nyswander's long-term methadone maintenance program between January 1964 and December 1971. They identified four cohorts by date of admission, which defined changes in admission criteria over time, and a shift from inpatient to outpatient induction to the methadone program. Outcome was evaluated by changes in social productivity, arrests for predatory crime, and mortality rates.

The demographic characteristics of patients entering the program changed over the period of study. The average age declined from 33 to 29 years; the proportion of women increased from 15% to 23%; and the percentage of whites decreased from 40% to 32%, while the percentage of Hispanic persons increased from 19% to 26%. Despite these changes in patient characteristics, retention in treatment was high and relatively constant across the first three cohorts who had been enrolled for sufficiently long for it to be assessed, namely, 90% after one year, 80% after two years, and 75% after three years.

Retention in treatment was associated with improved social productivity, reduced crime and a reduced mortality rate. The percentage who were employed, attending school or homemakers increased with treatment for all three cohorts, although less so for later cohorts. The three cohorts showed similar decreases in rates of arrest with increasing time in treatment, namely, 6.5% in the first year, 4.6% in the second year, 3.1% in the third year, and 2.9% in the fourth year.

The only comparative component of the study was a comparison of mortality rates among 3 000 patients while in treatment, 850 patients who left methadone, 100 patients entering detoxification in 1965, and the general New York population in 1969 to 1970 in the age range 20 to 54 years. The rates among patients while in treatment (7.6 per 1 000 population) were not substantially higher than those in the general population (5.6 per 1 000 population) which is impressive given that the mortality rate among opioid users is generally higher than that in the general population. The mortality rate among those entering detoxification was almost 11 times higher than that of those in treatment (82.5 per 100C population), while those who had left treatment had a rate that was almost four times higher than that of those who remained in treatment (28.2 per 1 000 population). The percentage of deaths that were judged to be probably or possibly drug-related was 50% among those in treatment, 80% among those who died after leaving treatment, and 100% among those who entered detoxification.

Gearing and Schweitzer's study is uncontrolled and, with the exception of mortality, there is no comparison group with which to compare outcome in the absence of treatment. Nonetheless, their results are noteworthy in replicating the positive results for drug use and crime reported by Dole and Nyswander in their early reports, and showing that these positive outcomes were sustained over four cohorts of 17 500 patients who were admitted to their program over a period of eight years. The outcomes assessed were relatively objective, and the advantage in favour of methadone maintenance was substantial in the case of mortality where some comparative data were available.

Ball and Colleagues

Ball and his colleagues (Ball et al., 1988; Ball & Ross, 1991) have recently reported the results of a large-scale outcome study of methadone maintenance treatment involving six methadone maintenance programs, two in each of Baltimore, Philadelphia and New York, over a three-year period between 1985 and 1987. During the winter of 1985–86, 633 male patients were interviewed, and 506 were re-interviewed a year later about their drug use history, their last period of injecting drug use, and their past and current criminal activity. The initial sample consisted of 113 new admissions and 520 patients who had been in treatment for at least six months. At follow-up 388 remained in treatment and 107 had left treatment at some time during the intervening year. The characteristics of the methadone maintenance programs were also extensively assessed to determine if there was any relationship between program characteristics and outcome.

The findings suggested that methadone maintenance had a dramatic impact on injecting drug use and crime among the 388 patients who remained in treatment during the follow-up year: 36% had not injected since the first month on methadone maintenance,

22% had not injected for a year or more, and 13% had not injected in the past one to 11 months. In all, 71% had not injected in the month prior to interview, and the rate of injection among the 29% who had injected in the past month was substantially less than before treatment.

The results also suggested that some programs were more effective at eliminating drug use than others: four of the programs reduced drug use by between 75% and 90%, whereas around 56% of patients in the other two programs were still injecting. Among the 107 patients who had left treatment by the time of follow up, 68% had relapsed to injecting drug use. The relapse rate increased linearly over time reaching a maximum of 82% among patients who had been out of treatment for more than 10 months. Those patients who had been in the less successful programs had higher relapse rates than those who had been in the more successful programs. Overall, these results suggested that methadone maintenance was effective at substantially reducing injecting drug use among the majority of patients, and that some methadone maintenance programs were more effective than others in achieving this goal.

The reduction of crime associated with retention in methadone maintenance also appeared impressive. The study sample had an extensive criminal history prior to entering methadone: a total of 4 723 arrests, with a mean of nine arrests for the 86% of the sample who had been arrested. Sixty-six per cent of the group had spent some time in gaol, 36% having been incarcerated for two years or more. Although these figures indicate extensive criminal involvement, they seriously underestimate criminal activity which is better estimated by self-reported crime.

The sample admitted to 293 308 offences per year during their last period of addiction. Among those who admitted committing criminal acts, each person committed an average of 601 crimes per year (range 1 to 3 588), and had committed criminal offences on an average of 304 days per year during their last addiction period. After entry to methadone, the number of self-reported offences declined to 50 103 crimes per year and the mean number of 'crime days' per year decreased from 238 in the year prior to entry to 69 crime days during the early months of methadone maintenance. The number of crime days continued to decline with the number of years spent in treatment. In terms of the number of crimes committed, the reduction during methadone maintenance was 192 000 offences per year. As Ball and Ross (1991) remark, such a substantial reduction in criminal activity among heroin users is usually only achieved by incarceration. As might be expected, given the relationship between drug use and crime, some programs were more successful than others in reducing crime.

According to Ball and Ross (1991) and Ball et al. (1988) the more effective programs in their study were characterised by the following features: they prescribed higher doses of methadone and had maintenance rather than abstinence as their treatment goal (see Chapter 6); they offered better quality and more intensive counselling services (see Chapter 8); they provided more medical services; they retained their patients in treatment and managed to achieve compliance in terms of regular clinic attendance; they also had close, long-term relationships with their patients; and they had low staff turnover rates.

Two important points emerge from this study. The first is that methadone maintenance treatment programs differ in effectiveness. The second is that, on average, methadone maintenance treatment is effective for the majority of patients while they are maintained on methadone; they relapse quickly once they leave treatment. The fact that the sample in this study was restricted to inner-city males with long histories of dependence (mean = 11.2 years), and long-standing criminal involvement, provided a stringent test of methadone maintenance treatment. It is reasonable to assume that if methadone maintenance treatment is effective in this difficult population, then it would also be effective with a less troubled group. As was the case with the DARP study, however, there is some concern about the reliance upon retrospective self-reports about drug use and crime. In the case of crime, the study may have over-estimated the impact of methadone maintenance in that it compared crime during the last period of addiction with that during treatment. This may have exaggerated the difference between the amount of crime reported before and during methadone maintenance.

General Accounting Office Study

In 1989 the Chairman of the Select Committee on Narcotics Abuse and Control asked the General Accounting Office of the United States Congress to evaluate the effectiveness of methadone maintenance treatment programs in reducing heroin and other drug use. The General Accounting Office staff selected 24 methadone maintenance programs in California, Florida, Massachussets, New Jersey, New York, Texas, and Washington State which had at least 200 patients enrolled, and had operated for at least five years. They obtained data on heroin and cocaine use by urine analysis from 5600 patients who had been enrolled for at least six months in methadone maintenance treatment. This included all patients from 21 programs and a random sample of patients from the other three programs. The effectiveness of the programs was evaluated in terms of whether less than 20% of patients who had been enrolled for at least six months were still injecting heroin. By this standard 10 of the 24 programs were judged to be ineffective.

The General Accounting Office study confirms Ball and Ross's (1991) findings that there was substantial variability between the programs' policies. The programs varied widely in the frequency with which urinalyses were conducted, in the consequences of continued drug use, and in the average dose of methadone. The majority of the programs (21 out of 24) provided sub-optimal doses of methadone, as defined by the minimum dose recommended by the National Institute for Drug Abuse, namely, 60 mg per day (Schuster, 1989). The mean dose in all 24 programs was 48 mg of methadone per day.

Given these differences in policies it is not surprising that there were also substantial differences in patient outcomes between programs. The proportion of patients in each program who had been retained in treatment at six months varied between 83% and 4%, with an average of 54%. The proportion that continued to inject heroin ranged between 13% and 67%, and the proportion who injected cocaine varied between 0% and 40%. Secondary analyses of the grouped data by Newman and Des Jarlais (1991) suggested that the mean dose of methadone in each program predicted both retention and continued illicit heroin use.

Overall, the results of the General Accounting Office study provide evidence that many methadone maintenance treatment programs in the United States are relatively ineffective in terms of reducing injecting drug use among those they retain in treatment. Nevertheless, the results also provided suggestive support for the Dole and Nyswander model of treatment in that the treatment programs that used adequate doses of methadone had the best outcomes in terms of patient retention and the frequency of injecting heroin use in treatment (Newman & Des Jarlais, 1991).

A COMPARISON OF RESULTS: RANDOMISED CONTROLLED TRIALS AND OBSERVATIONAL STUDIES

The observational studies of the effectiveness of methadone maintenance treatment generally support the results of the small number of randomised controlled trials in showing that methadone maintenance decreased heroin use and criminal activity. These studies also revealed two other features of contemporary methadone maintenance treatment. The first was that there was substantial variation between different programs in outcomes as measured by treatment retention and continued heroin and other illicit drug use, which most clearly emerged in the studies by Ball and Ross and the General Accounting Office. The second was that the average results of methadone maintenance treatment in recent observational studies are not as impressive as those reported from the randomised controlled trials. For example, the retention rates from the randomised controlled trials are usually of the order of 70% or more after one year whereas the retention rate in the DARP and General Accounting Office studies is approximately 50% after six months. Similarly, the early randomised controlled trials reported very little continuing heroin use among those who remained in treatment whereas the proportion who continued to use heroin in the General Accounting Office study, for example, was as high as 67% in some programs.

There are a number of candidate explanations for the differences in the apparent effectiveness of methadone maintenance between the randomised and observational studies. First, it is likely that randomised controlled trials have provided a somewhat optimistic estimate of treatment effectiveness. In order to produce clear results, such studies usually exclude some of the more difficult patients from entry, and they often have greater degree of control over the quality of the treatment that is provided than usually occurs under the ordinary exigencies of clinical practice. In addition, in many of the initial randomised controlled trials, patients who were denied access to methadone maintenance treatment were unlikely to receive it or any other form of treatment elsewhere. The comparison of methadone maintenance treatment with control treatment in such studies was not attenuated by the effects of treatment obtained elsewhere, as has more often been the case in recent observational studies, such as that of Bale and his colleagues.

Secondly, there is clear evidence that many current methadone maintenance treatment programs in the USA (and, as we shall see, in Australia) have departed from the original model of Dole and Nyswarder in directions that are likely to reduce average effectiveness. As the data presented by D'Aunno and Vaughn (1992) and in the General Accounting Office report show, many programs have reduced average methadone dose and put pressure on patients to become abstinent from all opioids, including methadone. There has also been a wide variation in the practices that different programs follow, and an absence of any interest in evaluating their impact on treatment outcome.

Thirdly, there have been important historical changes in patterns of illicit drug use between the time when methadone was introduced and when the more recent observational studies were conducted. The most obvious of these has been the spread of poly-drug use among people presenting for treatment. In the USA, cocaine use in particular has become widespread among methadone patients. Methadone has no specific effects on cocaine use, neither blocking the effects of cocaine nor avoiding withdrawal symptoms, so it has had minimal impact on the use of non-opioid illicit drugs.

Fourthly, the context within which methadone maintenance treatment has been provided has changed dramatically in the past 20 years. The Federal financial support for methadone maintenance treatment in the mid-1970s has given way in the USA to fiscal restraint on program budgets with consequent reductions in the quality of treatment services, and to a steady decline in the number of treatment places on methadone maintenance, with no new clinics having opened during the past 10 years. This decline in the quantity and quality of treatment in the USA has been accompanied by an increase in Federal government regulations that have encouraged the reduction in average methadone dose and the introduction of time limits (usually two years) on treatment.

SUMMARY

The findings of the comparative observational studies of methadone maintenance are consistent with the results of the small number of randomised controlled trials in showing that methadone maintenance retained patients in treatment and substantially reduced illicit opioid drug use and involvement in criminal activity in comparison with those patients who did not enter treatment. The pre-post-studies generally agree with the results of the comparative studies in showing that the longer patients remain in treatment, the less likely they are to inject heroin or to engage in criminal activity. In those studies that have used a quasi-experimental strategy to evaluate rival explanations, these results have proved robust.

The observational studies also indicate that there is substantial variation between different programs in their effectiveness in retaining patients in treatment, and reducing their drug use and criminality while they are in treatment. Analyses of the characteristics that predict the variations between programs in retention, drug use and criminality have generally supported the original model of Dole and Nyswander in showing that programs with higher doses, a maintenance goal and ancillary services have better outcomes than programs that use lower doses and aim to achieve abstinence.

The *average* effects of methadone maintenance treatment in the observational studies have been lower than those observed in the randomised controlled trials. Among the more important reasons that can be identified for the decline in the average effectiveness of methadone maintenance have been: a systematic departure from the model of methadone maintenance proposed by Dole and Nyswander in the direction of lower dose and time-limited treatment; a decline in the quality of methadone maintenance programs in the face of fiscal restraint and federal regulations in the USA; and changes in the patient population of methadone maintenance treatment programs with the rise in poly-drug use.

TREATMENT EFFECTIVENESS III: AIDS AND OTHER INFECTIOUS DISEASES

INTRODUCTION

An important aspect of the effectiveness of methadone maintenance (MM) is the extent to which it prevents the spread of infectious diseases among injecting drug users. The massive expansion of methadone maintenance programs in Australia and other countries in the latter half of the 1980s has taken place as an attempt to prevent the rapid increases that have been seen in some major urban centres throughout the world (e.g. New York, Edinburgh, Milan, Bangkok) in rates of infection with the human immunodeficiency virus (HIV) among injecting drug users. The two variants of the human immunodeficiency virus are known as HIV-1 and HIV-2. The most common variant infecting drug users throughout the world is HIV-1, although HIV-2 infection, which is more common in African countries, has also been reported (for a full discussion see Grmek, 1990). In this book, we use the generic term HIV which, at the time of writing, means HIV-1.

Although they have received less attention, other infectious diseases such as hepatitis B and C are also important in any consideration of protecting the health of drug injectors. For an interesting account of why the hepatitis B epidemic received much less attention than HIV see Muraskin (1988). Our discussion will focus on HIV because there is a large and rapidly growing literature on this topic. While the acquired immune deficiency syndrome (AIDS) poses a public health problem without precedent in recent times, we emphasise that it is only one of a number of serious health consequences associated with illicit drug use (Selwyn, 1991; Selwyn et al., 1989b). A more detailed description of the health consequences of injecting drug use is given in Chapter 5 where we consider ways in which harm associated with opioid dependence might be assessed.

In this chapter we outline the basic facts about HIV and AIDS, and the epidemiology of HIV infection among injecting drug users. We then review the research to date on what is known about the sharing of injecting equipment and unprotected sex which are the specific risk behaviours associated with HIV transmission in this group. Finally, we consider the evidence for the effectiveness of methadone maintenance treatment in preventing HIV infection among injecting drug users and its further spread to other sectors of the community. As will be seen from this evidence, there is good reason to believe that methadone maintenance is the best available treatment option for preventing HIV infection among opioid-dependent drug users. The implications of the advent of HIV and AIDS for methadone maintenance treatment are discussed in Chapter 11.

THE ACQUIRED IMMUNE DEFICIENCY SYNDROME

AIDS results from a person being infected with HIV. After being infected with HIV, the first clinical manifestation, known as seroconversion illness or acute HIV syndrome, usually occurs after a period of 3–6 weeks and consists of a relatively mild illness of brief duration, the symptoms of which include fever, sore throat, swollen lymph nodes, night sweats and headaches. This acute HIV syndrome is usually followed by a period during which few or no symptoms are observed. After this latency period, which varies between one and ten or more years, a progressive deterioration of immune functioning is observed which manifests itself in a variety of infections which are usually resisted by a healthy individual. As Sobel (1991) points out, it is too early in the course of the epidemic for the maximum length of the latency period to have been determined.

Although the clinical course is different in each case, some people may develop a series of relatively minor infections like oral thrush or candidiasis, and a range of other symptoms, typically fatigue and weight loss, as their immune system progressively loses its capacity to resist infection. A person is said to have AIDS when they manifest one of a number of serious illnesses such as pneumocystis pneumonia or Kaposi's sarcoma. Death usually results from a combination of such infections (for more detail about the clinical manifestations of AIDS among injecting drug users see Glasner & Kaslow 1990; McCutchan, 1990; Sobel, 1991).

AIDS first came to the attention of physicians in Los Angeles and New York in 1980, although it has now been established through retrospective searching of medical records and testing of stored sera that there were cases before 1980. Epidemiological research to date suggests that HIV has been present in human populations for some time, but that a number of societal and technological changes have created the conditions for its global epidemic spread. According to Grmek (1990), these changes include: the invention of the hypodermic syringe; the discovery of blood types early this century and the ensuing ability to transfuse blood; the increase in international travel afforded by developments in transport; and the liberalisation of sexual life and drug use during the 1960s. At the time of writing, infection with HIV has been reported among injecting drug users in 30 countries throughout the world (Des Jarlais, 1992a).

The Epidemiology of HIV Among Injecting Drug Users

There are three main modes of transmission of HIV: through the introduction of HIV-infected blood or blood products into the body by practices such as transfusing blood products and injecting with HIV-contaminated needles and syringes; through the exchange of HIV-infected body fluids during unprotected sex; and by being passed from mother to child during pregnancy or birth, and perhaps via breast milk during feeding (Glasner & Kaslow, 1990). Certain practices such as sharing injection equipment and unprotected sexual intercourse have been shown to be important risk factors in the spread of HIV (Turner et al., 1989).

After homosexual men, injecting drug users constitute the second largest infected group in most Western countries, and in some countries (e.g. Italy and Spain) are the largest group (Friedman & Des Jarlais, 1991). As a group, they are potentially at risk for both sexual and parenteral HIV transmission. Their sexual partners are at risk if they practise unsafe sex, and children born of these relationships are also at risk for perinatal transmission. As will be seen below, there is ample evidence to suggest that injecting drug users are a potential source for HIV infection for the non-injecting drug-using population via sexual transmission of the virus.

Des Jarlais et al. (1989) have divided the introduction of HIV into a defined risk group into three phases: an *introductory phase* in which HIV is introduced and begins to spread; a *rapid spreading phase* during which the virus spreads rapidly among the group members (if facilitating conditions exist); and a *stabilisation phase* during which the incidence of HIV infection levels out. In New York, for example, HIV was probably introduced among injecting drug users as early as 1975. After that, the incidence of HIV increased slowly until 1978 (introductory phase), when it spread rapidly among the group until 1981 (rapid spreading phase), after which the rates of HIV infection levelled out. During the rapid spreading phase, the percentage of infected drug users went from approximately 20% to 50% (Des Jarlais et al., 1989). The seroprevalence rate has since remained at around 50–60%. Similar rates of spread among injecting drug users have been observed in many other areas throughout the world (see Des Jarlais, 1992a). Des Jarlais et al. (1989) have argued that it is important that attempts to prevent the spread of HIV be put in place before the onset of this rapid spreading phase, because it appears that once infection reaches a critical level in a given population of drug injectors, and given the right conditions, it only takes a short period of time for it to reach epidemic proportions.

According to Des Jarlais (1992a), two conditions that allow for the rapid spread of HIV are: a) low levels of appreciation of the risks associated with AIDS and injecting behaviour; and b) frequent sharing of injecting equipment with multiple sharing partners, such as occurs in 'shooting galleries' and the houses of drug dealers who provide injecting equipment at the time of purchase. Friedman and Des Jarlais (1991) have noted that those areas where HIV has spread most rapidly are those where heroin is the major drug of injection, though they also note that this may simply be due to a lack of information about the epidemiology of HIV among injecting drug users in countries where cocaine is the major drug of injection.

Rapid spread of HIV is by no means inevitable. In some cities, infection rates appear to have stabilised at much lower levels (e.g. San Francisco where it remains at around 12%). Friedman and Des Jarlais (1991) suggest a number of reasons why these differences have occurred: the differential effectiveness of HIV prevention efforts; the extent to which injecting drug users have changed their risk behaviours; the time at which HIV was introduced to a given population of drug users and, more critically, its relationship to the discovery of the transmission characteristics of the virus and the ensuing risk reduction campaigns; and local variations in the rituals and lifestyle associated with drug injecting.

Socio-economic factors and ethnicity are important in any characterisation of the HIV epidemic among injecting drug users. In the USA, for example, black and Hispanic users have far higher rates of HIV infection than do white drug users (Friedland, 1989). The association between membership in these two groups and socio-economic deprivation is important. As Friedman and Des Jarlais (1991) observe, socio-economic disadvantage is not only a discernible risk factor for HIV infection but for injecting drug use as well. Ultimately, reducing injecting drug use, and therefore risk of HIV infection, among disadvantaged populations requires larger scale interventions than drug treatment programs can offer.

In Australia, HIV infection among injecting drug users has been surveyed in a number of ways. Wodak et al. (1987) in a study to determine the presence of HIV antibodies in needles and syringes exchanged in Sydney in late 1986 and early 1987 found that 1% contained infected blood. In a similar study conducted in the same city during July and August 1987, 3% of the syringes returned were found to be contaminated (Wolk et al., 1988). More recent estimates suggest that around 3% to 6% of injecting drug users in urban centres in Australia are HIV seropositive (Darke et al., 1992; Morlet et al., 1990; Ross et al., 1991). Finally, 4% of reported AIDS cases in Australia have injecting drug use identified as a risk factor (National Centre on HIV Epidemiology and Clinical Research, 1991).

There is as yet no cure for AIDS. The only means available to deal with HIV, therefore, is by eliminating or modifying the risk behaviours involved in its transmission (Becker & Joseph, 1988; Kelly & Murphy, 1991). In the case of injecting drug use, these changes amount either to abstinence or, if that goal is not feasible, to either changing the route of ingestion of the drug (say to smoking or swallowing) or to safer injecting, which means not sharing injecting equipment or properly cleaning this equipment if the user continues to share. As Becker and Joseph (1988) have pointed out, abstinence for life might seem an attractive option, but encouraging modification of injecting practices is more likely to be effective for many drug users. They argue that the consequences of not adopting measures that take into account likely behaviour change could be disastrous. It is possible that a limited number of quite active, infected individuals could maintain and perhaps increase the incidence of infection among injecting drug users.

Methadone maintenance is an intervention that takes into

account what is achievable with this population. It provides an orally ingested alternative to injected opioids such as heroin, which makes it an attractive option for opioid users who are not prepared, or who are unable, to become abstinent. This means that a reduction is achieved in the risks associated with the use of opioids without requiring abstinence on the part of the drug user. Other advantages are that methadone maintenance programs can also function as dissemination points for education about HIV and AIDS and provide contact with the health care system for those injecting drug users who are already infected.

HIV RISK BEHAVIOURS: INJECTING AND NEEDLE SHARING

HIV is transmitted via injecting drug use through the sharing of injection equipment that has been contaminated with HIV-infected blood. As we have already stated, needle sharing has been and remains a common practice among injecting drug users, albeit at a lower prevalence than was the case before HIV. With the advent of HIV and the ensuing public health campaigns to reduce HIV risk-taking behaviours, reductions in needle sharing have been reported in both the USA and in Europe (e.g. Des Jarlais et al., 1989; Durante. 1991; Harris et al., 1990; Käll & Olin, 1990; Klee et al., 1990a; Power et al., 1988; Ronald et al., 1992; Selwyn et al., 1987). Contrary to popular images of being irresponsible, out-of-control individuals, injecting drug users have responded positively to AIDS awareness and risk reduction campaigns (Friedland, 1989). However, as the evidence below shows, some drug users continue to share needles and therefore continue to expose themselves and others to the risk of being infected. In this section, we consider under what circumstances injecting risk behaviours occur and what, if anything, can be said about those users who continue to engage in these risk behaviours.

In Australia, studies that have surveyed the needle sharing practices of injecting drug users have found it to be a common practice. Morlet et al. (1990), in a survey of users attending the Albion Street (AIDS) Centre in Sydney, found that 87% of the sample had shared injecting equipment at some time in their lives. Wolk et al. (1990a) found similar rates, with 80% having shared in their current drug use period and 74% of these having shared with more than one person. Darke et al. (1990) report a rate of 40% having shared in the month prior to interview and 24% of these having shared with more than one other person. These figures are consistent with prevalence studies of hepatitis B and C among this population, where high rates (89% and 86% respectively) suggest that most injecting drug users have shared needles at some time in the past (Bell et al., 1990c).

If drug users do share needles, then the cleansing procedures they use are an important determinant of the probability of transmitting HIV. Rinsing the injecting equipment with bleach has been the most commonly recommended decontamination procedure if it is necessary to share at all (e.g. see Newmeyer, 1988). It is disturbing then to note that Wolk et al. (1990a) found that even though 86% of the needle sharers cleaned used needles before injecting with them, 80% of this group rinsed at some time with water, 8% with alcohol, and only 30% boiled the equipment. The authors note that the interviews were conducted before the campaign to educate users about the need to rinse shared needles with bleach. However, the Darke et al. (1990) study, which was conducted after this campaign, found that even though 89% of sharers rinsed before injecting, only 15% of this group had used bleach. Darke (in press), in a review of the literature on HIV and injecting drug use, has found that the low levels of cleaning with bleach found in Australia are similar to findings in the USA (with the exception of San Francisco) and Europe.

Risk Factors Associated With HIV Infection

A number of factors have been associated with an increased risk for contracting HIV through needle sharing. The frequency with which the user injects has been found to be associated with HIV seropositivity (e.g. Chu, et al., 1989; Schoenbaum et al., 1989). Duration of injecting drug use has also been associated with being HIV positive (Chu et al., 1989; Schoenbaum et al., 1989), although this presumably reflects the relationship between the time of beginning injecting and the advent of risk reduction campaigns among injecting drug users. Related to frequency of injecting is the issue of poly-drug use. Dolan et al. (1987), in an American study, found that drug users who used multiple drugs were more likely to share, as did Klee et al. (1990b) in an English study. Darke et al. (1990) also found that poly-drug use was associated with greater needle sharing in their study of Sydney injecting drug users. One drug that has been associated with more frequent injecting and needle sharing is cocaine (Chaisson et al., 1989; Darke et al., 1992; Schoenbaum et al., 1989; Torrens et al., 1991). Cocaine has a much shorter elimination half-life than heroin, meaning that it has to be injected more frequently to maintain its effects. A history of cocaine use has been found to be associated with being HIV positive in the United States (Chaisson et al. 1989; Schoenbaum et al., 1989).

The Dynamics of Needle Sharing

Injecting drug users share injection equipment for a variety of reasons. Not being in possession of a new needle and syringe at a time when illicit drugs are available leads users to either share their equipment with each other, or to use old equipment that they already have in their possession (Klee et al., 1990a; McKeganey et al., 1989; Selwyn et al., 1987). Users who report greater difficulty in tolerating withdrawal symptoms are also more likely to share (Magura et al., 1989a). This group of users appears to be willing to inject with used equipment rather than tolerate the period of withdrawal necessary until clean equipment can be obtained. As might be expected, the easy availability of clean injecting equipment has been found to be associated with reductions in needle sharing (e.g. Calsyn et al., 1991a).

A number of social factors have also been found to increase the incidence of needle sharing. Having a partner or friends who inject has been a factor associated with needle sharing (Klee et al., 1990a; Magura et al., 1989a). A number of important features of this variable have also been isolated. Sharing needles with family members, sexual partners and friends has been shown to function as a sign of bonding (Magura et al., 1989a; McKeganey et al., 1989). With sexual partners, who often do not regard their sharing as 'true' sharing, injecting each other may be an expression of intimacy (Turner et al., 1989). Peer pressure is an important component of the renewal of family and friendship bonds and has been reported to contribute to continued needle sharing (Magura et al., 1989a). Peer pressure is also reported to be felt by some users in the form of a duty to help other users who need their equipment to inject (McKeganey et al., 1989). In a study of the impact of needle exchanges on sharing in north west England, Klee et al. (1991a) found that injectors who did not use the exchanges put pressure on those who did to share their used equipment.

New users and irregular injectors are two groups who are also at risk because clean injecting equipment is usually unavailable at the time of use even in areas where such equipment is available through needle and syringe exchanges. New users are usually initiated into injecting by experienced users who teach the injection skills necessary to successfully inject oneself (Turner et al., 1989). Usually the skilled injector will inject the new initiate. Lacking their own equipment, new injectors are dependent upon the equipment of experienced users. Irregular injectors are unlikely to have equipment in their possession because their drug use is often unplanned and dependent on circumstance. In a study of drug users who use needle exchanges and those who do not, Hartgers et al., (1989) found that irregular drug use was associated with not using needle exchanges and with more needle sharing. This is consistent with the evidence above concerning the unavailability of injection equipment as a reason for sharing. In the Wolk et al. (1990a) study, 19% of those who shared said they did so because of an unplanned decision to use drugs. As well as these two kinds of users, Klee et al. (1990a) found that homeless drug injectors tended to share more than other drug users, a finding that has been reported elsewhere (Siegal et al., 1991).

Characteristics of Needle Sharers

There is growing evidence that a sub-group of drug users continue to share injecting equipment even though they know the risks associated with it (Selwyn et al., 1987; Wolk et al., 1990a). Some research has tried to determine if there are any definable characteristics of this group. Dolan et al. (1987) interviewed 224 males to identify variables that discriminated between sharers and non-sharers. They found that those subjects who had more severe drug problems and who used more drugs were more likely to share needles, even though they knew the risks involved. They rejected the notion that sharers had a particular personality profile or any specifiable psychopathology because of an absence of an association between sharing and subjects' scores on the Minnesota Multiphasic Personality Inventory, an instrument that is used for measuring personality variables.

Studies using more specific diagnostic criteria have, however, suggested otherwise. Nolimal and Crowley (1989) and Brooner et al. (1990) found that users with a diagnosis of antisocial personality disorder, a disorder frequently associated with illicit drug use, were more likely to share than other users. This finding suggests that users who fit into this diagnostic category may be less responsive to AIDS education aimed at changing behaviour when it is considered along with other evidence that has found that clients with antisocial personality disorder do not respond well to treatment (Brooner et al., 1990). Metzger et al. (1991) have also found psychiatric diagnosis to be associated with needle sharing, with methadone maintenance patients who were more depressed or who had more severe psychiatric problems overall being more likely to share. Antisocial personality disorder and other co-morbid psychiatric states are discussed in more detail in Chapters 8 and 13.

One other factor that has been found to be related to needle sharing is the concomitant use of benzodiazepines. In a study of HIV risk behaviour recently conducted in the north west of England, it was found that the tranquilliser temazepam was associated with needle sharing (Klee et al., 1990b). Temazepam users used more types of drugs, shared more often and had shared more recently than other drug users, including those who used tranquillisers other than temazepam. Temazepam users also had less friends and were involved in criminal activity to a greater extent. This association between the use of benzodiazepines has been found in other studies (Darke et al., forthcoming; Metzger et al., 1991).

HIV RISK BEHAVIOURS: SEX

The sexual transmission of HIV takes place through the exchange of body fluids that occurs during unprotected penetrative sex — that is, penile penetration of the vagina or anus (and perhaps the mouth if ejaculation takes place) without a condom. In the general population, the type and number of unsafe sexual contacts is known to be important in the spread of HIV (Turner et al., 1989). Injecting drug users who engage in needle-sharing behaviours are an important risk factor for their sexual partners. This risk of heterosexual transmission was identified early on in the epidemic (Sobel, 1991) and confirmed in findings like those of Schoenbaum et al. (1989) who found in a New York study that heterosexual contact with an injecting drug user was a risk factor for being infected with HIV.

Almost nothing is known about the sexual behaviour of injecting drug users as a group. This reflects a similar state of affairs concerning the general population (Turner et al., 1989). The frequency of specific types of sexual behaviours and the number and frequency of sexual contacts for most definable social groups is unknown. This lack of knowledge makes the prediction of the spread of HIV difficult. What is known to date concerning the sexual behaviour of drug users and the risk for HIV is reviewed below, outlining first the risk factors associated with sexual behaviour and then factors that have been found to be associated with increased or continued risk taking.

The Sexual Behaviour of Injecting Drug Users
Injecting drug users have been found consistently to be a sexually

active group in the USA, Europe and Australia (Darke et al., 1990; Donoghoe et al., 1989; Feucht et al., 1990; Klee et al. 1990c; van den Hoek et al., 1990; Wolk et al., 1990a). Sexually active injecting drug users report high levels of unsafe sex, considerable casual sex, and high rates of sexually transmitted diseases (STDs). Focusing on the Australian evidence, 69% of the sexually active subjects surveyed by Wolk et al. (1990a) reported very low or no use of condoms. Many of the subjects had had more than one sexual partner in the recent past. This finding is consistent with overseas findings concerning low condom usage and multiple sexual partners among many injecting drug users (e.g. Donoghoe et al., 1989; Durante, 1991; Lewis et al., 1990; Magura et al., 1990a).

Prostitution

Prostitution is a common way for female, and to a lesser extent male, drug users to support their drug use. Wolk et al. (1990a) found that 13% of males and 41% of females had worked as prostitutes since 1981, and 13% of the subjects interviewed were currently engaged in prostitution. Ten per cent of the Darke et al. (1990) sample and 15.5% in the Morlet et al. (1990) study reported current prostitution. Because prostitutes tend to have high numbers of sexual contacts, the use of condoms by this group is of interest. Overall the evidence suggests that sex industry workers have responded to the advent of HIV, and groups organised by sex workers themselves have been important in the widespread adoption of safe sex practices at work (see Donoghoe, 1992). It has been found, however, that drug injecting prostitutes use condoms at work but not with their regular sexual partners (Darke et al., 1990; Klee, et al., 1990a; Turner et al., 1989; van den Hoek et al., 1989; Wolk et al., 1990a). Van den Hoek et al. (1989) pointed out, however, that in their study most of these private sexual partners tended to be injecting drug users themselves, which may constitute a high risk if either party has been sharing injecting equipment.

Two findings suggest that prostitution may still be of concern. Bellis (1990) found low condom use by drug injecting prostitutes who worked the streets in five southern Californian cities. None of the subjects in this study was in any form of drug treatment. It may be that it is those prostitutes who are not in any form of drug treatment, and who work at the lower end of the market (e.g. on street corners), who may be under more pressure to engage in unsafe sex. The other finding of concern is that of van den Hoek et al. (1989) who, in their study of drug injecting prostitutes in Amsterdam, found that although the group as a whole reported reasonable use of condoms at work, 81% had reported contracting an STD in the six months prior to interview. This anomaly suggests that self-reported rates of unsafe sex may not always be accurate. The main risk factor for HIV infection among the prostitutes in their study remained injecting drug use.

Other Sexually Transmitted Diseases Among Injecting Drug Users

A high incidence of sexually transmitted diseases (STDs) within a group is a strong indicator that the group is engaging in high levels of unsafe sex (van den Hoek et al., 1990). Injecting drug users in Sydney have high rates of reported infection with STDs (Morlet et al., 1990; Ross et al., 1991). Half of the Morlet et al. (1990) sample and just over one-third of the males and one-half of the females in the Ross et al. (1991) study reported having an STD at some time in their life. Besides indicating high levels of unsafe sex, these findings are of concern because ulcerative genital lesions are thought to heighten the risk of HIV transmission during sexual intercourse and have been found to be associated with HIV seropositivity among injecting drug users (Morlet et al., 1990; Trapido et al., 1990; van den Hoek et al., 1989).

Homosexual and Bisexual Males

Homosexual and bisexual male injecting drug users who engage in unsafe sex are at greater risk for infection with HIV. They have higher rates of HIV infection and STDs than male heterosexual and female drug users who have approximately equal rates (Morlet et al., 1990; Ross et al., 1991). The differential rates of infection for HIV for each of these groups are similar to those found in the general population. Homosexual men tend to have higher rates of infection with HIV than bisexual men, who in turn have higher rates than heterosexual men (Ross et al., 1991).

Factors Associated With Unsafe Sex

Some factors have been found to be associated with an increase in unsafe sex. Darke et al. (1990) found that younger injecting drug users tend to engage in more unsafe sex than older users. Both Klee et al. (1990a) in the United Kingdom and Loxley et al., (1991) in Western Australia have found that younger users also tend to have more casual sex. As with needle sharing, the use of temazepam (Klee et al., 1990b), antisocial personality disorder (Brooner et al., 1990; Nolimal & Crowley, 1989) and being homeless (Klee et al., 1990a) are associated with having more sexual partners and not using condoms. Partner pressure has been found to be another important factor in condom use. The extent to which a patient perceives their partner to be receptive to suggestions about safe sex has been found to be related to level of condom use (Magura et al., 1990).

Although injecting drug users are, at this point in time, primarily at risk because of their injection practices, they do provide the most important transmission bridge to the heterosexual population at large. In the USA, just over 60% of AIDS cases reported in women for the two years April 1987 to March 1988 and April 1988 to 1989 had heterosexual contact with an injecting drug user as the suspected route of HIV transmission (Feucht et al., 1990). In New York, which has the highest concentration of injecting drug users in the USA, sexual contact with an injector was the source of 90% of cases of heterosexually transmitted AIDS and of 80% of the cases of maternal transmission (New York City Department of Health, 1988 cited in Des Jarlais et al., 1990). Many injecting drug users have non-injecting sexual partners and, given the above evidence about high rates of unsafe sex, could become the major source for heterosexual transmission in other parts of the world (Abdul-Quader et al., 1987; Donoghoe et al., 1989; Klee et al, 1990c). Reports concerning the differences in risk for males and females with regard to heterosexual transmission of HIV are misleading when it comes to prevention. The risk to males when compared with females would have to be inconceivably low before such differences would matter (Kaslow & Francis, 1989).

It is a common finding that drug treatment and education campaigns are more effective at reducing needle sharing than they are at reducing unsafe sex (Donoghoe, 1992). The continued practice of unsafe sex by injecting drug users in spite of education campaigns and contact with drug treatment programs presents a challenge for methadone maintenance programs to develop more effective ways of modifying risky sexual behaviour. This challenge is important not only for the patients in methadone treatment but also for their sexual partners and their children.

METHADONE MAINTENANCE AND THE CONTAINMENT OF HIV

As is evident from the previous two chapters of this book, methadone maintenance treatment is effective in reducing illicit opioid use and therefore is also likely to be effective in reducing those behaviours associated with injecting opioid use that are involved in HIV transmission. This substantial body of evidence has to be considered as part of the case for the role of methadone maintenance treatment in HIV prevention. For the purposes of this chapter, the focus is on the impact of methadone maintenance on the frequency of injecting and sharing. As already stated above, methadone maintenance treatment has not as yet had any substantial effect on the levels of unsafe sex among its patients. Ways in which methadone treatment might contribute more in this regard are considered in Chapter 11.

Methadone Maintenance and HIV Infection

One indicator of the success of methadone treatment in protecting its patients from infection with HIV is whether it has protected them from infection in places where HIV has already spread rapidly among injecting drug users. As already noted, Des Jarlais et al. (1989) have observed that prevention attempts are most likely to be effective during the rapid spreading phase of HIV infection. Retrospective studies have found an association between length of time in methadone treatment and low rates of seropositivity. Patients who entered methadone treatment in New York before 1982 were found to be less likely to be HIV positive than those who had entered treatment after that year (Abdul-Quader et al., 1987). Schoenbaum et al. (1989), again for injecting drug users in New York, found that there was an inverse relation between total months of methadone treatment since January 1978 and the presence of HIV antibodies.

In a group of long-term, stable patients who entered treatment before the spread of HIV in New York, Novick et al. (1990) reported that none was seropositive, even though 91% had been exposed to hepatitis B, indicating that nearly all of them had shared needles at some time. Two other studies have found that patients in methadone treatment were less likely to be HIV positive than those in detoxification programs (Marmor et al., 1987) and those not yet receiving methadone (Chaisson et al., 1989). Similar findings suggestive of the effectiveness of methadone maintenance in preventing HIV infection among its patients have been reported for Italy and Sweden (see Des Jarlais, 1992a).

Although the studies discussed in the previous paragraph are consistent with the evidence for the overall effectiveness of methadone treatment, there are other plausible explanations for many of these findings (Ward et al., 1992). It could be the case, for example, that those patients who remain in methadone maintenance are less likely to engage in risk behaviours than either patients who leave methadone treatment early or injecting drug users who do not enter treatment. The finding of lower rates of HIV seropositivity among methadone patients would then be due to naturally occurring selection between those who enter treatment and those who do not.

The Swedish study (Blix & Grönbladh, 1988; described also by Des Jarlais, 1992b) is of special interest in this regard, because the way in which patients were accepted into methadone treatment approximated a random selection procedure. The important point to be made about this study is that nearly all the patients who entered treatment after 1983 had previously applied and been refused. Applicants for methadone maintenance were accepted or refused treatment in an almost random fashion which depended on whether there was a place available at the time of application or not. Three per cent of patients who entered methadone maintenance before 1983 were found to be HIV positive, compared with 16% of those who entered treatment during the years 1984 to 1986 and 57% of patients who entered treatment after 1987. There had been no seroconversions of any patients who had tested negative for HIV antibodies on entry since 1984. This study provides stronger evidence in that it demonstrates that methadone maintenance protects its recipients from HIV infection and that this appears to be independent of selection bias. The following section reviews evidence that methadone maintenance treatment specifically affects risk behaviours associated with injecting. There is still, however, a need for better controlled prospective studies to confirm the findings that methadone maintenance protects its recipients from HIV infection.

The Effectiveness of Methadone Treatment in Reducing Injecting and Needle Sharing

The largest study to date of whether methadone treatment reduces injecting and needle sharing has been the Three Cities Study conducted by Ball and his colleagues, which is reviewed in detail in Chapter 3 (Ball & Ross, 1991; Ball et al., 1988). The outcomes relevant to HIV were the number of subjects that reported injecting and the number of days per month that they had injected. For sharing, the same measures were employed — the number of subjects sharing and the number of sharing days as an indicator of frequency of sharing.

For injecting, methadone treatment had a marked effect on both injecting and on the frequency of injecting for those who did inject. Of the 388 subjects who had remained in methadone maintenance until the end of the study period, 36% had not injected again after one month of treatment. A further 22% had not injected in the past year, and a further 13% had not injected for a period of between one and 11 months. The remaining 29% had injected in the last month. Overall 71% had not injected in the month prior to being interviewed. These data are consistent with the notion that methadone treatment leads to a slow reduction in injecting and its eventual cessation for most patients while they remain in treatment.

Similar results were found for needle sharing — both the number of sharers and the frequency with which they shared were reduced. Those who shared during their last period of injecting shared less than those whose last period of drug use occurred before or during the admission phase of treatment. Twenty-nine of the group who had injected in the previous month (9% of the overall sample in treatment) had shared needles.

These results are supported by a number of other findings. Selwyn et al. (1987) found that being in methadone treatment was associated with a decrease in both needle sharing and injecting drug use. The subjects in the Abdul-Quader et al. study (1987) who had been in methadone treatment longest had the lowest levels of these risk-taking behaviours. In their Sydney study, Darke et al. (1990) found that of the 20% of their subjects in treatment (the majority of whom were in methadone treatment) reported needle sharing in the month prior to interview compared with 68% of the subjects who were not in treatment. In this case it was unlikely that drug users in treatment were less likely to report such behaviour, as it was demonstrated through collateral interviews with subjects' sexual partners that patients in treatment were reasonably truthful about their risk-taking behaviour when interviewed by independent researchers (Darke et al., 1991). Klee et al. (1991a) report similar findings in an English study, finding that long-term methadone maintenance was associated with a reduction in needle sharing, but only for older patients who had been long-term injecting drug users. Younger patients had the same levels of risk taking as patients out of treatment. Finally, in terms of injecting safely, Hartgers et al. (1989), in a Dutch study, found that needle exchange users tended to have had more contact with methadone mainten-ance programs over the previous five years than did injectors who did not exchange, suggesting that methadone maintenance programs may be effective as dissemination points for information about safe injecting practices.

Although all of the studies reviewed here have been observational studies without control groups, the evidence is reasonably consistent that methadone treatment is effective in reducing the HIV risk behaviours associated with injecting. This consistent finding — supported by the evidence reviewed in the previous two chapters — that methadone treatment is effective at reducing injecting drug use is difficult to ignore. In the absence of evidence to the contrary, it is reasonable to conclude that methadone maintenance is an important HIV prevention measure among opioid-dependent injecting drug users.

Are Some Methadone Programs More Successful Than Others?

As we have observed in the previous chapters, much of the research concerned with the effectiveness of methadone treatment has focused on the issue of whether the treatment works at all. Methadone maintenance programs, however, differ from each other in substantially important ways, and very little research has looked at what types of programs are the most successful (Ball & Ross, 1991). Knowledge of this sort is important to the issue of HIV containment so that methadone maintenance programs can respond in the most effective way possible. Two aspects of treatment that are important in delivering effective treatment are dosage and the duration of methadone maintenance, both of which are dealt with in detail in Chapters 6 and 9 respectively.

It is worth noting briefly that two studies have looked specifically at dosage in relation to HIV. Brown et al. (1989a), in a study of 454 methadone patients in New York, found that low methadone doses were associated with being HIV positive. This held true even after total time spent in drug treatment was controlled for — a variable that was also predictive of HIV status. In the Ball et al. study (Ball & Ross, 1991; Ball et al., 1988), patients on lower methadone doses were more likely to be currently injecting. These findings suggest that lower doses of methadone (<60 mg) may be less effective than higher doses in preventing HIV infection, a conclusion that is consistent with the evidence reviewed in Chapter 6. Although by themselves these two studies do not provide strong evidence for a causal relationship between methadone dose and HIV infection, taken together with the evidence in Chapter 6 they are strongly suggestive of one.

Cocaine

As mentioned above, methadone treatment is primarily a treatment for opioid dependence. The treatment situation for methadone maintenance programs has been complicated recently in the USA by the advent of the widespread use of cocaine, and to a lesser extent in Australia by the use of amphetamines. Methadone does not provide cross-tolerance for cocaine and would not be a recommended treatment for someone with primary cocaine dependence. Two studies have tried to separate the effects of methadone on injecting heroin and injecting other drugs. Magura et al. (1989a) found that of 110 methadone patients who continued to inject, very few were injecting heroin, leading them to conclude that methadone maintenance was effective in eliminating heroin use. Chaisson et al. (1989) also found an association between being in methadone treatment and a substantial reduction or cessation of heroin use. They also found methadone treatment was associated with a reduction in cocaine injection for more than half the methadone patients. Cocaine injection, however, remained a major problem for these programs. In Australia, a recent increase in the availability of amphetamines is comparable to that seen with cocaine in the USA. The extent to which amphetamine use in Australia is associated with HIV infection has yet to be established, although some research suggests that Australian amphetamine injectors were less likely to engage in risky behaviour than heroin injectors (Hall et al., in press).

The Fate of Methadone Treatment Drop-outs

While injecting decreases over time for most patients in methadone maintenance programs, leaving a program is associated with an increase in injecting drug use. In the Ball et al. study (Ball & Ross, 1991), the subjects who had dropped out of treatment during the year to follow-up interview were much worse off than their counterparts who remained in treatment. By the time of the interview 68% of drop-outs had relapsed to injecting drug use, with 27% of the relapsers having shared needles. Although it could be argued that these figures are inflated because treatment drop-outs differ from other patients, this does not appear to be the case in the Ball et al. study. The patients who dropped out of treatment only differed on three of the characteristics assessed: they had received less methadone maintenance treatment overall; more were unemployed; and they were slightly younger than those that stayed in treatment. However, although the drop-outs did not differ in terms of the aspects of their drug dependence on which they were assessed (age of onset, length of dependence etc.), data were not provided that compared rates of injecting among the drop-out group while they were in treatment with those of the patients who remained in treatment. Murphy and Rosenbaum (1988) also claim that clients who were mandatorily withdrawn from methadone after two years because of a change in treatment policy were at greater risk for HIV infection due to relapse, but they present no data to support these conclusions. Findings like these are difficult to ignore and have important implications for treatment duration and dismissal of patients from programs. Uchtenhagen (1990a), for example, suggests that expectations about patients and the regulations of methadone maintenance programs should be relaxed in an attempt to keep patients in treatment.

Low Threshold, Low Intervention and Interim Methadone Programs

Increasing the effectiveness and the attractiveness of methadone treatment may necessitate offering different kinds of services and trying to reach a wider range of opioid users, and accordingly a number of innovative programs have been proposed and implemented (Uchtenhagen, 1990a). Low intervention methadone maintenance programs are those in which methadone is dispensed with minimal ancillary services. Such programs may or may not be 'low threshold', implying that there are few restrictions in terms of entry criteria. Dispensing low doses of methadone by bus in The Netherlands is another innovation (Buning et al., 1990). The interim maintenance program for people on waiting lists for methadone treatment discussed in Chapter 2, which existed for a brief time in New York, is another variant of these new post-HIV forms of methadone maintenance (Yancovitz et al., 1991).

These new forms of methadone treatment have a number of rationales. One is that making treatment easier to access will mean that more injecting drug users at risk will be treated. Another is that treatment might be more attractive to drug users if less therapeutic demands are made and might therefore encourage subsequent entry to more change-oriented forms of treatment. Such programs also have an economic attraction for governments. Low intervention methadone maintenance programs are a much cheaper option than the more intensive variants of methadone treatment, and a broad move to low threshold treatment would mean that more patients could be maintained on methadone for the same cost.

Schuster (cited in Nathan & Karan, 1989), however, has warned that a danger associated with low intervention programs is that they may be seen as a cheap alternative to traditional methadone treatment if this means compromising the quality of care being delivered. This point is important, because these new variants of methadone treatment have yet to be properly evaluated and, although there is reason to believe that they may reduce injecting drug use, there is little direct evidence at present that they are effective.

SUMMARY

The advent of HIV has meant a new life threatening addition to the existing risks associated with injecting drug use. Evidence from New York and other cities throughout the world suggests that once HIV is introduced to the injecting drug using population it can spread rapidly. The main mode of transmission that initiates and maintains this spread among drug injectors is the sharing of contaminated injecting equipment. HIV is also spread sexually and perinatally, thus putting at risk the sexual partners and children of injecting drug users. There is as yet no cure for HIV infection, so the only way in which the pandemic will be stemmed will be through the permanent modification of behaviours known to be routes of transmission.

Some of the dynamics of needle sharing have been identified. The frequency with which a person injects, the type of drugs they use, and having a long history of injecting drug use have all been found to be significantly associated with being HIV positive. The sharing of injecting equipment is influenced by peer pressure, having family and friends who are users, the absence of easily available injecting equipment, being unable to tolerate withdrawal symptoms, injecting irregularly, being homeless, having a diagnosis of antisocial personality disorder, and the use of benzodiazepines.

HIV is transmitted sexually via the exchange of body fluids that occurs during unprotected penetrative sexual intercourse. This mode of transmission in combination with the sharing of injecting equipment means that the sexual partners of injecting drug users are also placed in a high risk category. Little is known about the sexual behaviour of the general population or the population of injecting drug users which makes predicting the spread of HIV difficult. The little research available suggests that drug injectors are a sexually active group and that the incidence of unsafe sex among this group is quite high. This evidence is confirmed by studies which have shown that having a sexual partner who injects is a discernible risk factor for HIV infection.

The high incidence of STDs among injecting drug users suggests that unsafe sex is common among this group. Research to date suggests that drug users who work as prostitutes engage in safe sexual practices at work but do not do so when not working. Homosexual and bisexual male injecting drug users are at greater risk if they engage in unsafe sex due to the higher rates of infection among these groups in general. Unsafe sex among injecting drug users has been found to be associated with being younger, with using benzodiazepines, with being homeless, with having antisocial personality disorder, and with being unable to resist partner pressure about the use of condoms. As yet, methadone treatment has had little influence on the unsafe sexual practices of its patients.

Being in methadone treatment has been associated with lower rates of HIV infection for opiate injectors than not being in treatment in cities where the incidence of infection is quite high. Evidence also suggests that methadone treatment is effective at reducing injecting drug use and needle sharing. Successful methadone programs retain their patients in treatment, have higher maintenance dosages, have low staff turnover, and develop close, long-term relationships with their patients. Patients who drop out of methadone treatment have been found to have higher levels of HIV risk-taking behaviour than those who remain in treatment. Attracting HIV positive injecting drug users into methadone treatment is also important. Low threshold methadone programs may be a way of widening the appeal of methadone treatment, thereby reaching members of the injecting drug using population who would not otherwise consider treatment as an option.

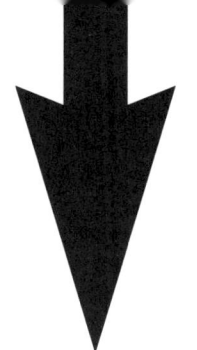

SECTION II

PROCESS

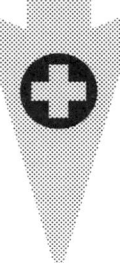

5

ASSESSMENT FOR METHADONE MAINTENANCE

INTRODUCTION

rug maintenance regimens involve exposing patients to certain risks that have to be weighed against the benefits to be gained from ameliorating the condition being treated. Diagnosis is very important in deciding who should receive treatment in such cases, so that individuals who do not have the condition are not exposed to unnecessary dangers. For example, psychosis can often be treated successfully with a range of anti-psychotic medications, each of which has specifiable risks associated with them (Dawes et al., 1989). Methadone maintenance is similar in that it uses a prescribed opioid to manage a dependence on illicit opioids (usually heroin). In this chapter, we examine the criteria that should be used to decide who should receive methadone maintenance. Put simply, these criteria seem non-controversial: methadone maintenance is suitable for individuals who are opioid dependent, or for whom the risks associated with continued illicit opioid use outweigh those associated with being maintained on methadone. Difficulties arise, however, in defining what constitutes dependence, and in assessing the balance of costs and benefits associated with methadone maintenance.

Diagnosing that a condition is present and sufficiently severe to warrant an intervention is often only one step in deciding whether a particular treatment is indicated or not. One other important issue is whether a particular type of patient will respond to the treatment under consideration. This issue is especially important in the treatment of drug dependence where there are often long waiting lists. Though an applicant may fulfil the criteria for entry to a treatment program, it may be considered a waste of time for all concerned if it can be predicted that he or she will not respond positively (Baekeland & Lundwall, 1975). It is well known that there is a minority of patients who continue to use illicit drugs heavily after entering treatment and then leave or are expelled quickly. If early drop-outs from methadone maintenance, and patients who from any viewpoint would be considered failures, could be somehow identified prior to admission, then methadone maintenance programs would be freed from their disruptive influence, applicants who would benefit from methadone maintenance could be given places, and the overall performance of methadone maintenance programs would be improved.

The evidence reviewed in Chapter 9, which is concerned with the duration of methadone maintenance, provides some direction on how to identify applicants who probably would not respond to methadone maintenance treatment. Individuals who use opioids more heavily, who have used them for more time, and who have longer and more extensive criminal histories tend not to respond to methadone maintenance. However, there are two immediate problems associated with this statement. Firstly, such individuals are those who are most in need of methadone maintenance, and they are the population that the treatment was originally introduced to treat. Secondly, the statement is very general and applies equally to a greater proportion of patients who have similar backgrounds but do respond to methadone maintenance. At this stage there are no reliable criteria to distinguish these two groups of patients. The matter of exclusion criteria is further complicated by recent research findings which suggest that methadone maintenance programs differ substantially in their treatment practices and that this is reflected in their effectiveness. A difficult patient may therefore respond well to methadone maintenance in one program and fare poorly in another. For all of the above reasons, it is not possible on the basis of existing knowledge, therefore, to specify at the assessment stage which applicants will or will not respond to methadone maintenance.

The word 'assessment' perhaps also suggests to some readers a broader process of devising a treatment plan. Depending upon the range of services available within a methadone maintenance program, attempts might be made to determine the needs of each individual and then design measures to meet them, either by providing services within the program or by referring them to an outside agency. This aspect of assessment — a form of treatment matching — falls outside the scope of this chapter.

This chapter examines the criteria used to define an individual's suitability for methadone maintenance, and discusses the way in which these criteria can be assessed. This requires a discussion of the nature of opioid dependence, its assessment, and the definition of what constitutes harm reduction. Research on the effect of the assessment process on retention in methadone maintenance is also examined. For details about determining initial methadone dose at the beginning of treatment see Chapter 6.

ADMISSION CRITERIA FOR METHADONE MAINTENANCE

Dole and Nyswander (1965) established fairly stringent criteria for entry when they established the first methadone maintenance program in New York some 30 years ago. To be considered suitable for methadone maintenance, applicants had to be at least 21 years of age, had to have been dependent on opioids for at least four years, have no serious psychopathology, alcohol or other non-opioid drug problems, and had to have failed repeatedly in other forms of treatment for their opioid dependence. These criteria reflected specific concerns at the time about maintaining individuals in a drug dependent state, which were addressed by restricting methadone treatment to applicants considered to be untreatable by other methods. This ensured that patients admitted to methadone maintenance would be recidivist addicts whose primary problem was their opioid addiction.

In the three decades since the introduction of methadone maintenance, a variety of forms of methadone maintenance have emerged and a range of admission criteria have been developed. In general, these criteria have been liberalised, with programs reducing the patient's age and the length of dependence necessary for entry, although some countries have maintained strict restrictions on access to methadone maintenance (Gossop & Grant, 1991; Uchtenhagen, 1990b). For example, the minimal age for entry has been reduced to 16 in the USA, although it remains at 22 in Switzerland. Similarly, the length of opioid dependence necessary for admission is six months in The Netherlands, but in Switzerland there is a stricter requirement of three years (Uchtenhagen, 1990b).

Changing patterns of illicit drug use have also meant that excluding individuals who use drugs other than opioids has come to be seen as impractical in many countries. Twenty to 30 years ago, it was common for applicants to present for admission with a clearly defined opioid dependence which was not complicated by the frequent use of other illicit drugs. In the intervening period this has changed and the applicant for methadone treatment in recent years is more likely to use a variety of illicit drugs (e.g. Bell et al., 1990a). Accepting poly-drug users into methadone maintenance programs is problematic in that methadone replaces opioids but not other drugs and the continued use of some other drugs (e.g. benzo-diazepines) may be considered unsafe in combination with methadone. For these reasons, poly-drug use is still considered a reason for exclusion in some programs, while others are willing to accept such patients and interpret their poly-drug use as a reason for special attention. Uchtenhagen (1990b) observes that in most countries the final decision about whether to accept any individual or not lies with the treatment provider, suggesting that it is their interpretation of policy that ultimately matters.

Another recent factor that has influenced assessment policy in some countries is the advent of HIV. For example, in The Netherlands, admission criteria have been reduced to a minimum in some programs as a specific measure to try to reduce the spread of HIV among the injecting drug using population (Gossop & Grant, 1991). Such programs that have little or no admission criteria have become known as 'low threshold' programs.

OPIOID DEPENDENCE

The basis for methadone maintenance as an intervention is the phenomenon of cross-dependence which refers to the capacity of one drug of a class to replace another drug upon which an individual is dependent without inducing a withdrawal syndrome (Jaffe, 1985). A person who is dependent on heroin can, for example, successfully substitute methadone for heroin and not experience any discomfort; they will thereafter be dependent on methadone. Given this rationale for the use of methadone, there has always been an understandable concern about iatrogenic dependence — that is, inducing opioid dependence in individuals who may be using heroin but who are not dependent in the sense that they would not manifest a significant withdrawal syndrome if they ceased their sporadic use of heroin.

Physical Dependence

According to Jaffe (1985), the term 'physical dependence':

refers to an altered state (neuroadaptation) produced by the repeated administration of a drug, which necessitates the continued administration of the drug to prevent the appearance of a stereotypical syndrome, *the withdrawal or abstinence syndrome,* characteristic for the particular drug (p. 533).

Physical dependence is closely related to the phenomenon of tolerance where after repeated administration of a drug, increasing doses are necessary in order to achieve the desired effect. Opioids have their main effects on the body within the brain by acting on specific receptor sites in certain clusters of neurones, and the phenomenon of tolerance is thought to be a result of these neurones adapting to the chronic effects of opioids. The term neuroadaptation refers to this adaptive process and is responsible, through a rebound effect, for the withdrawal syndrome when the use of the drug ceases or the dose is sharply reduced. The extent to which neuroadaptation has been established in an individual is assessed by the severity of the withdrawal syndrome that occurs when use of the drug is suddenly stopped (Jaffe, 1985).

Edwards et al. (1981) have pointed out that the term 'physical dependence' is imprecise and have suggested that it be replaced by the more correct and specific term 'neuroadaptation'. The word dependence has connotations that suggest that the person concerned finds the drug in question necessary for the conduct of their life. Edwards et al. point out that some patients become neuroadapted to opioids when they are used for the purposes of pain management and experience a withdrawal syndrome when they are stopped, but neither wish to continuing taking, nor seek out the drugs. Such patients, while certainly neuroadapted to opioids, would not by any criteria be considered dependent in the sense that the term heroin dependence is used. It is useful, therefore, to conceptually distinguish between the physiological adaptive processes induced by the chronic administration of opioids and the drug-seeking behaviour that also characterises dependence.

The Opioid Dependence Syndrome

A major implication of the observation that a person can be

neuroadapted to opioids and not be dependent in the usual sense is that neuroadaptation, by itself, cannot account for the typical clinical picture seen in cases of opioid dependence. That is, the fact that a person has taken enough heroin for neuroadaptation to take place is not a sufficient explanation for their inability to cease its use, or to avoid relapse after withdrawal, even though the person concerred may attribute their problems to being physically addicted (Edwards, et al., 1981; Jaffe, 1985). In order to provide a more adequate characterisation of the phenomenon of drug addiction, Edwards et al. (1981) developed a definition and a model of the drug dependence syndrome which has been extremely influential in the development of definitions of drug dependence by both the World Health Organization and the American Psychiatric Association (Koster et al., 1987).

The drug dependence syndrome was defined by Edwards et al. (1981) as a cluster of phenomena that would need to be established by thorough research but which would probably include:

- neuroadaptation as evidenced by tolerance or withdrawal;
- a compulsive desire to use the drug, especially when trying to reduce or stop use of the drug;
- being unable to stop use of the drug even though wanting to;
- a well-developed narrow repertoire of behaviours associated with use of the drug;
- using the drug of dependence to prevent or relieve withdrawal;
- drug-seeking behaviour having become more important than other previously more important activities;
- early relapse after withdrawal.

Edwards et al. emphasised that neuroadaptation should not be given special importance. It was acknowledged that it would not be possible, given the little that is known about drug taking, to clearly make a distinction between dependent and non-dependent drug use. At the same time, it was pointed out that a person need not be dependent to be beset with difficulties as a result of their drug use, nor need they necessarily experience such difficulties if they are dependent. A dependent physician, for example, need not experience any of the drug-related problems that usually beset the street addict (Rounsaville et al., 1987). Rounsaville et al. (1986) point out that although drug-related problems are often the reason that treatment is sought, it is still important to maintain a clear distinction between a disorder and the social problems that arise through having the disorder. Psychotic individuals, for instance, experience many problems within society but these problems are not included in the definition of their disorder. Problems as a result of drug use were therefore not included in the definition of the drug dependence syndrome proposed by Edwards et al. (1981).

The most important implications of these definitions of the drug dependence syndrome are that a diagnosis of drug dependence does not require the presence of all of these phenomena, and that dependence is a condition that can be more or less severe, rather than simply present or absent. Some individuals who do not currently use the drug of dependence, and who are therefore not neuroadapted, could be considered to be dependent, if the presence of cues associated with drug taking evokes an overbearing desire to take the drug.

The extent to which the proposed elements of the dependence syndrome constitute a unidimensional phenomenon (i.e. that the elements do cluster together as a syndrome), and the independence of the syndrome from drug related problems, have both been investigated. There is consistent evidence from around the world that for opioids the proposed elements of the syndrome are unidimensional (Burgess et al. 1989; Hasin et al., 1988b; Kosten et al., 1989; Kosten et al., 1987; Phillips et al., 1987; Skinner & Goldberg, 1986; Stripp et al., 1990; Sutherland et al., 1986; Sutherland et al., 1988). The evidence for the independence of the drug dependence syndrome from drug related problems is less well established empirically (see Hasin et al., 1988a; 1988b; Kosten, et al., 1987; Skinner & Goldberg, 1986). This may be because it is less amenable to empirical validation than the unidimensionality hypothesis in the biased samples of individuals with problems who present at treatment agencies.

THE ASSESSMENT OF OPIOID DEPENDENCE

This section looks at the procedures that have been proposed and/or used to assess dependence in individuals applying for methadone maintenance.

Naloxone Testing

Opioid substances can be classified according to whether they are agonists or antagonists (Jaffe & Martin, 1985). Opioid agonists (e.g. morphine and methadone) act by occupying and stimulating receptor sites within the brain, thereby producing their well known effects of analgesia, sedation etc. Opioid antagonists have the capacity to reverse these effects because of their ability to displace opioid agonists from their receptor sites. Naloxone is a pure opioid antagonist and is widely used to reverse the effects of opioid agonists in cases of overdose. When it is administered by injection to individuals who are neuroadapted to opioids, it produces a withdrawal syndrome in a matter of minutes which is not unlike the withdrawal that occurs after abrupt cessation of opioid use. Naloxone-induced withdrawal lasts for about two hours.

The first use of naloxone in combination with a scoring system for assessing physically dependent (neuroadapted) individuals was reported by Blachly (1973) and there have been a number of other tests developed since (Judson et al., 1980; Peachey & Lei, 1988; Wang et al., 1974; Zilm & Sellers, 1978). The procedure involves scoring for the presence and intensity of signs (and at times symptoms) associated with the opioid withdrawal syndrome. These signs include gooseflesh, sweating, rhinnorrhea (running nose), vomiting, lacrimation (tears in the eyes), restlessness, yawning, and increased blood pressure. Some tests weight these items and priority is usually given to the first four listed. Patients are usually assessed before and then 20 to 30 minutes after intramuscular/ subcutaneous administration of naloxone. If there is no response to the first injection, it is usual to proceed with a second injection given intravenously followed by another assessment for withdrawal signs.

There is some debate concerning what is an adequate dose of naloxone for use in these tests. Judson and Goldstein, who reviewed the literature on naloxone testing in 1983, argued that the use of 0.18 mg of naloxone should be a sufficient dose for both the first and second injections. They suggested that individuals who required higher doses should not be considered as dependent. Recently, however, Jacobsen and Kosten (1989; see also Kosten et al., 1989) have argued that a dose of 0.8 mg may be necessary, because previous studies had found that when doses lower than 0.8 mg were used, fewer patients were assessed as opioid dependent.

The contradictory advice about the dose of naloxone raises the vexed issue of just what constitutes a significant level of neuroadaptation to opioids. There is a demonstrable quantitative relationship in both animals and humans between the chronic dose of an opioid and the severity of the naloxone-induced withdrawal syndrome (Judson & Goldstein, 1983; O'Brien et al., 1978; Wang et al., 1974), but this relationship may become unreliable at the lower end of the scale. As Jaffe (1985) notes, an individual who has been administered therapeutic doses of morphine for two to three days will manifest a withdrawal syndrome when administered naloxone, but would not do so if administration of the drug was suddenly stopped.

Resnick (1983), in a commentary on Judson and Goldstein's 1983 review raised what now seems to be the most serious problem with the naloxone test. Using the term 'psychological dependence', he suggested that there may be individuals who use opioids compulsively for their psychotropic effects without becoming neuroadapted. He wonders whether, when refused methadone maintenance, these people would not increase their heroin use so that they would be accepted. Kanof et al. (1991) point out that even without escalating their drug use, such individuals will continue to be at risk for the social, legal and health problems associated with habitual illicit drug use. Moreover, it is clear from the discussion earlier in this chapter that the use of naloxone to test for neuroadaptation as an indication of extent of drug dependence is overly focused on the physiological aspects of compulsive drug use.

Another proposed use for naloxone test results is in the determination of methadone dose. Wiesen et al. (1977) reported that there was a good relationship between naloxone test scores and initial holding dose of methadone (the dose that kept the new applicant comfortable) among applicants who had a clear reaction to their first of two naloxone injections. Wang et al. (1982), in a double-blind, randomised controlled trial, assessed high, medium and low initial methadone doses as predicted by naloxone test scores on their ability to hold patients without inducing intoxication or withdrawal. Although the authors claimed that they found the medium doses to be the most satisfactory and that initial methadone dose could be predicted from the naloxone test scores, it is difficult to accept this conclusion without reservation because of the relatively small sample size (n = 76) in relation to the number of sub-groups of patients (9 levels of naloxone scores × 3 dose levels = 27 cells). Inspection of the data table also makes this interpretation difficult to accept. Although it is reasonable to conclude that initial methadone dose can be determined on the basis of naloxone test scores, there are no published data tables for this to be easily done by an inexperienced clinician. It is doubtful that an experienced clinician would need them in any case (see Chapter 6).

An important disadvantage of naloxone testing is the discomfort involved for the patient. Kreek (cited in Cooper et al., 1983a) opposed naloxone testing because she believed the discomfort involved to be unnecessary (along with the cost) when a careful history and physical examination would be sufficient. Although some authors have claimed that the discomfort involved is minimal (e.g. Judson & Goldstein, 1983), as will be seen below, the naloxone challenge may be the first step in the construction of a hostile and suspicious therapeutic relationship.

Sanchez-Ramos and Senay (1987) attempted to obviate the discomfort involved in the procedure by administering naloxone in eye drops unilaterally to methadone maintenance patients and measuring the change in pupil diameter (the expected response being mydriasis). However, four out of the five patients in this case study experienced bilateral mydriasis and dysphoria. They concluded that administering naloxone to the eye in opioid-dependent individuals can induce a typical withdrawal syndrome and therefore is not indicated as a routine assessment procedure.

Methadone Challenge

Higgins et al. (1985) report a procedure for assessing level of neuroadaptation to opioids by measuring the amount of miosis (pupil constriction) in response to a 20 mg dose of methadone. They found a strong relationship between amount of pupil constriction and reported current levels of heroin use and length of time since first opioid use (these two measures together accounted for 60% of the variance in pupillary response). The authors of the study argue that this relationship demonstrates that pupillary response to a challenge dose of methadone is a valid measure of dependence. Given the necessary equipment (Polaroid camera with 3X magnification) and the time involved (a two-hour wait for maximum response to methadone), a more utilitarian interpretation of these results would be that the methadone challenge test provides evidence for the validity of a careful history as a measure of dependence.

Urinalysis

Urine samples are sometimes taken at assessment and tested for the presence of opioids. An opioid positive urinalysis result establishes recent opioid use but does not reveal any information about the extent of use or dependence. It is apparently common knowledge among drug users that the production of an opiate-positive urine at the assessment interview (if the unit concerned takes a urine sample) for methadone maintenance will help in establishing suitability (Bell et al., 1990a). Judson et al. (1980) concluded that since a urine sample only establishes recent use, and not dependence or pattern of use, urinalysis had no place in assessment for methadone maintenance. However, one possible use for urinalysis during assessment other than establishing dependence is to determine the range of other drugs currently used by the applicant (e.g. benzodiazepine use may require special attention).

The Severity of Opiate Dependence Questionnaire

The Severity of Opiate Dependence Questionnaire (SODQ) was developed to assess the drug dependence syndrome for opioids as developed by Edwards et al. (1981). Accordingly, the SODQ consists of five main sections, each devoted respectively to quantity and pattern of opiate use, physical symptoms of withdrawal, affective symptoms of withdrawal, withdrawal relief drug-taking and the rapidity with which withdrawal symptoms recur after returning to opioid use after a period of abstinence (Sutherland et al., 1986). However, as Burgess et al. (1989) point out, the SODQ does not assess compulsion or salience which were included in the original dependence syndrome model. The SODQ has been trialled on British, American and Australian samples and found to have good psychometric properties (Burgess et al., 1989; Phillips et al., 1987; Sutherland et al., 1986; Sutherland et al., 1988).

DSM-III-R

The Diagnostic and Statistical Manual of the American Psychiatric Association (American Psychiatric Association, 1987) in its revised third edition (DSM-III-R) has been influenced by the Edwards et al. (1981) model. In the section on psychoactive substance use disorders, a diagnosis of psychoactive substance dependence is made if any three of the nine criteria listed below have been present for at least one month or longer:

'1. substance often taken in larger amounts or over a longer period than the person intended;
2. persistent desire or one or more unsuccessful efforts to cut down or control substance use;
3. a great deal of time spent in activities necessary to get the substance (e.g., theft), taking the substance..., or recovering from its effects;
4. frequent intoxication or withdrawal symptoms when expected to fulfil major role obligations at work, school, or home..., or when substance use is physically hazardous...;
5. important social, occupational, or recreational activities given up or reduced because of substance use;
6. continued substance use despite knowledge of having a persistent or recurrent social, psychological, or physical problem that is caused or exacerbated by the use of the substance...;
7. marked tolerance;
8. characteristic withdrawal symptoms;
9. substance often taken to relieve or avoid withdrawal symptoms.' (pp. 167–8)

As Stripp et al. (1990) have pointed out, these criteria differ from the Edwards et al. model in two ways: narrowing of repertoire is not included; and the nine criteria emphasise relative salience of drug use to other activities and compulsion by having three items covering the first and two the second, compared with one item for each of the other elements assessed. Although Edwards et al. thought that the items might eventually be weighted in a manner suggested by research results, as Stripp et al. go on to say, the DSM-III-R provides no reasons for giving more weight to salience and compulsion than to the other criteria.

The other way in which the DSM-III-R departs from the original definition of the dependence syndrome is the inclusion of drug-related problems (6) as part of the criteria. Despite the problems outlined above, the DSM-III-R (and the SODQ) may be useful in establishing criteria for suitability for methadone maintenance.

Clinical Assessment

Clinical assessment, as used in this chapter, refers to the assessment of applicants for methadone maintenance by a clinician experienced in working with opioid-dependent people. A clinical assessment for opioid dependence involves the taking of a drug use history, an examination for physical signs of injecting drug use (e.g. puncture marks and scars), and noting any signs of opioid intoxication or withdrawal. The main criticism of this procedure is that it is not possible to objectively determine if the person concerned is neuro-adapted to opioids, primarily because it is believed that applicants for methadone maintenance will exaggerate the severity of their problems so that they may be more certain of being admitted. This criticism makes two independent points: that applicants exaggerate, and that neuroadaptation is a necessary condition for entry to methadone maintenance. The second point will not be discussed any further because, as argued above, it does not take into account the compulsive aspect of opioid use and the harm associated with it.

In relation to the possibility that clinicians might be duped and non-dependent individuals might be accepted into methadone maintenance, Jaffe (1985) draws a useful distinction between purposive and non-purposive behaviour associated with the withdrawal syndrome that can be applied to assessment. According to Jaffe, some of the behaviours associated with the withdrawal syndrome are only apparent in specific places (e.g. methadone clinic, doctor's surgery) in the presence of certain other people (person who has power to dispense opioids) and have the sole purpose of obtaining drugs. These behaviours, which include a manipulative communication style and simulated withdrawal symptoms, run the full gamut of behaviours possible in the situation. However, other behaviours (and signs) are not dependent on place and the presence of an observer (e.g. puncture marks, gooseflesh, pinpoint pupils). Experienced clinicians are fully aware of this distinction and through their knowledge of the opioid-using lifestyle would usually be able to select out a person with little or no history of opioid use. This kind of clinical assessment by experienced clinicians is, at this time, probably the best method for assessing opioid dependence in methadone maintenance programs.

It would, however, be useful for basic assessment criteria to be established for use by clinicians and this could be based on well-researched instruments like the SODQ and well-developed criteria like those outlined in the DSM-III-R (and the forthcoming DSM-IV). We have, however, emphasised the importance of experience because of the possible consequences that may result from inexperienced clinicians inadvertently overdosing non-tolerant individuals (see Chapter 6 for a full discussion of this issue). The practical solution to this problem is to make available appropriate training for future methadone prescribers.

ASSESSING DRUG-RELATED HARM

Although the drug dependence syndrome is considered to be independent of the problems associated with drug use, the latter are important in assessing applicants for methadone maintenance. Opioid dependence is often associated with serious negative consequences for both society and the individual. The illegality of opioids in combination with the presence of an extensive black market for high-priced, impure heroin means that society must bear a range of costs, some of which include significant levels of drug-related crime, extensive corruption and a loss of respect for legitimate authority. More recently, the cost of providing care for HIV-infected injecting drug users has added another dimension to the cost associated with opioid dependence for society.

For the individual, being opioid dependent may have a range of medical, social, legal and psychological costs associated with it. According to Jaffe (1985):

> The medical complications common among drug users include infections (e.g. septicemia, endocarditis, hepatitis, AIDS, tetanus, and pulmonary, cerebral, and subcutaneous abscesses) due to shared needles and unhygienic

procedures, foreign body emboli, granulomata due to
injection of contaminants, and a variety of neurological,
musculoskeletal, and other lesions that may be due to
hypersensitivity reactions or to toxic impurities in drugs
produced in illicit laboratories (p. 542).

People who inject opioids are also at risk of dying through overdose
or toxic reactions to contaminated drug supplies (for a detailed
discussion of the health complications of injecting drug use see
Levine and Sobel, 1991). Social complications include
unemployment, poverty and disruption to personal relationships,
while the legal complications include arrest and imprisonment for
both drug and drug-related (e.g. breaking and entering) crimes.
Psychological difficulties associated with opioid dependence would
include a range of reactions to the stress associated with
maintaining a drug-dependent lifestyle.

An approach to the assessment of suitability for methadone
maintenance that incorporates a harm reduction perspective (see
Chapter 11) takes into account the risks associated with the
applicant's current lifestyle and state of health. This means that as
well as assessing for the presence of the opioid dependence
syndrome, the problems associated with the syndrome are also
assessed. Just as an individual does not have to be neuroadapted to
opioids to be diagnosed as being dependent, he or she does not have
to be neuroadapted to experience serious drug-related problems.

There is a growing body of evidence that methadone
maintenance can be an effective intervention in the lives of many
drug users (see Chapters 2 to 4). If there is a concern on the part of
the clinician concerning the possibility of iatrogenic opioid
dependence, then the harm associated with not taking the person
into methadone maintenance has to be weighed against this
consideration.

There is no established procedure for assessing the harm
associated with opioid dependence and there is no necessary
relationship between the level of harm and the level of dependence.
For example, a street-dwelling, sporadic (but compulsive) heroin
user who injects himself with syringes he finds on the street may
suffer more harm from his drug use than a heroin dealer who
injects with relatively pure heroin five or six times a day with a
clean needle every time. Assessing drug-related harm need only be
considered an added dimension to a clinical assessment of opioid
dependence.

A physical examination (which may involve laboratory tests, e.g.
liver function tests) and taking a history of infections and other
drug-related medical problems would establish the extent to which

the applicant has suffered physical harm as a result of his or her drug use. Questions concerning the applicant's involvement in prostitution, crime, loss of employment, broken relationships and loss of housing, etc. would indicate the extent to which his or her social life has been disrupted. Past and current involvement in HIV risk-taking behaviours is another important area of potential harm that needs to be assessed. Psychological harm as a result of drug use would involve the extent to which the applicant's drug use and the problems just outlined have led to anxiety and depression. Through this process the consequences of accepting or rejecting the applicant would be weighed in a cost-benefit analysis. If the predominant drug of choice is an opioid and there is significant harm, then methadone maintenance would be indicated.

There is a need perhaps to formalise the assessment of drug-related problems for both research and clinical purposes. Two assessment instruments currently exist that have been developed for this purpose. Both the Addiction Severity Index (McLellan et al., 1980) and the Opiate Treatment Index (Darke et al., 1992a) assess a range of outcomes (health, involvement with crime, psychological and social functioning) as well as estimates of current drug use. The Opiate Treatment Index also assesses extent of recent HIV risk behaviour. The use of such instruments would help to systematise and standardise the assessment process and would be useful for program evaluation (e.g. to what extent methadone treatment reduces drug-related harm).

THE INFLUENCE OF ASSESSMENT ON RETENTION AND HEROIN USE

There has been little research on the influence of the assessment process on applicants for methadone maintenance. In this section we look at the few studies that have been done and try to answer three questions: 'Who seeks methadone maintenance?' 'What is the fate of applicants who are refused methadone maintenance?' and 'How does the assessment process itself affect those who are accepted into methadone maintenance?'

Drug Use Patterns of Methadone Maintenance Applicants

Bell et al. (1990a) describe the characteristics of 767 individuals who applied for methadone maintenance in Western Sydney between 1986 and 1988. Fifteen per cent either did not complete the assessment process or were unsuccessful in gaining a place.

Most of the applicants were either poly-drug users or had used a range of different drugs at different times in their lives. Bell et al. suggest that their patterns of drug use point to a wish to be intoxicated as the central phenomenon in compulsive drug taking rather than neuroadaptation. They also point out that if the drug dependence syndrome as formulated by Edwards et al. (1981) had been used as the assessment criteria, then nearly all the applicants would have been suitable for methadone maintenance.

The Fate of Unsuccessful Methadone Maintenance Applicants

In a follow-up study of 84 applicants who either did not complete the assessment process (n = 26) or who were not accepted (n = 58) for methadone maintenance, Bell et al., (in press) found that the fate of unsuccessful applicants was poor. When the decision process of whether to accept an applicant or not was examined, it was found that daily opioid use, producing an opiate-positive urine, and having an extensive criminal record were the distinguishing criteria for acceptance into the program. This implies that as a group, the unsuccessful applicants had less reported drug use at the time of assessment and less extensive criminal histories.

Just over half of the unsuccessful applicants subsequently entered methadone maintenance at an average of 16 months after being rejected for methadone treatment in Western Sydney. When the group was examined as a whole it is found that a significant proportion of the group (44%) spent quite a deal of their time in prison (46 terms) and drug treatment (37 subjects were admitted 59 times to detoxification units or residential treatment and spent 1760 in-patient days there). One of the applicants who did not complete assessment and three of those who were rejected died in the period to follow-up. Two each of the two sub-groups were considered to be successfully abstinent — a proportion that is to be expected from studies of the natural history of opioid dependence (Wodak, 1985).

The two sub-groups of individuals in this study raise two sets of issues. For those who were rejected, Bell et al. (1990a) argue that the main consequence of their rejection was a 16-month delay in their entry to methadone maintenance. For the applicants who did not complete the assessment process, the question arises as to whether the assessment process itself discouraged them from entering methadone maintenance.

How Much Assessment?

It is often claimed that a protracted assessment process will select out the unmotivated applicants from those who wish to change.

This proposition was investigated by Woody et al. (1975) who compared the retention rates of patients who went through a one to three day assessment process and those who were accepted or rejected after a first assessment interview. The patients who went through the minimal assessment procedure had significantly better retention rates at two and five months suggesting that, rather than selecting out the more motivated individuals, the protracted assessment procedure had negative consequences. As Woody et al. pointed out, this result makes sense in that opioid-dependent individuals typically lack impulse control, tend to be passive, and do not tolerate frustration and postponement of gratification well.

In the only other study reported in the literature on the effect of the assessment process on retention, Bell (1990) compared the retention rates of two groups of patients, one of which went through a long assessment process (up to nine weeks) and another group which had virtually no assessment. This natural experiment was made possible when a private methadone unit was closed because it was thought that the patients were not being assessed properly. These patients were then referred to the public methadone unit that had the protracted assessment process. There were no differences between these two groups on any of the characteristics assessed, nor in retention rates over a three-year follow-up.

On the basis of the two studies reviewed in this section it is concluded that there is no evidence in support of the proposition that a protracted assessment process for admission to methadone maintenance results in the selection of a more motivated group of patients. Both of these studies failed to support this notion. In fact, the Woody et al. study (1975) suggests that a long assessment process may alienate prospective patients, a finding that was supported by Bell's (1990) data which showed that patients who went through the protracted assessment process were more likely to drop out or be expelled from methadone maintenance during the first six months on the program.

WHAT IS THE PURPOSE OF ASSESSMENT?

Assessment is an important part of most long-term treatments and can have a range of purposes (Miller & Rollnick, 1991). It can be used for evaluating the needs of the applicant, for diagnosis, for devising a treatment plan, and for determining suitability. This paper has essentially addressed the last of these purposes. Bell et al.

(in press have argued that policy concerning assessment has been dominated by the perceived necessity to prevent iatrogenic physical dependence at all costs. They go on to suggest — and this is consistent with the evidence reviewed above — that this concern is misplaced, is inconsistent with a harm reduction approach, and does not take account of the compulsive nature of opioid use.

According to Miller and Rollnick (1991), in the worst case the assessment process becomes a set of hoops that the applicant has to jump through in order to be allowed to receive treatment. The assessment process described by Bell et al. (1990a; in press) seems typical of this type of assessment. In order to be accepted for methadone maintenance, applicants had to attend two interviews at each of which they had to provide a urine specimen. If the patient was suspected of not being dependent, he or she had to attend an appointment for a naloxone test. Due to the low numbers of applicants turning up to these tests, they were soon dropped. A set of procedures like these, with relatively long delays before the actual treatment (dispensing of methadone) is begun, consists of a set of tests that the applicant has to pass in order to gain entry.

An applicant's first contact with a treatment agency is very important and has a strong influence in defining the nature of the future therapeutic relationship (Bell, 1990; Miller & Rollnick, 1991; Woody et al., 1975). Opioid-dependent people who feel in need of help for their drug problems are not unusual in often being reluctant to seek out treatment (Woody et al., 1975). Methadone maintenance, in particular, has a poor image among the drug-using subculture and many patients remain ambivalent about methadone while in treatment (Hunt et al., 1985–86; Rosenblum et al., 1991). The motivational interviewing technique of dealing with ambivalence about drug use could usefully be applied in such cases by helping the applicant/patient to think about the positive and negative aspects of being 'on' or 'off' methadone (see Miller & Rollnick, 1991).

Prochaska and DiClemente's (1986) stages of change model (which characterises a drug user's motivational state in relation to their drug use as pre-contemplative, contemplative and action) may be useful when considering the applicant for methadone maintenance. The three terms 'pre-contemplative', 'contemplative' and 'action' refer to whether the person concerned has not thought about stopping or controlling their drug use, wants to stop or control their drug use, or wants to stop or gain some control and is ready to do something about it. Importantly, there is no natural progression through these three states and a person may switch back and forth between them, e.g. a legal crisis may lead to thoughts about wanting to stop heroin use but, when it passes, the person concerned may no longer think about it. An applicant for methadone maintenance is, by definition, in the action stage. As Woody et al. (1975) point out, the forces in a person's life that result in them making the decision to seek help may dissipate if the assessment is protracted. This would be compounded if the applicant experienced the assessment process as something other than the help they were seeking.

Bell (1990) emphasises the need to be aware of what the applicant is seeking by turning up at a methadone maintenance unit when he suggests that:

> Rather than testing whether the applicant 'really' wants to change, clinicians should welcome the opportunity to demonstrate to clients the benefits of treatment. The challenge in drug treatment should not be to test motivation, but to foster it, and to maximise the likelihood that the individual will benefit from treatment.

Bell et al. (in press) also suggest that rather than screening people out, assessment for methadone maintenance would be more usefully seen as a procedure in which the applicant is assisted to make an informed, rational decision about whether he or she would benefit from treatment, thus shifting the responsibility for the decision on to the applicant. It is also important to assist the applicant to try and understand what they expect and want from a treatment program.

While one of the major purposes of assessment is to decide about the suitability of the applicant for methadone maintenance (whether this is the clinician's, a joint or the applicant's decision), the process itself is also important in defining a therapeutic relationship and might also be a potentially important moment in reconfiguring the patient's motivation concerning their drug use (Miller & Rollnick, 1991). Assessing dependence and suitability for methadone maintenance need not be in contradiction with these goals.

SUMMARY

Admission criteria for methadone maintenance programs reflect concerns about maintaining individuals in a drug-dependent state, the extent to which they are treatable, and the safe management of patients once they are in treatment. Over the three decades since the introduction of methadone maintenance programs there has been a tendency towards relaxing the criteria for entry.

Physical dependence refers to the adaptive changes that take place in the body due to the chronic administration of a drug. Its presence is indicated by the onset of a withdrawal syndrome when the use of the drug is abruptly terminated. In the case of opioid dependence, these physiological changes are primarily thought to involve the adaptation of neurones (neuroadaptation) to drug effects. Physical dependence is an imprecise term because some individuals may be neuroadapted to opioids but not be dependent in the usual sense of this term, e.g. patients who are administered morphine for pain relief and who experience a withdrawal syndrome when it is stopped but who do not then experience any impulse to take morphine again or exhibit drug-seeking behaviour.

The requirement that patients show evidence of physical dependence as a criteria for admission to methadone maintenance is inconsistent with contemporary conceptions of the nature of opioid dependence. According to the drug dependence syndrome, as formulated by Edwards et al. (1981), opioid dependence consists of some or all of the following: neuroadaptation (marked tolerance and withdrawal); a compulsive desire to use opioids; a loss of control over opioid use; an habitual and routine pattern of opioid use; the use of opioids (and other drugs) to prevent withdrawal; a preoccupation with drug use to the exclusion of other activities; and rapid relapse after withdrawal. Neuroadaptation is neither necessary nor sufficient for a diagnosis of opioid dependence.

Neuroadaptation to opioids can be assessed by three methods: abrupt cessation of the drug of dependence and observation of the ensuing withdrawal syndrome; the use of naloxone to induce an immediate withdrawal syndrome; and by measuring the extent of pupil constriction in response to a low dose of methadone. Although there is a demonstrable quantitative relationship between chronic opioid dose and the severity of a naloxone-induced withdrawal syndrome, the procedure is not useful for assessing prospective methadone patients because at lower dose levels it is unreliable, and because obvious neuroadaptation is not always a necessary feature of opioid dependence. Bringing assessment procedures for methadone maintenance into line with contemporary thinking about opioid dependence means abandoning the reliance on the single criterion of neuroadaptation (physical dependence) and assessing applicants for all the syndrome elements listed above.

When used for the purposes of assessment, urinalysis

demonstrates recent drug use but not extent or pattern of use. It provides no information concerning presence or extent of dependence, and therefore serves no useful purpose in the assessment of dependence. The SODQ and the DSM-III-R, on the other hand, provide useful guidelines for the assessment of the opioid dependence syndrome by establishing criteria for diagnosis based on the Edwards et al. model. However, at present a clinical assessment by an experienced clinician probably remains the best, albeit imperfect, method of assessing opioid dependence in methadone maintenance programs.

Illicit drug use is associated with a range of medical, legal and psychosocial problems which entail serious costs to both to the individual and society. From a harm reduction perspective a person is suitable for methadone maintenance if these individual and social harms can be reduced by entry to methadone maintenance.

Assessment for methadone maintenance should be more than a series of barriers that the applicant has to pass through in order to be allowed entry to the program. An assessment interview is the applicant's first experience of the program and probably lets the applicant know what to expect as a patient in the future. As well as a process in which the applicant's suitability for methadone maintenance is assessed, assessment may also be seen as an opportunity to establish the beginnings of a working relationship. There is a need to shift the emphasis away from exclusion criteria to viewing assessment as part of the treatment process.

6

METHADONE DOSAGE

INTRODUCTION

In this chapter we examine the following issues related to methadone dosage: initial dosing at the commencement of treatment; the debate about the comparative effectiveness of high versus low dose methadone maintenance; what studies of methadone plasma levels can tell us about dosing; whether or not there are definable patient characteristics that are associated with high or low dose methadone maintenance; and who should be involved in setting and changing dose levels.

INITIAL DOSING AT THE COMMENCEMENT OF METHADONE MAINTENANCE

A patient commencing methadone maintenance is usually given a relatively low dose of methadone which is increased slowly until a satisfactory maintenance dose is achieved, at which point the patient is said to have been stabilised. There has been very little experimental research on this aspect of methadone maintenance, because the major pharmacological effects of methadone are known and there has always been a basic consensus about dosing during the induction phase of methadone maintenance. In this section, we summarise the clinical literature about initial dosing procedures. We also consider two coronial investigations in which overdosing during induction into methadone maintenance was found to have contributed to death, and discuss the lessons that might be learned from these deaths.

The Pharmacology of Methadone

Aspects of the pharmacology of methadone relevant to initial doses are as follows. The usual oral analgesic dose for non-tolerant individuals is in the range of 5 to 15 mg (Jaffe & Martin, 1985). Methadone has a long half-life in comparison to other narcotics (24 to 26 hours) and on repeated administration its effects can be cumulative in individuals with little or no tolerance. A lethal dose for a non-tolerant individual is generally considered to be around 70 to 75 mg (Blum, 1984; Gardner, 1970). Toxicity is related to blood plasma concentrations and at very high levels may be due to effects other than the narcotic actions of methadone (Wu & Henry, 1990). Some effects, like respiratory depression, have been found to persist for longer than the usual half-life after one dose in non-tolerant individuals (Olsen et al., 1981).

Deaths at the Commencement of Treatment

Though nearly 20 years apart, two investigations into deaths associated with the commencement of methadone maintenance came to very similar conclusions about which aspects of the induction process contributed to the deaths of the individuals concerned. Gardner (1970) inspected coroner's records in London for the period January 1965 to March 1969 and found 12 cases of methadone overdose-induced death. In the cases where the individuals concerned had just commenced treatment and the initial dose was found to have been too high, the following factors were considered to be of concern: seven non-tolerant or minimally tolerant individuals were prescribed methadone doses greater than 70 mg; there had been a lack of adequate assessment of individuals at induction; there had been a lack of understanding on the part of prescribers of the cumulative effects and lethal dose levels of methadone; and there was no evidence that patients who were given prescriptions for several days had been informed about the dangers of overdosing.

The commencement of methadone maintenance has also been associated with deaths in Victoria during 1989 (Drummer et al.,

1990; State Coroner of Victoria, 1990). In five of these deaths no life threatening anatomical abnormalities were found. In a coronial inquest into four of these deaths, methadone toxicity or overdose was found to be the cause of at least two of the deaths (State Coroner of Victoria, 1990). Liver disease can lead to a slowing down in the elimination of methadone from the body and, after repeated doses, can lead to toxic methadone plasma levels (see p.). While this may not be a problem in the tolerant individual with liver disease, it can be in an individual who has little or no tolerance (Novick et al., 1981). Chronic persistent hepatitis was present in all of the 10 cases of death in Victoria and, even though this is not unusual in the injecting drug using population, it was a matter for concern (Drummer et al., 1990; Wu & Henry, 1990). The Coroner found that at the time of the deaths, there was little information easily available to guide clinicians in selecting starting doses of methadone. He concluded that there was a need for more careful assessment of potential methadone maintenance patients, as well as a need to carefully monitor new patients' responses to methadone, especially during the first week of treatment (State Coroner of Victoria, 1990).

Extent of Illicit Opiate Use and Initial Methadone Dose

Because of the unknown actual quantity of heroin in street doses and the tendency on the part of potential methadone maintenance patients to exaggerate their drug use, it is difficult to use this equivalence to determine an initial dose. Johns and Gossop (1985), in a study designed to investigate this issue, found there was no relationship between self-reported heroin dose (adjusted to take into account purity of prevailing street doses) and the oral methadone dose needed in each case to prevent withdrawal. In contrast, Holman and Brown (1989) claimed there was a relationship between initial starting dose and the average daily heroin intake of the Melbourne heroin user, though no research was reported to support this contention. Johns and Gossop (1985) suggest that monitoring the effects of initial doses may be the 'least unreliable method' of meeting the needs of the opioid-dependent patient in replacement therapy and there would seem to be considerable agreement on this point. As we have seen in the previous chapter, naloxone testing to establish the level of physical dependence is no more reliable than titrating dose against patient response and has a number of unpleasant features associated with it.

The First Doses

Recommendations for initial dosing have not varied since the inception of methadone maintenance. There is considerable agreement that, based on a careful assessment of the patient, it should be somewhere in the range of 10 to 40 mg (e.g. Aylett, 1982; Blum, 1984; Dole & Nyswander, 1967; Gardner, 1970; Goldstein, 1971; Holman & Brown, 1989; Lowinson & Millman, 1979). Those authors who recommend lower first doses tend to encourage serial or split dosing on the basis of careful observation of the reaction of the patient. For example, Lowinson and Millman (1979) suggest that a starting dose should not exceed 40 mg unless the patient has been transferred from another program. They argue that ideally the initial dose should be set at a level that prevents withdrawal without intoxication. Split dosing is often found to be useful, where 10 to 20 mg is administered and the patient is observed for three to four hours to see what his or her response to the initial dose is. New patients should be carefully monitored for sedation. Given that methadone usually reaches peak plasma concentrations within two to six hours after being administered orally (Kreek, 1979), careful assessment for withdrawal or intoxication based on this time frame can be used to ensure patient comfort and maintain a safety margin. Because of the possibility of cumulative effects, the dose should be increased with care. Lowinson and Millman (1979) suggest that after patient comfort has been achieved, increases of 10 mg every three to four days until maintenance dose level is achieved should be sufficient. The immediate goal of administering methadone at the commencement of methadone maintenance is to suppress withdrawal symptoms without intoxicating or overdosing the patient. This immediate goal should not be confused with what is considered to be an adequate maintenance dose of methadone, an issue considered in detail in the next section.

To summarise, the first dose of methadone at the commencement of methadone maintenance treatment should be based on a careful assessment of the patient, which is preferably carried out by someone experienced in working with opioid addicts (see Chapter 5). Important factors concerning the effect of methadone are that it has a long elimination half-life of 24 to 36 hours, that a lethal dose for non-tolerant individuals is around 70 to 75 mg, and that methadone can accumulate in the body over successive doses and result in overdose, even though each single dose by itself may be less than toxic. The first dose should be between 10 to 40 mg. Split or serial dosing may be useful where there is doubt about the degree of tolerance. Patients with severe liver dysfunction should be dosed with care.

HIGH AND LOW DOSE METHADONE MAINTENANCE

In this section, the vexed question of what is an appropriate dose range for adequately maintaining individuals on methadone will be examined. In order to place our discussion in context, we will review some aspects of the history of methadone maintenance as a treatment modality before examining the research evidence on the effects of high and low dose methadone maintenance. We suggest that the two outcome measures of direct relevance to this issue are retention in treatment and the suppression of heroin use. They are the two measures most commonly reported across the studies that we will review.

Retention in treatment is an accepted indicator of program functioning, given that it is important to keep patients in treatment in order for change to occur. Successful maintenance on methadone is also *the* goal of treatment according to some practitioners (e.g. Dole & Nyswander, 1965; Newman, 1991). The amount of heroin use is an important outcome that might be expected to exhibit a dose-response relationship to methadone dose given. The provision of an 'adequate' dose of methadone should therefore lead to the cessation of, or a dramatic reduction in, heroin use. The debate about high versus low dose methadone maintenance has revolved around the meaning of the term 'adequate'.

Rationales for High and Low Dose Maintenance

As we have explained in the previous chapter, tolerance to a drug is said to occur when repeated, chronic ingestion at the same dose leads to a reduction in the drug's effects on the body. A person who is tolerant to a drug will require increasing doses of that drug to achieve the sought after effect. Cross-tolerance refers to the phenomenon of tolerance to one drug producing tolerance to another drug of the same type (Blum, 1984). For example, for opioid drugs such as heroin, morphine and methadone, developing tolerance to the effects of one will mean that the person concerned is tolerant to the effects of others.

Dole and Nyswander (1965) argued that one of the reasons why methadone maintenance is effective at reducing illicit opioid use is because when high doses (>80 mg) are used, the substantial level of tolerance to methadone that develops induces sufficient cross-tolerance to heroin, preventing it from producing its desired effects should a patient relapse. They referred to this high level of cross-tolerance as 'narcotic blockade' (see also Dole et al., 1966). Dole and Nyswander (1967) believed that opioid dependence was a metabolic disease and argued that high, blockading maintenance doses of methadone for long periods of time were a necessary component of successful methadone maintenance. This high dose model of methadone maintenance treatment was shown to be effective in a series of case reports and observational studies (e.g. Dole & Nyswander, 1965; Dole et al., 1968), and was subsequently supported in the randomised controlled trials discussed in detail in Chapter 2.

During the 1960s Dole and Nyswander developed protocols for an opioid maintenance program using high dose methadone and published research attesting to its effectiveness. By the end of the decade, the necessity of such high doses of methadone began to be questioned for a number of reasons and low doses (around 30 to 40 mg) were experimented with. The main reasons for changing what had been shown to be an effective treatment were that:

- the metabolic disease model of opioid dependence was implausible and hence the necessity for long periods of *blockade* methadone maintenance was questioned;

- lower doses of methadone sufficient to prevent withdrawal and craving for heroin would serve most patients' needs;

- lower doses of methadone would be just as effective as higher doses in suppressing heroin use, with fewer side effects (e.g. Berry, 1972; Goldstein & Judson, 1973);

- effective lower doses of methadone might allow easier withdrawal at the end of treatment which would be possible after relatively brief periods of methadone maintenance (Berry, 1972; see also Jaffe, 1970);

- there was a pharmacological principle involved of the least effective dosage being the best (Berry, 1972; Goldstein & Judson, 1983);

- concern about the morality of prescribing a drug of dependence to dependent individuals was translated into a concern about how much was being prescribed (Attewell & Gerstein, 1979; D'Amanda, 1983; Schuster, 1989).

Because of the controversy about the necessity for high doses of methadone, a significant amount of research effort in the 1970s addressed the question of what might be the optimum dose for methadone maintenance. Unfortunately, this question was primarily addressed by research which evaluated the relative effectiveness of 'high' and 'low' *fixed* dose methadone regimens. The researchers who undertook this work perceived the issue as one of whether a fixed low dose regimen was equivalent in effectiveness to a fixed high dose regimen. When they failed to find a difference in treatment outcome (measured by treatment retention and heroin use) they usually concluded that high and low dose regimens were of equivalent effectiveness. In so doing they were trying to prove the null hypothesis.

There are circumstances in which it is reasonable to act as if a null hypothesis was true (Hall & Einfeld, 1990). In the case of high and low dose methadone regimens these require that: a) there was no statistically significant difference between the two dose regimens and b) alternative explanations of a failure to find such a difference had been ruled out. When the research design was a randomised controlled trial, the most plausible alternative explanation that needed to be excluded was that insufficient numbers of cases were observed to ensure a reasonable chance of detecting a difference of the expected magnitude.

The second of these conditions has rarely been addressed in the research on methadone dose because researchers have not posed the question of what the expected size of the difference would be between high and low fixed dose regimens, and so have not designed studies with a specified sample size to detect the nominated difference. Judged by the relatively small sample sizes that have typically been used in these studies, and the categorical outcome measures used to assess outcome, many of these researchers have implicitly assumed that the difference would be a large one. This seems a doubtful assumption when a fixed dose regimen is used — a dosing practice that bares little resemblance to clinical practice. It is perhaps all the more remarkable then that many of these studies found differences in outcome in favour of higher dose regimens.

The State of the Art Symposium: The Hargreaves' Review

In 1983, the United States National Institute on Drug Abuse published a substantial monograph entitled *Research on the Treatment of Narcotic Addiction: State of the Art* (Cooper et al., 1983c), which consisted of literature reviews on the treatment of heroin addiction, critical commentaries on each of the reviews by appointed experts, and summaries of the ensuing discussions that took place at a symposium convened to discuss the reviews. This book has relied extensively on the *State of the Art*, as evidenced by the numerous citations that appear throughout.

The review of research on methadone dose in *State of the Art* was prepared by Hargreaves (1983) and a critical commentary was prepared by Goldstein and Judson (1983). Hargreaves provided a comprehensive coverage of the literature that had been published up until that time, especially of the experiments that had compared high and low dose methadone maintenance. In the symposium devoted to this topic it was decided that research that compared patients maintained on fixed methadone doses (e.g. 50 mg versus 100 mg) should not be pursued in the future. Since that time there has not been any further research of this kind, although as we will see the dose issue has been investigated using other research designs.

Hargreaves used stringent criteria in assessing the relevant research for his review. He took the view that double-blind, randomised controlled trials were the gold standard for research concerned with drug effects and found that most of the reported studies had little to offer as evidence. He argued from a clinical drug trials perspective that in order to isolate the effects of dose, experiments had to be double-blind (i.e. neither patients nor staff should know what dose had been used) in order to rule out the influence of expectancy effects. It is only through employing double-blind methods in combination with the random allocation of subjects to high and low dose groups that one can confidently draw causal inferences concerning the relative impact of different dose levels. Both patients' and staff knowledge of dose, their interactions concerned with setting dose levels, and a range of other factors that will become apparent in this chapter, probably interact with the effect of dose on treatment outcome. For example, knowledge of dose enhances the effects of higher doses (Bickel et al., 1986; Goldstein et al., 1975).

Hargreaves (1983) concluded that for a small proportion of patients (10% to 30%), higher doses of methadone (>50 mg) would be needed to eliminate heroin use, especially in the early stages of treatment. However, in a much less quoted conclusion, he also suggested that:

> In summary, we have virtually no evidence that a 30 mg maintenance regimen is inappropriate to use for a large group of patients, so long as all patients are not rigidly restricted to this dose level. This contrasts with the opinion among many clinical leaders that 30 mg is not adequate during early maintenance. In view of the widespread use of this dose, I suggest that this is an important issue for further research (p. 55).

This latter conclusion was, contrary to the way in which Hargreaves is often cited, broadly consistent with the low dose approach to methadone maintenance that had become popular in the early 1970s as a result of the influence of researchers like Goldstein and his colleagues (e.g. Goldstein, 1971; 1972a; 1972b).

We read the research literature from a slightly different perspective to that adopted by Hargreaves (1983)* because we believe that double-blind, fixed dose, randomised controlled trials lack external validity. Such an approach assumes that the effects of heroin or methadone are specific to the physiological effects of opioids on the body, which almost certainly means the receptor sites within the brain. While not denying that the physiological effects of opioids play an important role in the initiation and maintenance of opioid dependence, we argue that social and psychological factors also play an important role — a point that is supported by research which shows that treatment factors other than dose are important in affecting outcome (e.g. Ball & Ross, 1991; Caplehorn et al., in press; Garbutt & Goldstein, 1972; Ling et al., 1975 — see Chapters 8, 9 and 13).

The Evidence for Low Dose Maintenance

In a series of influential review articles published in the early 1970s, Goldstein and his colleagues (1971; 1972b; Garbutt & Goldstein, 1972; Goldstein & Judson, 1974) made the claim that low dose methadone maintenance (30 to 40 mg) was adequate for most patients. A careful examination of the studies on which this claim was based revealed fundamental flaws in their interpretation of the data. There are methodological, statistical and logical problems in these articles which make it difficult to accept this conclusion. In fact, the results of the two studies where data is reported in any detail, if anything supported the reverse of the conclusions drawn by the authors.

The first study was reported in the USA in 1972 to the Fourth National Conference on Methadone Treatment by Garbutt and Goldstein. They compared 30 mg, 50 mg, and 100 mg in a randomised single-blind trial, assessing retention and heroin use at 13 weeks, 27 weeks and 53 weeks. (A single-blind trial is one in which staff know the dose being administered but the patient does not.) In terms of retention, there were two significant results reported. They found that subjects on 50 mg had higher retention rates than those on 100 mg when assessed at 13 weeks (p < 0.04) but not on the other two occasions. The second significant

---

* Even though we have adopted a different reviewing strategy to the one adopted by Hargreaves (1983), we believe that his review still provides the most comprehensive assessment of the literature to that date. We have not reviewed all the studies that Hargreaves (1983) covers and we would refer the interested reader to his work for more detail and for a slightly different point of view.

difference relating to retention was that patients on 50 mg showed higher retention than those on 30 mg when assessed at 27 weeks (p < 0.02). Thus there were two significant differences out of the nine comparisons presumably made. Adjusting for the number of statistical tests conducted, these results are no longer significant and possibly are chance results. It is usual in cases where multiple tests are conducted to adjust the test statistic for the number of tests conducted. In the current case, given that nine tests were presumably conducted, the appropriate probability for the experiment is .05 divided by 9 (p < 0.006), which means that both of these findings cease to be statistically significant.

Adding to this problem is the inconsistency of the direction of the significant retention findings. It is unclear, if we accept these findings at face value, why both less than 50 mg and more than 50 mg should be inferior to 50 mg in retaining patients in treatment. This becomes even more difficult to accept when the data on heroin are considered. There was a tendency for less heroin use for the higher doses, but methodological problems in the handling of the urinalysis data on which the result is based casts doubt on the robustness of the finding (see Hargreaves, 1983).

In 1973 Goldstein and Judson reported a second study to the Fifth National Conference on Methadone Treatment. Again the study was single blind and compared 40 mg, 80 mg, and 160 mg methadone maintenance for 120 randomly allocated subjects. All patients were stabilised on a dose of 80 mg over nine weeks. The three groups then had their dose raised or lowered, or left the same over the next eight weeks, depending upon which group they were in. Subjects continued for 10 weeks on their experimental dose. Although no tests of significance were reported, Hargreaves analysed the data and found that retention was significantly poorer in the low dose (40 mg) group. Goldstein and Judson argued that the poorer retention rates in the 40 mg group may have been influenced by staff being more ready to drop the low dose patients from the study if they complained of inadequate dosing. They supported their argument for the equivalent efficacy of the doses with data showing that heroin use was not different across the three doses. However, there were more drop-outs from the low dose group which may have suppressed the difference between this group and the higher dose groups. Also, there was very little heroin use in the study sample at the beginning of the study, so the finding that dose did not differentially influence heroin use was to be expected. In conclusion, it is difficult to see how the results of these two studies were used to support Goldstein's contention that doses of 30 to 40 mg were as effective as higher methadone doses

(Goldstein, 1971; 1972b). Indeed, in hindsight, it is difficult to see why these two studies had such a major impact on subsequent clinical practice.

Another study that supposedly provided evidence for the adequacy of lower doses was reported by Berry and Kuhn (1973) at the Fifth National Conference on Methadone Treatment. They conducted a double-blind, randomised controlled trial to investigate whether there was any difference in retention or treatment outcome between two groups of stabilised patients, one of which was maintained on 100 mg, while the other had their dose reduced from 100 mg at a rate of 10 mg every four weeks until it reached 50 mg. The study period was for six months. They found no differences between the two groups of 26 patients for the six-month period, and concluded that there was no difference between 50 mg and 100 mg maintenance doses in terms of retention or patient drug use during treatment. However, the relatively short study period meant that there was only one month during which these two dose ranges were actually compared, and more importantly that the study period may not have been long enough to detect any changes that might have taken place. Further, the level of illicit drug use was very low for both of the groups for the whole duration of the study, meaning that there were very few differences to detect. Hargreaves (1983) has also pointed out that the sample size by the final stages of the experiment was probably too small to reliably detect the kind of differences that were being assessed.

Methadone Dose and Retention in Treatment

A number of studies using a variety of designs have found high dose methadone maintenance to be associated with longer retention in treatment. As we have seen, the data from the Goldstein and Judson (1973) study revealed that low dose methadone maintenance had significantly poorer retention rates than high dose methadone maintenance (Hargreaves, 1983).

Siassi, Angle and Alston (1977a) in a retrospective study of 86 patients admitted over a two-year period to a methadone unit looked at the relationship between dose and treatment success defined quite stringently as: having been employed or in school for three months; having no illicit drug use or criminal acts; and having successfully withdrawn from methadone with the approval of the treatment staff. They found that higher dose (80 mg or more) was associated with longer retention in treatment and with greater treatment success. The authors argued that their findings provided evidence against the notion that withdrawal from maintenance was easier on lower doses and therefore leads to more successful treatment completions.

McGlothlin and Anglin (1981a) conducted a retrospective study of patients graduating from three methadone maintenance programs in California. Two of the programs were high dose, long retention programs and the other was a low dose, abstinence-oriented program. As expected, given the difference in retention policy, the high dose programs retained their patients in treatment for longer periods than the low dose programs. However, as Hargreaves (1983) has pointed out, when the differences between the programs in terms of termination types are examined, the results consistently favour the high dose programs. In the high dose programs, more patients completed their treatment course, fewer dropped out and fewer were expelled for illicit drug use. While it is difficult to disentangle the effects of dose and policy on retention and discharge in this study, the finding is consistent with the other findings in this section. The McGlothlin and Anglin (1981) study is also discussed in Chapter 9, where we make the point that the differences observed between high and low dose programs in this study reflect the differences found in two broad approaches to methadone maintenance.

Caplehorn and Bell (1991) inspected the records of 238 patients admitted to two Sydney methadone units during 1986 and 1987 to determine if there was any evidence of a relationship between maximum daily dose of methadone recorded for a patient and retention in treatment. Methadone dose was found to be significantly associated with retention in a regression analysis that controlled for clinic (which was correlated with dose) and a range of patient variables. Compared to patients who received a maximum dose of less than 60 mg, the relative risk of leaving treatment was halved for those whose maximum dose was between 60 and 79 mg, and halved again for those whose maximum dose was over 80 mg. That is, patients who always received less than 60 mg were twice as likely to leave treatment as those in the mid-range quoted above, and four times as likely to leave treatment as those in the highest range.

In another recent article that quantified the relationship between dose and retention in methadone maintenance, Joe et al., (1991) report an analysis of the TOPS data for 606 patients who were in treatment during 1979–1981 at 21 clinics in 10 cities across the USA. A full discussion of the TOPS study is found in Chapter 3. Using survival analysis and controlling for differences between clinics in retention, Joe et al. found that higher methadone doses significantly predicted longer stays in treatment. This was true for all three of the dose variables that were entered into the analysis (dose at admission, at one month, and at three months). Dose at three months proved to be the best predictor when all three recorded doses were used in the analysis. The size of the effect was reported for the analysis of dose at one month, and it was found that each increase in methadone dose of 1 mg was associated with a 0.6% increase in the survivorship rate (the number of patients remaining in treatment).

In a number of additional studies, an association has been observed between low dose ranges and high treatment drop-out rates. In an extensive review of the literature to determine factors that contribute to treatment drop-out across a range of treatments, Baekeland and Lundwall (1975) found that for methadone maintenance one of eight predictive variables was dose, with lower doses of methadone being associated with poorer retention in treatment. In this section we examine further evidence for the association between low dose methadone maintenance and high attrition rates from treatment. In order to provide a comparative baseline for interpreting the retention rates reported in the studies below, it should be kept in mind that average retention rates for 21 methadone maintenance programs recently surveyed in the USA by the General Accounting Office (1990) were 78% at three months (range: 45% to 91%) and 62% at six months (range: 42% to 83%).

In a study designed to compare LAAM (a long-acting alternative to methadone) and low dose methadone (42 mg or less per day), Freedman and Czertko (1981) found their study foiled by high drop-out rates in the low dose methadone group. By week 24 of the study only one patient remained in treatment out of the original 24 subjects in the methadone condition; inspection of the graph representing drop-out over time reveals that half the patients had dropped out by around week 13. This high rate of attrition seems even more unusual given that the initial sample was chosen in a way to select employed, stable patients.

Craig (1980) compared patients on a low dose program (average dose = 30 mg) at six months and one year to patients who had dropped out in the first month of treatment. Craig claimed improvement for the patients who remained in treatment, arguing that low dose methadone maintenance can be effective for some patients. However, inspection of the data reveals that this turns out to be for a very small proportion of patients that began treatment. By six months 87% of patients had left the program and by one year the drop-out rate had increased to 90%. Most of the drop-outs occurred in the first two months of treatment. It would seem that for a very few patients low doses might, as Craig argues, be suitable, although it is questionable whether comparing first month drop-outs with patients who stay in treatment does anything more than demonstrate that the sample of patients who leave treatment in the first month are different to those who stay in treatment, and that the ways in which they are different account, at least in part, for the apparent difference between the two samples.

Overall, when the research findings on the relationship between methadone dose and retention in treatment are surveyed, there is a consistent relationship demonstrated in studies using different types of designs between higher doses of methadone and better retention rates in treatment and, in a few studies, of lower doses of methadone being associated with less than average retention rates. In the next section we review studies that have investigated the relationship between methadone dose and heroin use.

Methadone Dose and Heroin Use

Using a range of experimental and quasi-experimental designs, a number of studies have found that higher doses of methadone are associated with less heroin use during treatment. These studies suggest that when adequate sample sizes are employed and/or dose is not arbitrarily fixed for each group of patients, this relationship is apparent.

Ling et al. (1976), in a study on which Hargreaves (1983) based his major conclusion, conducted a double-blind, randomised controlled trial to compare LAAM with two fixed dose (50 mg and 100 mg) methadone maintenance regimens. The study was conducted in 12 Veterans Administration hospitals across the USA and the subjects were restricted to male war veterans attending these hospitals. Only comparisons between the low and high dose methadone maintenance groups will be discussed here. The high dose methadone maintenance group had less heroin use — as measured by morphine-positive urine test results — than the low dose group, and the low dose group was judged by staff, who used a global measure of improvement during treatment, to be less improved than the high dose group.

In an earlier double-blind, randomised controlled trial, Jaffe (1970) reported on a study in which 63 patients were randomly allocated to low (<45 mg) and high (100 to 110 mg) dose methadone maintenance. The findings were less certain than might otherwise be the case because of the brief duration of the study (14 weeks — with the high dose group only reaching their maintenance dose mid-way through) and the substantial drop-out from both the high and low dose groups (approximately 50% by 14 weeks), which was apparently due to a strict clinic policy with regard to heroin use. A significant difference was observed in favour of the high dose group at 13 weeks in amount of heroin use (as measured by urinalysis), although this was the only week in which this difference was found to be statistically significant. Jaffe (1970) reported that the difference between the two groups was not significant when compared at 17 weeks, although no data were reported.

Handal and Lander (1976), in a retrospective observational study, found that higher doses of methadone (>80 mg) were more effective than lower doses during the early months of treatment in reducing heroin use as measured by urinalysis results. We are not convinced by Hargreaves' (1983) contention that the results reported in this study may be due to a spurious correlation generated by the concomitant tendency for doses to increase and heroin use to decrease in the early months of treatment. This assumes that all subjects were on the same increasing dose regimen, whereas Handal and Lander (1976) state that methadone dose was determined by history and extent of heroin use. We believe it more likely that the disappearance of the effect of dose on heroin use is due to selective attrition, an interpretation that is supported by the substantial drop-out rate from the samples being studied (79% for one sample and 54% for the other).

McGlothlin and Anglin (1981a) in their retrospective study of three methadone units in California (discussed in the previous section and in Chapter 9) also found a significant difference between the high and low dose methadone maintenance units in terms of self-reported daily heroin use. Again in the USA, the Three Cities studies conducted by Ball and his colleagues (Ball & Ross, 1991; Ball et al., 1988), which we have discussed in more detail in Chapter 3, found, as can be seen from Figure 2,* that as methadone dose increased the rate of current heroin use (during methadone maintenance) decreased (Ball & Ross, 1991). Some indication of the size of this effect is given by the estimate that patients maintained on low doses of methadone (45 mg or less) were approximately five times more likely to have used heroin in the past 30 days compared with patients who were on higher doses (>46 mg; Relative Risk = 5.16). Results of the regression analyses reported in Ball and Ross (1991) confirm this finding, with the results suggesting that patients maintained on lower doses of methadone were more likely to have used heroin in the past 30 days than patients maintained on higher doses of methadone and that this relationship remained when patient and other treatment variables were controlled for. Ball et al. (1988) also reported the results of a discriminant function

---

* We would like to acknowledge Dole (1989) who first provided a graphic representation of these data.

analysis for injecting drug use and found methadone dose to be the most important predictor of injecting, with those patients on lower doses of methadone injecting at a higher rate during treatment than those on higher doses.

FIGURE 2: RELATIONSHIP BETWEEN METHADONE DOSE AND HEROIN USE
(Adapted from Ball & Ross, 1991)

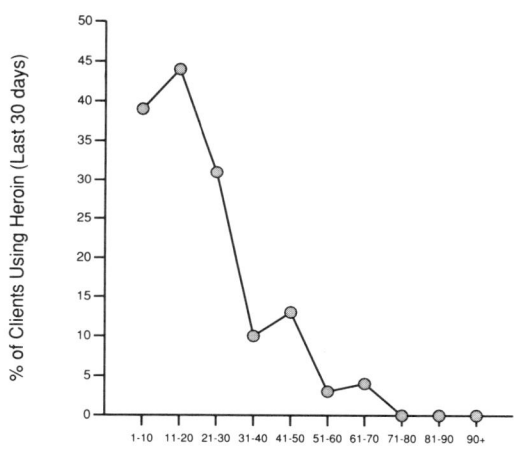

Dose of Methadone (mg)

In a recent Australian study, Caplehorn et al. (in press), report on the analysis of data for 62 subjects to determine the relationship between methadone dose and heroin use. They found that when time spent in methadone maintenance and a range of patient characteristics were controlled for, the patients who were maintained on lower doses of methadone were more likely to have used heroin than patients who were maintained on higher doses. The size of this effect was estimated: patients on 40 mg of methadone were 1.64 times as likely to submit a urine specimen positive for morphine as patients maintained on 65 mg. These findings are consistent with an earlier Australian study reported by Reynolds and her colleagues (Reynolds & Magro, 1975; Reynolds et al., 1976) which also found higher doses to be significantly associated with less heroin use at two- and four-year follow-up.

One contrary finding suggesting that patients on higher doses of methadone (>80 mg) are more likely to use illicit opioids is reported by Seow et al. (1980). This study reports the relationship between daily methadone dose and urinalysis results for a three-month period in 1978 in Western Australia for three groups of patients: a group on a short-term methadone withdrawal program who never received more than 50 mg per day; a group who at some time during the study period received doses between 51 and 79 mg per day; and a group who at some time in the study period received doses between 80 and 100 mg. Contrary to previous findings, Seow et al. reported an association between receiving a higher dose of methadone on any given day during the study and using illicit drugs.

This finding is not surprising once it is acknowledged that this dosage range was solely for patients who continued to experience withdrawal at lower doses or claimed that their dose was not adequate. It is probable that such patients would be more likely to use illicit opioids. The high dose group also appears to have been a very small proportion of the total sample (9% of the total number of urine samples) and since four days of treatment was sufficient for inclusion in the study, there are doubts about how well 'stabilised' patients were on the higher doses. We believe that these and other confounding variables such as duration of methadone maintenance treatment are highly likely to have produced a spurious difference in favour of patients on doses lower than 80 mg.

Maddux et al. (1991) have published the results of a cross-sectional study of 395 patients who were in treatment in a low dose methadone maintenance program in Texas during December 1989. They failed to find a correlation between dose and heroin use as indicated by urinalysis results. The only variable they found that predicted heroin use was length of time spent in treatment, a finding which Maddux et al. correctly suggest may, in part, be accounted for by selective attrition. The authors claim that their findings suggest that low dose methadone maintenance is adequate for the majority of patients on their program. However, it is difficult to see how a finding from a study like this can overturn the bulk of evidence suggesting otherwise. Maddux et al. themselves point out that it was the practice of the program to increase the doses of patients using heroin and encourage the lowering of those who did not. As in the Seow et al. (1980) study, this reduces confidence in the conclusion drawn by the authors, especially given that the high dose (>60 mg) patients comprised less than 5% of the overall sample.

High and Low Dose Maintenance: Conclusions

The conclusions we draw from this evidence are different from those drawn by Hargreaves in 1983. We believe that there is evidence that methadone doses below 60 mg are less than optimal for the majority of patients. We believe that the advent of the HIV epidemic among injecting drug users changes the meaning of the often quoted statement that there is 'a wider margin of safety' in prescribing higher doses of methadone (Lowinson & Millman, 1979).* We therefore reject Hargreaves' (1983) conclusion that there was no evidence to suggest that 30 mg is unsuitable for most patients.

We base our overall conclusion on the following interpretations of the evidence:

- low dose methadone maintenance (<50 mg) is associated with treatment drop out;
- high dose methadone maintenance (>60 mg) is associated with retention in treatment;
- higher doses of methadone are associated with greater reductions in heroin use.

As with other topics in the area of methadone maintenance research, the literature is not as clear as we might wish. The research on methadone dose has not been as well controlled as it might have been, and many results are open to alternative interpretation. Nonetheless, it is not an issue on which one can afford to await better information because it is unlikely to be forthcoming. The conclusions we have drawn about the desirability of higher doses in the range of 60 to 100 mg a day are similar to those of recent reviewers (e.g. Gerstein and Harwood, 1990; Schuster, 1989; Sisk et al., 1990), and they are not substantially different from the views of Goldstein and Judson (1983) who concluded that most patients could be adequately managed with doses in the range of 50 to 100 mg per day, a view that Goldstein (1991) has recently reiterated. The consensus at the *State of the Art* symposium (Cooper et al., 1983b) was that higher doses in the range of 50 to 100 mg (and individualised for each patient) led to better treatment retention and less heroin use than lower doses. We have emphasised the consensus that now exists about high dose methadone maintenance because there is evidence that many methadone clinics in the USA and Australia do not prescribe adequate doses of methadone (Baillie et al, 1991; D'Aunno & Vaughn, 1992).

To avoid misunderstanding, we stress that we are not advocating a fixed dose of 60 mg for all patients. We agree with the point made by Ling et al. (1976) that:

Clinical experience tells us that dosage of many drugs needs to be individualized not only during the induction phase but in the search for the optimal stabilization dose... It seems hardly

---

* For a full description of the implications of HIV for methadone maintenance treatment see Chapters 4 and 13.

necessary to stress the importance of individualization of dosage in clinical practice. However, the hard-line advocates of low-dose methadone maintenance might reconsider their position in the light of these findings (p. 719).

METHADONE PLASMA LEVEL STUDIES

During the 1970s one field of research of general relevance to methadone dose was concerned with the levels of methadone actually present in body fluids, especially blood plasma. Using new analytic technology that allowed the precise measurement of methadone in plasma, researchers were able to determine many of the physiological dimensions of methadone metabolism (Kreek, 1979). This ability to determine methadone plasma levels also enabled researchers to ask whether the level of methadone in plasma might be a more sensitive indicator for a range of variables than ingested dose. Studies have been done that relate methadone plasma level to dose, treatment outcome, cross-tolerance for heroin, and inexplicable signs and symptoms of withdrawal in some maintenance patients. In this section we examine this evidence to see what light it might shed on the role of dose in methadone maintenance.

Methadone Metabolism

The major aspects of methadone metabolism of relevance to methadone dose have been reviewed by Kreek (1979). The major site for the biotransformation of methadone is the liver. Peak plasma levels of methadone have been found to occur two to six hours after oral ingestion. Methadone remains in the body for long periods of time and can accumulate in body tissue during chronic administration, resulting in higher than expected levels of methadone in the blood. Considerable individual differences have been observed in both the bioavailability after oral ingestion (an average of 80% with a range of 41% to 99%) and in the elimination half-life, ranging from 8.5 to 75 hours (Nilsson cited in Säwe, 1986), although the more usual cited range for the half-life is 24 to 36 hours (Jaffe & Martin, 1985). Methadone is eliminated from the body by biotransformation and excretion in urine and faeces (Säwe, 1986). Important factors that influence the pharmacological effectiveness of methadone are hepatic dysfunction, the effects of some drugs, and variations in individual metabolism rates (Kreek, 1983a).

Liver Disease and Methadone Metabolism

Severe liver disease has been shown to influence the rate at which methadone is eliminated from the body; the same is suspected in the case of renal dysfunction but has yet to be demonstrated by research (Kreek, 1983a; Säwe, 1986). As we have indicated at the beginning of this chapter, this has important implications for assessment for methadone maintenance and for the setting of an initial dose of methadone.

The Influence of Other Drugs on Methadone Metabolism

A small number of drugs have been shown to have an influence on the amount of methadone present in blood plasma due to their ability to speed up the elimination of methadone from the body. Most drugs are transformed in the body by the microsomal enzyme systems located in the liver (Benet & Sheiner, 1985). Some drugs are known to induce the activity of these enzymes, thus speeding up the rate at which the elimination of methadone takes place. The effect of this faster than expected metabolism of methadone is to produce seemingly inexplicable signs and symptoms of withdrawal in patients who are being maintained on an apparently adequate dose.

Rifampin, a drug used in the treatment of tuberculosis, and the anticonvulsant phenytoin are associated with withdrawal in the majority of maintenance patients to whom they are administered (Brockmeyer et al., 1991; Kreek, 1979, 1983a; Bell, et al., 1988). Phenobarbital (barbiturates) leads to lowered methadone plasma levels and is also associated with the same withdrawal effect (Bell et al., 1988; Kreek, 1983a). Benzodiazepines and another anticonvulsant, carbamazepine, are suspected of producing similar effects but there is no experimental evidence to support this conclusion (Bell et al., 1988; Bell et al., 1990b; Kreek, 1983a; Wolff et al., 1991b). Another drug suspected of enhancing methadone metabolism is disulfiram, a drug used in the treatment of alcohol dependence (Wolff et al., 1991b). A recent report has also found the anti-viral agent zidovudine (AZT) produces symptoms of withdrawal in patients being maintained on an otherwise adequate dose of methadone (Brockmeyer, et al., 1991).

Methadone Plasma Levels and Withdrawal Symptoms

Although the drugs discussed above seem to precipitate both low methadone plasma levels and withdrawal, it does not necessarily follow that low plasma levels always cause withdrawal. A number of studies have tried to resolve this and other issues concerned with the relationship between methadone plasma levels and a range of behavioural indicators. Some of these studies have shown no relationship between plasma levels and patients' subjective perceptions of withdrawal (e.g. Horns & Goldstein, 1975; Tennant et al. 1984). It has been suggested that this may be due to the amount of methadone available in the blood not being related to activity at the relevant receptor sites associated with the opioid effects of methadone (Säwe, 1986; Horns & Goldstein, 1975). However, two studies have found that withdrawal symptoms are likely when methadone plasma levels fall below 50 ng/ml (nanograms per millilitre) (Bell et al., 1988; Wolff, 1990 cited in Wolff et al., 1991b).

Methadone Plasma Levels and Dosage

There would seem to be no simple relationship between oral dose and methadone plasma levels. As Bell et al. (1988) have remarked, well controlled studies conducted on inpatients on closed hospital wards have established that there is some consistency between dose and plasma levels over time in individuals (Holmstrand et al., 1978; Verebely et al., 1975). Outpatient studies (e.g. Horns & Goldstein, 1975) where there is no control over illicit methadone ingestion, diversion of dose, and other perhaps influential but unknown factors that might affect plasma levels, do not displace this conclusion. Wide variability in plasma levels has been observed between individuals on the same dose (Horns & Goldstein, 1975; Holmstrand et al., 1978; Tennant et al., 1984). Finally, it has been consistently found that stable plasma levels within individuals decrease over time with repeated methadone administration (Holmstrand et al., 1978; Verebely et al., 1975). The rate and extent of this decrease also varies widely across individuals (Holmstrand et al., 1978). However, Wolff et al. (1991b), using more sensitive methods of estimating methadone plasma levels and determining dose per kilogram of body weight as a measure of dosage, found a linear relationship between dose and concentrations of methadone in plasma.

Atypical Methadone Metabolism

One outcome of research on methadone plasma levels is the confirmation of the clinical observation that some methadone patients have a fast or atypical methadone metabolism and that for these patients the usual dose and dosing schedule may not be appropriate. Walton et al. (1978), in a case study of two individuals with apparent atypical methadone metabolism, used methadone plasma levels to develop individually tailored dosing schedules using much higher and more frequent doses than usual, claiming that patient comfort and satisfaction was achieved in this way.

Evidence that such patients exist is difficult to assess because they are usually the odd patient out in experiments designed to research other related issues (Holmstrand et al., 1978; Horns & Goldstein, 1975; Tennant et al., 1984).

Tennant (1987) attempted to assess whether a dosage increase from 80 mg to 100 mg would result in less illicit drug and heavy alcohol use. The dose increase only reduced such drug use in one subject (who also showed a marked increase in methadone plasma levels) out of 14, although there was an overall reduction in signs and symptoms of withdrawal in the group. However, one problem with the way in which this study is reported is that the authors did not report the incidence of heroin use as distinct from other illicit drug use. Heroin, and other opioids, are the only class of drugs that methadone is specifically a replacement for and therefore for which one would expect a dose response relationship. Though methadone maintenance treatment as a whole (i.e. methadone plus counselling etc.) could be expected to have some impact on both illicit drug use and heavy drinking it would seem an unreasonable expectation that an increase in dose by itself should affect the use of other types of drugs. The increase in dose used in this study is perhaps also not sufficient to have had a marked effect on subjects with an atypical methadone metabolism. Although only suggestive because of the descriptive nature of the study, Walton et al. (1978) had to increase the overall daily dose, that is, the sum total of the split doses used, of their two patients to 180 mg and 260 mg respectively. Kreek (cited in Cooper et al., 1983b) suggests that doses in excess of 100 mg may be necessary to achieve maintenance with such patients.

Methadone Plasma Levels and Treatment Outcome

Reasoning that methadone plasma levels are a more sensitive indicator of the effect of methadone than is dose, some researchers have tried to relate plasma levels to treatment outcome. Holmstrand et al. (1978) found that high plasma levels were associated with less illicit drug use and more successful rehabilitation. They concluded that patients on high doses (65 to 85 mg) who also had trough plasma levels greater than 200 ng/ml have a better chance of good outcome. Tennant et al. (1984), in an earlier study, found an association between heavy drinking and illicit drug use and lower mean plasma levels among a group of 24 subjects on a standard high dose (80 mg) of methadone. Although these two studies are suggestive it would be difficult to conclude that plasma levels are associated with outcome without further research. A number of commentators have, however, commented that in their opinion a minimum trough plasma level is necessary for successful methadone maintenance (e.g. Dole, 1988: 150 to 600 ng/ml; Loimer et al., 1991: >400 ng/ml).

Finally, Volavka et al. (1978) conducted a study which found that cross-tolerance from methadone to heroin was associated with duration of treatment and with increasing dose of methadone but was not related to plasma levels.

Methadone Plasma Studies: Conclusions

Measuring methadone plasma levels has been an important procedure in determining some aspects of methadone metabolism. Research in this area has resulted in an understanding of the dynamics of clinical observations concerning liver and renal dysfunction, the effect of other drugs, and the phenomenon of the patient with atypical methadone metabolism. The results of these studies have a number of clinical implications. Induction of patients with liver and renal dysfunction should be made with care. Drugs that induce microsomal enzyme activity like phenytoin, rifampin, phenobarbital, and perhaps zidovudine, disulfiram, carbamazepine and some benzodiazepines, will enhance methadone metabolism and may make the establishment of maintenance or the continuation of maintenance difficult. Increasing dose and perhaps split dosing may be solutions.

It would seem that there are some individuals who have atypical methadone metabolism for reasons which are not understood. Measuring trough methadone plasma levels (at the 24-hour low point before daily dosing) may be useful for managing these patients and patients who fall into the categories described in the previous paragraph. Wolff et al. (1991a) also suggest that monitoring plasma levels may useful in cases where high dose methadone is used to manage pain in heroin addicts or methadone patients, a procedure that may be complicated with HIV-infected patients who are also being prescribed other drugs to manage their condition (e.g. rifampin, zidovudine).

PATIENT CHARACTERISTICS AND FLEXIBILITY IN DOSAGE POLICY

Some researchers have examined the question of whether higher or lower doses of methadone are associated with any specifiable types of patients. In the absence of clear guidelines about which type of patient should receive which dose, some researchers have argued that doctors prescribing methadone operate on unexamined or implicit hypotheses in making dosing decisions (Hargreaves, 1983; Roszell & Calsyn, 1986). Studies that attempt to describe, for example, which types of patients receive higher doses may contribute to an understanding of what these unexamined hypotheses are.

Patient Characteristics and Dose

Descriptive evidence gathered so far suggests that patients who tend to receive higher doses are those with certain kinds of psychiatric disorders and those who are in greater psychological distress (independent of psychiatric diagnosis) than other patients. This evidence is only suggestive, as we will see below, because methodological problems make these studies difficult to interpret. Of the four studies that have attempted to relate patient characteristics to dose, two have looked at psychopathology, and two at a range of other patient variables.

In 1980, Meltzer and Katz attempted to examine whether psychopathology was related to maintenance dose of methadone. They concluded that there was no relationship between these two variables. However, the study was seriously compromised by very small sample sizes (n = 20) and the use of inappropriate statistical procedures to analyse the data.

Treece and Nicholson (1980) did find a relationship between personality disorder and dose level using DSM-III criteria. The three groups of subjects of interest for this discussion were Type A patients, classified as having schizoid, schizotypal, or paranoid personality disorder and generally described by the authors as appearing withdrawn, odd and eccentric; Type B patients, classified as having histrionic, narcissistic, anti-social, or borderline personality and generally described by the DSM-III as appearing dramatic and emotional; and a group with no diagnosed personality disorder. On a small sample of subjects (n = 31), the authors found that Type A subjects were more likely to be on a high dose (75 mg or more) than either Type B or the group with no personality disorder. The group with no personality disorder was more likely to be on a low dose (45 mg or less). On a larger group of subjects (n = 75), the frequency of Type A subjects increased as dose increased. However, this larger group was classified using less rigorous criteria than the sub-sample described above. This study suggests though that certain types of personality disorder may be associated with higher doses. This may be because, as the authors suggest, it is common clinical knowledge that high doses of methadone have therapeutic effects on some mental disorders. As might be expected, the suggestion that highly motivated, psychologically stable patients are appropriate for low dose maintenance has been made by others (e.g. Schut et al., 1973; Williams, 1971).

Metzger and Platt (1987) examined the relationship between a variety of patient characteristics and dose. The only significant findings out of the many variables the authors examined were that males and patients who have more contact with their fathers tend to be on a higher dose. They concluded that patients who see their fathers more often have better relationships with authority figures, and therefore get on better with clinic staff and are able to negotiate a higher dose for themselves. Besides the implausibility of this interpretation, the finding is questionable because of the large number of statistical tests performed, which means that the result may well have been due to chance.

Roszell and Calsyn (1986) set out to test the hypothesis that patient characteristics are an important part of any explanation why certain patients end up on certain dose levels. While acknowledging that individual differences in methadone metabolism are an important determinant of maintenance dose, they chose to examine the importance of a range of demographic, drug use, and psychological variables. The sample consisted of 106 male veterans on a program with a flexible dose policy. Stabilised dose, which was a result of negotiation between patients and program staff, was classified *a priori* as either high (60 mg or more), medium (36 to 59 mg), or low (35 mg or less). In comparison to the low dose group, the high dose group was found to be less stable and to be in greater 'psychological turmoil'; to exhibit greater anxiety; to have been prescribed psychoactive medications more frequently; to have more illicit drug use as indicated by urinalysis during the first months of treatment; and to have had a history of barbiturate, sedative, and amphetamine use. The authors suggest that their results may be compatible with those of Treece and Nicholson (1980). However, their results are based on two significant findings out of 29 statistical comparisons — findings that may be due to chance. Roszell and Calsyn concluded that patients who are anxious, in psychological turmoil or who continue to return drug-positive urines may benefit from being maintained in the high dose range.

These two studies (Treece & Nicholson, 1980; Roszell & Calsyn, 1986) have found a relationship between higher doses of methadone and psychological variables and confirm the impressions of clinicians working in the field of methadone maintenance. They are also consistent with research and case studies that suggest that methadone has anti-psychotic properties (Berken et al. 1978; Verebey, 1982) and with the well known anxiolytic qualities of opioids in general.

Flexibility in Dosage Policy

Roszell and Calsyn (1986) have suggested that their finding of a relationship between patient variables and different methadone dose ranges supports the findings of Brown et al., (1982–83) who found that a flexible dosage policy is associated with retaining patients in methadone maintenance programs. If there are important differences in patients' needs in terms of methadone dose, then presumably programs that vary dose according to the individual will more successfully meet those needs and hence increase retention in treatment.

Brown et. al. (1982–83) surveyed 113 methadone units who responded from a random sample of 154 units situated in 11 states of the USA. The 113 units participating in the study had 13 177 patients on stabilised doses in their programs. Patients were classified as being on a high (60 mg or more), medium (30 to 59 mg), or low (0 to 29 mg) dose. The differences in the States' policies concerning dose were reflected in State differences in numbers of patients in different dose ranges. Methadone units were classified into four categories of dosage policy according to the percentage of patients found in each dosing range. This resulted in high, medium or low dose policy programs and, in cases where there seemed to be no specific concentration of patients in any one range, flexible dosage policy programs.

In terms of patient characteristics, low dose policy programs tended to have younger patients than high dose programs. These low dose patients had less years of heroin use than patients in either medium or high dose programs. Low dose patients had less prior treatment episodes than all the other groups, and medium dose patients had less than their high dose counterparts. Dose setting policy was significantly related to treatment retention in that programs with a flexible dosage policy retained patients longer in treatment than fixed dose policy programs. Dose itself was found to be unrelated to retention. Brown et. al. (1982–83) concluded that individualising treatment was associated with retaining patients in treatment.

These findings are apparently inconsistent with our conclusions that low dose methadone maintenance is associated with patients leaving treatment and high dose methadone maintenance is associated with retaining patients in treatment. However, given that the unit of analysis in the Brown et al. (1982–83) study was the methadone unit rather than the patient, that these units were classified as being high or low dose in the way described above, and that retention was determined as an average for the whole unit, we do not think that the findings of this study threaten the validity of those conclusions. The findings, for example, of studies like those of Caplehorn and Bell (1991), that dose predicts retention independent of clinic, are more compelling. Still, the results of the Brown et al. study are suggestive and are consistent with other findings that have found clinic policy to be important in terms of patient response to treatment (e.g. Ball & Ross, 1991; Caplehorn et al., in press; Fisher & Anglin, 1987).

Patient Characteristics and Dosage Policy: Conclusions

It would appear that certain patient characteristics are associated with dose levels. Patients who are older and have used heroin longer — the long-term 'junkie' — and patients who use more illicit drugs, are more likely to be on a higher dose, as perhaps is the patient who is more distressed or who has a schizoid-like personality disorder. These descriptive characteristics may be added to those of the patient with atypical methadone metabolism to describe types of patients who may benefit from a higher dose in one way or another. It may be the case, as Roszell and Calsyn (1986) have suggested, that atypical methadone metabolism and these other patients characteristics may be related.

PATIENT SELF-REGULATION OF DOSAGE

Another question that has attracted the attention of researchers concerns who should set and control methadone doses. There are three simple alternative answers to this question: the prescribing doctor, either alone or in consultation with unit staff; the prescribing doctor and/or unit staff in negotiation with the patient; and finally, within certain constraints, the patient without the aid or interference of clinic staff. The first two options may have negative therapeutic consequences in that they perpetuate the patient's belief that ingesting a drug will solve their problems. It can also result in a great deal of conflict with unit staff when the patient claims that his or her dose is not 'holding' (sufficient to prevent withdrawal). Goldstein et al., (1975) claimed that when these conflicts result in an increased dose, the patient was often satisfied with the increase, but that the same increase when made 'blind' had no effect on patient satisfaction, suggesting that non-pharmacological factors are important in defining a satisfactory dose for the patient.

Goldstein et al. (1975) decided to investigate the effect of giving patients some control over their own dose on dose levels and illicit drug use as measured by urinalysis. Fifty-nine subjects, who were attending a methadone unit that operated on a single blind basis in which only staff knew and controlled dose, were studied for five weeks to provide a baseline. Then an open-dose, self-regulation policy was instituted for 25 weeks. Patients could change their dose up or down once a week by 5 mg, the maximum possible dose being 120 mg. If their dose at any time exceeded 50 mg their take-home privileges were withdrawn. The important finding was that patients did not opt for the highest dose possible. Moreover, patients who increased their dose had significantly less drug use as measured by urinalysis than at baseline, and both patients and staff were satisfied with both the policy changes and the limitations imposed on self-adjustment of dose. The findings of this study suggest that if patients are allowed to control their dose (within certain constraints), they will do so responsibly, and that this may have a positive effect on their drug use and on clinic life in general.

The issue of self-regulation was tested more thoroughly in a randomised clinical trial by Havassy and Hargreaves (1979, 1981). Of interest here are the comparisons made between an experimental group who had control of their dose (with limitations similar to the Goldstein et al. study) and the control group who were constrained under the usual program conditions of having to negotiate their dose. The self-regulating group, consistent with the Goldstein et al. study, did not increase their dose to any great degree. After initially increasing the dose slightly, this group tended to subsequently stabilise. On the whole, except for a significant improvement for a four-week period early in the study period, there was no change in the amount of illicit drug use as measured by urinalysis for the self-regulating group compared to baseline. Unexpectedly, however, the control group showed a significant increase in illicit drug use during the study period. The authors attributed this to stresses that the program was put under during the experiment which had nothing to do with the study.

In trying to explain the unexpected findings, Havassy and Hargreaves related the outcome to evidence concerning the perception of control. They argued that having control over their dose protected the patients in the self-regulation group from the vicissitudes that the program went through during the study period, while the 'ordinary' patients may have dealt with these stresses by supplementing their methadone with illicit drug use. Although these interesting speculations are not directly supported by the evidence provided by this study, Havassy and Hargreaves have provided, as they themselves argue, good evidence that giving patients control of their own dose does not undermine stabilisation.

There seems, on this evidence, little basis to the fear that if patients are given control over their own methadone dose that they will raise it irresponsibly in an attempt to achieve intoxication. It has to be emphasised, however, that these studies had constraints in place to guard against the possibility of overdose. The evidence is contradictory with regard to the contribution of self-regulation to reducing illicit drug use. On the one hand the Havassy and Hargreaves experiment used a superior methodology (randomised experiment), but there were apparently historical factors that make the findings difficult to interpret. It has been argued that self-regulation may, independent of its effect on illicit drug use, contribute to the process of methadone maintenance by enhancing patient trust and responsibility and that this outcome is worthwhile in and of itself (Havassy & Tschann, 1983). As with many aspects of methadone maintenance, there is a need for more research on the possible benefits of patients regulating their own methadone doses.

SUMMARY

The induction phase of methadone maintenance involves, among other things, the commencement of a daily methadone dosing regimen. The relevant pharmacological details concerning methadone are that it has long elimination half-life (24 to 36 hours), that a lethal dose for a non-tolerant individual is approximately 70 to 75 mg, and that methadone accumulates in body tissue, which means that over a series of successive doses overdosing may occur, even though each single dose by itself may be within the individual's tolerance range. Most clinicians recommend initial doses of between 10 and 40 mg and split or serial dosing is often used to achieve patient comfort. Patients with severe liver dysfunction may not tolerate methadone well and should be dosed with care.

The research evidence suggests that maintenance doses of methadone should be individualised to suit each patient and that no ceiling should be established on the range of possible doses. Restricting the dosing range to below 50 mg (low dose) is associated with losing patients from treatment. The evidence to date suggests that higher doses of methadone (>60 mg) are associated with longer stays in treatment and greater reductions in heroin use.

An alternative to using dose ingested as an indication of exposure to methadone is to measure the actual concentration of methadone found in blood plasma. Research using this method has led to an understanding of the way in which methadone is metabolised and the factors that can alter this process. Liver disease, the concurrent administration of some other drugs, and variations between individuals are all factors that may influence methadone metabolism.

Research suggests that patients with more severe psychological problems are more likely to receive higher doses of methadone during methadone maintenance and that adopting a flexible dosing policy is associated with better retention in treatment. Finally, patients are capable of responsibly managing their own methadone dose levels (within certain constraints) and doing so may have positive benefits for the way they feel about their treatment.

7

MONITORING ILLICIT DRUG USE WITH URINALYSIS

INTRODUCTION

The term urine testing, or urinalysis, describes a variety of methods used to determine if any given drug or its metabolites are present in a sample of urine. According to De Angelis (1972), large-scale urine testing for illicit drug use was developed during the occupation of Japan after World War II because American military personnel serving there began to use opiates in substantial numbers. The need to develop reasonably inexpensive and accurate urine tests resulted in paper chromatography procedures that were able to detect small amounts of opiates in urine. Derivatives of this procedure — for example, thin layer chromatography — are still in use today.

Since its inception, methadone maintenance treatment has played a unique role in the history of the use of urine testing to detect illicit drug use. Urinalysis was first used regularly on a reasonably large scale by Dole and his colleagues in New York in the first methadone maintenance program (De Angelis, 1972). Since that time, urinalysis has been a familiar and important component of methadone maintenance treatment. As Trellis et al. (1975) have pointed out, most clinical and administrative decisions in methadone maintenance programs are based in part on urinalysis results. In this chapter we assess the role urinalysis has played in methadone maintenance treatment and discuss what role it might play in the future on the basis of what has been learnt after nearly three decades of its use.

The Rationale for the Use of Urinalysis in Methadone Programs

Patients in methadone maintenance treatment are tested for drug use using urinalysis for two reasons: to ensure that they are ingesting the methadone they are being dispensed; and to detect whether they are taking any other non-prescribed drugs. Urinalysis results are also sometimes used to establish daily heroin use during assessment for methadone maintenance (although its usefulness in this regard is debatable — see Chapter 5). When patients are tested, they are asked to provide a sample of their urine and the act of urination is often observed to ensure that the sample provided is the patient's own and has not been tampered with (e.g. diluted with water to reduce the concentration of any drug that may be present). The sample is then sent to a laboratory to be tested for methadone and a range of other drugs. A report is returned after the urinalysis has been completed. In some countries (e.g. USA) urinalysis is stipulated as a necessary component of methadone maintenance treatment by government regulations (Calsyn et al., 1991b).

Urinalysis results are essentially used for three purposes: as part of patient management, for program evaluation and research and, more broadly, as a deterrent against unsanctioned drug use on the part of patients. In terms of patient management, drug-positive urine results are an indication of illicit drug use which is responded to in a variety of ways. They might lead to a session in which a staff member expresses concern that the patient has relapsed; an increase or decrease in methadone dose; the loss of take-home methadone privileges; extra individual counselling; the drawing up and signing of a contract promising not to relapse again; and eventually discharge from treatment (Calsyn et al., 1991b). Urinalysis results are also often used for program evaluation by unit managers, government officials and researchers. Historically, this has been important in establishing the effectiveness of methadone maintenance as an intervention to reduce heroin use. Urinalysis results provide politicians and other interested parties with the hard data they need to convince them that methadone maintenance is a worthwhile intervention despite its controversial status.

The Accuracy of Urinalysis

The immediate goal of urinalysis is to determine whether or not a drug, or its metabolites, are present in a urine sample (Blanke, 1986). However, like all scientific procedures, urine testing is subject to a variety of sources of error. Because of the serious consequences of a positive result in the case of testing for illicit drug use, the way in which error is controlled for tends to favour the production of true positive results. This allows for the occurrence of false negative results in which the result of the test is negative even though in some cases the drug concerned was taken and is present in the sample. The usual procedure is to test all samples by an inexpensive and relatively insensitive method and then to confirm positive results by using more sensitive and more expensive procedures.

Apart from the sensitivity of the testing procedures, other factors also affect the interpretation of urinalysis results (Manno, 1986a). These factors include the type of drug being tested for, the dose taken, the number of times the drug has been taken recently, the delay between last ingestion and the taking of the urine, and the quality of the procedures used by the laboratory doing the tests. Different drugs are eliminated from the body at different rates, so, depending upon the drug, the time between ingestion and taking urine will affect test results. For example, cocaine is eliminated from the body very quickly and will be only detected in a sample of urine taken within a day of ingestion, whereas a drug like methadone can be detected for much longer periods. Higher doses and frequent use both increase the likelihood of detection by increasing the time period during which the drug will be present in urine. Finally, in the USA, different laboratories have been shown to have less or more likelihood of detecting drugs in a specimen because of differences in the quality control of laboratory procedures (Hansen et al., 1985).

A negative test result therefore does not mean that the subject being tested has not taken the drug. He or she may not have used the drug concerned, they may have used the drug recently but not recently enough to still have traces in their urine, or they may have interfered with the sample by substituting other urine for it, by drinking excessive amounts of water before urinating, or by adulterating the specimen with a diluent or some other substance (Manno, 1986a; Manno, 1986b; Montalvo et al., 1972). A positive result has more confidence associated with it and, in nearly all cases, means that the person has recently taken the drug indicated.

ADVANTAGES AND DISADVANTAGES OF URINALYSIS

n this section, we assess the arguments for and against the use of urinalysis to monitor drug use in methadone maintenance programs. Because many of the issues concerned with urinalysis are not amenable to research, the costs and benefits of urinalysis have to be considered when deciding what role urinalysis should play in methadone maintenance treatment.

The advantages and disadvantages of urinalysis that have been suggested are listed below in Table 4.

Table 4. The Advantages and Disadvantages of Urinalysis

Advantages:
- Able to monitor illicit drug use for program evaluation
- Objective measure of drug use on which to base clinical decisions
- Able to monitor patient compliance in taking methadone
- Reduces illicit drug use
- Results can be used for legal purposes
- Keeps patients in contact with the treatment program
- Provides a basis for staff–patient bond

Disadvantages:
- Implies distrust of patients
- Humiliating for patients and staff
- Inaccurate indicator of drug use
- Expense involved

The most important advantage of urinalysis is its objectivity in providing information about patients' drug use. Urinalysis results provide an objective index for monitoring the success of programs in reducing illicit drug use and for making clinical decisions concerning methadone dose, take-home privileges and treatment termination for continued illicit drug use (Magura & Lipton, 1988). One of the important advantages claimed for urinalysis is that it reduces unsanctioned drug use. Urinalysis results also allow program staff to ensure that patients are actually taking the methadone dispensed to them and they have also been used for legal purposes as evidence of compliance with treatment goals (De Angelis, 1972). De Angelis has also proposed that urinalysis keeps patients in contact with the program and that the inability to deceive staff about drug use fosters respect and honesty among patients.

The disadvantages of urinalysis fall into three categories: the negative effect it has on patients and treatment; the relative inaccuracy of the procedure; and the economic cost involved. It has been claimed that urinalysis has a negative impact on patients and treatment by conveying to patients that they are not to be trusted. The humiliation involved in having to urinate while being watched by staff members is also thought to affect staff–patient relationships and patients' attitudes to treatment (Gottheil et al., 1976). Proponents of this view argue that time and money would be better spent in trying to construct more cooperative relationships with clients in order to deal with their drug use.

Another disadvantage of urinalysis is the relative inaccuracy of the procedure. Although positive results indicate that a person is using a specified drug, the possibility of false negatives is quite high due to the insensitivity of the tests used, the short elimination half-life of many of the drugs being tested for, and the proven unreliability of some laboratories in blind studies (Gottheil et al., 1976; Hansen et al., 1985; Trellis et al., 1975). Attewell and Gerstein (1979) found, in a study of methadone maintenance clinics in California, that the inconsistent detection rate of urine monitoring has adverse consequences on patients' attitudes to treatment. Rather than seeing urinalysis as an objective, scientific procedure, they viewed it as a game of luck that depended on whether they would be caught out on a 'bad' day and, if so, a further round in the game as to whether the result would come back negative or not. According to Attewell and Gerstein (1979) patients:

> tended to respond to being caught with a dirty urine by becoming angry. Indeed, anger is a rational response to a situation where a series of low-probability outcomes (day urine requested, metabolism, accuracy of urinalysis, etc.) all coincide causing the addict to be caught. Yet anger was seen by staff as addicts' refusal to take personal responsibility for their actions (p. 322).

The other major disadvantage of urinalysis is the substantial cost involved. Cost, as will be seen in the section below, has always been an important factor in determining the frequency of urine testing in methadone maintenance programs. Urinalysis is a major component in the overall cost of methadone maintenance, although in Australia this seems to vary between public clinics that have access to relatively cheap government laboratories and private clinics that often test elsewhere (Baldwin, 1987; Swensen, 1989;

Wells & McKay, 1989). In government programs, the annual cost for regular testing is roughly equivalent to that of the methadone syrup itself (Baldwin, 1987; Swensen, 1989). However, the total cost of urinalysis for any methadone maintenance clinic will of course depend on the frequency with which patients are tested.

URINE SAMPLING SCHEDULES AND SUPERVISION

iven the short elimination half-life of most opioids, the only way to reliably detect unsanctioned drug use is to have a daily schedule of urine specimen collection. This was the option adopted in the first methadone maintenance program (Dole & Nyswander, 1965). A daily testing schedule removes the possibility that patients will have safe periods where they can risk drug use, because they do not expect to be tested in the near future (Harford & Kleber, 1978). However, daily testing is not feasible for a number of reasons. The first is the prohibitive costs involved (e.g. laboratory, transportation etc.). The second is that the daily testing of all patients takes up considerable time in staff supervision and the clerical work involved in processing the samples. Finally, providing a sample every day is inconvenient and irritating for patients (Harford & Kleber, 1978).

Fixed-day Collection Schedules

Given that collecting urine samples daily is not feasible, a compromise has to be sought that will allow the collection of the minimum number of samples while still allowing for a reasonable chance of detecting unsanctioned drug use (Harford & Kleber, 1978). A fixed collection schedule, where urine is taken on fixed days known in advance to the patients, is useless for reliably detecting most drugs because the patients know when they can and cannot use without being detected. The solution to this problem has been to adopt a variety of collection procedures where the taking or testing of samples will depend on some random factor.

Random Schedules

One possible solution to the cost involved in daily testing is to take samples daily but to select randomly from those samples the one or more to be tested each week. While this solves the problem of the cost involved in daily testing, it does not alleviate the considerable burden to staff and patients of having samples taken daily (Goldstein & Judson, 1974). More widely practised are a variety of collection procedures that randomly select patients to be tested each day. Harford and Kleber (1978) have described three possible random urinalysis collection schedules.

Fixed-interval Schedules

The first and, according to Harford and Kleber (1978), the most widely-used schedule for collecting urine samples is what they term a 'fixed-interval schedule'. According to this procedure, each patient is tested a specified number of times within a pre-determined period. For example, if the period is one week and each patient has to be tested once during that interval, then each week each patient is tested on a day that is randomly chosen for them. The problem with this method is that if the period is a calendar week beginning on Sunday and the patient is tested on Monday they will very quickly learn that they are free to take whatever drugs they like until approximately 24 hours before the time they show up for the first methadone dose of the next week. Harford and Kleber argue that a schedule like this might actually encourage drug use by allowing for periods when the patient knows that they will not be tested.

Goldstein and Brown (1970) proposed a possible solution to the problems set out above. They tried to provide an answer to the question 'If testing is less than daily, how often does it need to be done to adequately monitor drug use?' Using statistical procedures they devised a probability model to determine the consequences for a truly random schedule (i.e. the patients would neither know the time interval, nor be able to predict when a test would be). According to this model, for any time period, if there were 20 consecutive negative results, it would be reasonably certain that the patient had not used drugs on more than 13% of the days in the time period. The actual number of days would depend on the frequency of the tests. In the case of one test every five or so days, 20 negative test results would mean that the patient has used illicit drugs on less than 12 days out of 90 (i.e. 13% of 90). Harford and Kleber (1978) argue that this procedure still allows for relatively long periods without testing (e.g. if the patient is tested on the first day of a testing interval and the last day of the following interval it will mean that there will be an extended period when they will not be tested). As an alternative they proposed random-interval testing.

Random-Interval Schedules

The solution to the latter problem, according to Harford and Kleber, is to be found in what they call a random-interval schedule. This schedule was originally proposed by Kleber and Gould (1971).

Long periods without testing are eliminated by having a maximum period during which a patient will not be tested. For example, if a sample is taken on a Monday in a weekly testing schedule then the next testing period begins the next day (i.e. on Tuesday). The patient will then be tested again during the next week beginning Tuesday. Using this procedure, no more than six days can elapse without testing on a weekly schedule. Kleber and Gould point out that patients at different levels of functioning (doing well, doing poorly, etc.) can be managed on different testing schedules to accommodate their progress in treatment. New patients could be tested on a three-day schedule and stabilised patients could be tested on a more infrequent schedule (e.g. fortnightly or monthly). All that this procedure requires is a table of random numbers that includes the numerals for their period (i.e. one to three for the new patients and one to 14 for the well-stabilised group). The next number in the table would determine on which day in the next period the patient would be tested.

Harford and Kleber (1978) conducted a study to try to determine the impact of random-interval testing on illicit drug use in a methadone maintenance program. This retrospective case study attempted to assess the change from a fixed-interval to a random-interval schedule by looking at the rates of opiate-positive samples before and after the change. The authors argue that the data indicate an initial increase in detected drug use and then a permanent decline, showing that the random-interval schedule was more successful at detecting illicit drug use and therefore in controlling it. However, this conclusion is difficult to support on the basis of this study. It is difficult to conclude that the increase in detected drug use was due to the adoption of the new testing schedule because of the retrospective single-group design used in the study.

This problem is well displayed by the fact that there was a similar increase in detected drug use in the year before the beginning of the study. Such increases may reflect other influences such as the availability and price of heroin on the streets. Another confounding influence is that simultaneous with the introduction of the new testing schedules was the adoption of a stricter policy concerning unsanctioned drug use. Patients who gave drug-positive urine samples were punished by withdrawal of privileges and threat of expulsion from the program. The fall in drug use may have been due to this stricter policy rather than the testing schedule itself. However, if prolonged periods without testing are of concern when using random schedules, then, as Harford and Kleber argue, the adoption of random-interval collection would alleviate that concern.

Supervised Collection

It has become common practice to supervise the collection of urine samples in methadone maintenance programs to prevent patients from subverting the process (Calsyn et al., 1991b). A variety of procedures have been employed to make sure that patients do not interfere with or substitute their sample, including close observation of the act of urination, observing the client through a one-way mirror and monitoring the act by means of a video camera placed in the toilet. Goldstein and Brown (1970) suggested that every sample collected should be supervised, and that where this was not done there was no point in collecting the sample at all. According to this argument, the cost involved might as well be saved, and patients asked whether they had recently used any drugs or not. While not all patients will interfere with the collection procedure, it does seem to be the case that some patients will go to extraordinary lengths to avoid providing a proper sample of their urine if they know that it will return a positive result.

One alternative to observing the act of urination is taking the temperature of the sample (Judson et al., 1979). If the sample is around body temperature (37°C), then it can be assumed that it has not been diluted with water. However, as Manno (1986b) points out this does not solve the problem of adulteration. Ordinary table salt, detergent and many other household cleansing products can affect the sample and return a false negative result. Other solutions are to remove all soap and any other possible adulterants from the toilet room and dye the water in the cistern so that adding it to the sample will change its colour. Manno (1986b) warns that these measures are only suitable if there is a low possibility that the persons to be tested will bring other substances to the testing room (e.g. salt). As Judson et al. (1979) point out, it is impossible to conduct a foolproof sample collection procedure and the only real way to stop interference in the long term would be in cases where there were no negative consequences to handing in drug-positive samples.

Supervised collection is, then, probably a necessary part of monitoring drug use by means of urinalysis, because a proportion of patients will not provide a true sample of their urine under other circumstances. This supervision is also one of the most controversial aspects of urinalysis. According to one point of view, supervised urine collection means that in order to receive treatment methadone patients have to regularly humiliate themselves by urinating in front of clinic staff. According to Lewis et al. (1972), in summarising the results of a study of ex-addicts' attitudes to urine testing as part of parole surveillance:

> For the subject, urinalysis represents on the average a demeaning procedure designed by the state to determine with a certain accuracy whether or not he has reverted to drug use... For most subjects...the process is a further indication of the absence of control over important parts of their body and their existence. Given the shame associated with the evacuative functions in American society, such a finding should not be surprising (p. 306).

The most frequent responses reported by ex-addicts to supervised urine sample collection were that they were embarrassed, that it made them angry and upset, that they could not urinate while being observed, and that often the supervising officer was just as embarrassed as they were. It also has to be acknowledged that the usual outcome to the procedures used to ensure proper urine collection is that a proportion of those being tested come to see the collection procedure as a 'game' which they attempt to win. This has been shown to occur with American soldiers in Vietnam, ex-addict parolees as suggested above and, of course, methadone maintenance patients (Gottheil et al., 1976). The extent to which the negative effects of supervision on patients are worthwhile has to be weighed against the need for accurate urinalysis results.

CONTROLLING DRUG USE: THE RESEARCH EVIDENCE

n 1977, Goldstein et al. remarked that even though urinalysis was almost universal, there were no answers to the simple question of whether it played a useful role in methadone maintenance treatment or not. Subsequently, in a brief review of the literature in 1983, D'Amanda observed that little had changed since 1977 and that there was not much more information available with which to answer this question. Since then, there has been no further basic research into whether urinalysis *per se* contributes at all in any useful way to methadone maintenance treatment. The only research has been in the area of applying behaviour modification principles in the use of urinalysis results.

Does urinalysis reduce or control illicit drug use?

Three experiments have attempted to determine whether urinalysis has an effect on illicit drug use. In the first study, Grevert and Weinberg (1973) conducted a study in which 64 stabilised patients in a San Francisco methadone maintenance program were randomly allocated to receive feedback about their urinalysis results or not to receive any feedback. Feedback consisted of a preliminary discussion with a staff member and could result in revocation of take-home privileges, being put on 'probation', or finally being placed on a withdrawal regimen as a precursor to having treatment terminated. The study assessed the impact of feedback about urinalysis results on the incidence of unsanctioned drug use. The main finding was that there was no difference between the two groups in terms of drug-positive test results. Interestingly, unit staff were more likely to attribute drug use to patients in the feedback condition than in the no feedback condition. This finding was contrary to the initial expectations of the unit staff, who thought that not responding to urinalysis results would result in an increase in drug use. This study provides evidence against the notion that negative consequences contingent upon handing in a drug-positive urine sample lead to a reduction in illicit drug use among methadone patients.

In a second series of studies, Goldstein and Judson (1974) randomly assigned new methadone maintenance patients to monitored and unmonitored groups in a series of three experiments at three different methadone maintenance units to see if urinalysis monitoring had an effect on drug use. In the monitored group, take-home methadone privileges could be revoked if positive urinalysis results were returned (no other details of clinical response to positive results are given, nor is it stated whether there were differences in response across the three clinics). After three months, on a date unknown to patients and unit staff, the researchers appeared at the clinic and took a urine sample from each of the subjects in both groups. In the first experiment, a significant difference was found showing that the monitored group had less heroin use than the unmonitored group. In the second and third replications no significant differences between the two groups were observed, but the final sample sizes were so small (n = 22, n = 18) that they almost certainly undermined the capacity of the studies to find such a difference if it did exist.

Havassy and Hall (1981) argue that Goldstein and Judson's (1974) results only suggested that urinalysis does not deter drug use among methadone patients because the study was flawed by a high drop-out rate that resulted in small final sample sizes, marked variation between the three clinics used in the study, and too brief a study period. They conducted a further study that tried to overcome these flaws by randomly allocating 431 methadone patients in stratified blocks to a monitored and unmonitored condition for a year at five methadone clinics in northern California. No detail was given about response to positive urinalysis results in any of the clinics. The effect of monitoring was measured by two surprise collections of urine specimens at four and eight months after the commencement of the experiment. The data was analysed in two ways. Firstly, by not including subjects who refused to provide a specimen and, secondly, by including refusals as being drug-positive, which is the usual solution to this problem. The only significant difference between the two groups was for the eight month test when subjects who did not return a specimen were not included in the analysis. The monitored group returned slightly more drug-free specimens than the unmonitored group and this difference was significant. However, when refusals were included as drug-positive this difference was diminished and no longer significant. The latter result is the stronger evidence.

Havassy and Hall concluded that urinalysis does not reduce or control drug use for methadone patients as whole, nor does it do so for any definable subgroup of patients. The only unproblematic significant finding in the experiment was that being monitored was significantly associated with a higher treatment drop-out rate. The unmonitored group expressed more satisfaction with treatment, as well as a belief that they had improved in terms of the frequency of their illicit drug use.

The above three studies suggest that there is little to be gained by using urinalysis to monitor drug use, if the main purpose of the procedure is to deter patients from using illicit drugs. Unmonitored patients do not, according to these three studies, return more positive urine test results than patients who are monitored. On the basis of the *available* evidence, it has to be concluded that there is no compelling evidence that the absence of urinalysis leads to an increase in illicit drug use.

Are there ways to make urinalysis more effective at reducing drug use?

The three studies discussed in the previous section suggest that urinalysis contributes very little to reducing unsanctioned drug use during methadone maintenance treatment. However, perhaps the reasons why there are no discernible effects of urinalysis monitoring is because the results are not being used in an optimal fashion. More studies have tried to resolve this issue than the more general one of whether having urinalysis *per se* makes a difference or not in terms of patients' drug use. All of these studies have investigated ways of using urinalysis results that are based on behaviour modification principles.

Two studies have looked at whether immediate feedback on

urinalysis results is more effective than delayed feedback (Goldstein et al., 1977; Schwartz et al., 1987). The studies were based on the principle that immediate reinforcement is more effective than delayed reinforcement. In both studies, on-site testing (immediate feedback condition) was done using the EMIT system and off-site testing (delayed feedback condition) was done by thin layer chromatography. Goldstein et al. (1977) found no discernible differences between the two groups. Schwartz et al. (1987) also failed to find a significant difference in drug use. However, it has to be acknowledged that their study was confounded by having different schedules for the collection of urine samples for the two groups and by the fact that the so-called 'immediate' feedback was given after a four-day delay from the time the sample was taken. On the basis of these two studies, it has to be concluded that evidence for the efficacy of immediate versus delayed feedback about urinalysis results is lacking.

Most research in the area of applying behaviour modification techniques to methadone maintenance treatment has investigated contingency management procedures. According to the theoretical model on which such techniques are based, behaviour is determined by reinforcement contingencies found in the environment. Changing behaviour in any given environment, therefore, requires taking control of these reinforcement contingencies (Hall, 1983). In the methadone maintenance clinics, such contingencies include the use of positive reinforcers like increases in dose and take-home privileges contingent upon drug-free urine samples, and negative consequences like dose reduction and expulsion from treatment in response to drug-positive samples. Proponents of this view argue that most methadone clinics operate some form of contingency management, though the way in which the system is applied is neither well thought out, nor well enacted, according to the behaviourist model about the relationship between reinforcement, punishment and behaviour (e.g. Calsyn & Saxon, 1987). They also argue that the three tests of urinalysis described in the previous section attract this same criticism, although we would dispute this because in at least two of the three trials (Goldstein & Judson, 1974; Grevert & Weinberg, 1973) there were clearly stipulated consequences to continued illicit drug use and it seems likely that this was also the case in the third study (Havassy & Hall, 1981) because the practice has been found to be virtually universal in the USA (Calsyn et al., 1991b).

Stitzer et al. reviewed the literature in 1985 and concluded that although there was a small amount of suggestive evidence to support the use of dose increases and decreases in reducing illicit drug use among methadone patients, only the use of take-home methadone as a reward had been widely evaluated and found to be effective. Since that time, further studies have found that threatened expulsion is effective with some patients in reducing drug use (McCarthy & Borders, 1985), and that dose increases (positive reinforcement) contingent upon drug-negative urine samples are just as effective as dose decreases (punishment) in response to drug-positive samples (Stitzer et al., 1986). One contrary finding is that of Magura et al. (1988) who failed to find much value in the use of take-home privileges to reduce illicit drug use.

McCarthy and Borders (1985), in an influential report, describe a randomised controlled trial in which 69 subjects were assigned to either a 'structured' or 'unstructured' treatment stream for 12 months on entry to a low dose (<50 mg) methadone maintenance program in California. Subjects in both conditions had to provide a sample of urine for testing each week. Outcome for illicit drug use was measured in terms of months in which the subject was drug free and months in which the subject had returned one or more urine samples containing illicit drugs. After two consecutive months in which illicit drug use was detected, all subjects received a letter expressing concern about their drug use. In the unstructured condition, subjects were also invited to come in for extra counselling. In the structured treatment condition the subjects were warned that continuing methadone maintenance was contingent upon patients returning urine samples free of illicit drugs for at least one month out of every four and that if their urinalysis results indicated illicit drug use for the next two months, then they would be placed on a mandatory detoxification schedule which was irrevocable (psychiatric and counselling services would not be withdrawn). Six subjects had methadone maintenance terminated in this way.

McCarthy and Borders (1985) found that the patients in the structured treatment condition had more drug-free months than the patients in the unstructured condition and that this was achieved with better retention in the structured treatment group. This interpretation is a reasonable one. However, the authors do not present the data on urine test results in a way which allows checking. The transformation of this data to drug-free and drug-use months considerably reduces the sensitivity of the data as a measure of illicit drug use. The finding with regard to retention is problematic in that patients who transferred to another program (one structured, six unstructured) were regarded as non-completers, as were those who went to prison (two structured, six unstructured), although no indication is given as to whether these offences were committed before or after entry to treatment. Comparisons between the two groups are also threatened by the difference in subjects leaving or being expelled from the study (structured = 47% left study; unstructured = 70% left study). Finally although the authors claim that the randomisation was successful and that the two groups did not differ on any variable, none of these data is tabled in the report which is usual for a randomised controlled trial of this quality.

Despite the results of the McCarthy and Borders trial, the evidence available, according to two reviewers sympathetic to the use of contingency management, suggests that the use of punishment in this style of methadone maintenance treatment leads to high treatment drop-out rates (Iguchi et al., 1988; Stitzer et al., 1986). As Nolimal and Crowley (1990) point out, the recent advent of HIV means that the potential risk for patients lost to treatment must bring into question a treatment practice that entails losing a significant proportion of them (see also Iguchi et al., 1988). The use of expulsion from treatment in response to relapse also attracts the same criticism. The McCarthy and Borders (1985) trial notwithstanding, the evidence overall suggests that patients respond in an 'all or none' fashion to contingency management with only a small proportion stopping their illicit drug use and the rest not responding positively at all (Iguchi et al., 1988; Magura et al., 1988; Stitzer et al., 1986). No patient variables have been found to be associated with a positive response to contingency management procedures, so it is not possible to predict which patients will respond well in an attempt to avoid the high drop-out rate. A final problem is that clinic staff are concerned about the fate of patients who leave or are expelled from treatment and for this reason it is often difficult to introduce and to get staff to comply with contingency management systems (Calsyn & Saxon, 1987).

The use of punishment in contingency management as a way of responding to drug-positive urines has little experimental support and may have serious public and individual health consequences. However, the use of take-home methadone as a reward for drug-free urine samples does not seem to have any negative features associated with it and seems to be no less effective than punishment. It is important to add a patient perspective to the overall assessment of contingency management systems. As we have already noted, Attewell and Gerstein (1979) found that patients view urine surveillance for illicit drug use as an arbitrary system not that different from a game of chance. It is important to add to this that Attewell and Gerstein found that patients in the methadone maintenance programs they surveyed regarded the ultimate punishment of mandatory detoxification not as the termination of treatment but as the inflicting upon them of the pain of withdrawal. Programs that readmit patients after a stipulated period of time reinforce this view among patients.

Is urinalysis more accurate than self-report?

One important reason for the use of urinalysis to monitor drug use is the assumption that patients lie about their drug use. This assumption is confirmed often in clinics where urinalysis results will reveal drug use in the face of the vehement denial of some patients. Nevertheless, it could be argued that the use of urinalysis itself is partly responsible for a climate in which patients feel they have to lie about their drug use. If the consequences of telling the truth are going to be some form of punishment, even if this is only imagined, then it is highly likely that most patients will lie if asked about a recent relapse. The belief that patients will not be truthful may be a self-fulfilling prophecy based upon experience in methadone maintenance clinics that create the conditions within which such beliefs are always confirmed. There is some indirect support for such a proposition from the research literature on the veracity of self-report by methadone maintenance patients when interviewed by independent interviewers.

Magura et al., (1987; 1988) reviewed and reanalysed nine studies that reported on either former or current drug treatment patients and that had compared self-report with urinalysis data. They concluded that this evidence suggests that under certain conditions many patients will tell the truth about their drug use and that self-report, under these conditions, reveals as much drug use as does urinalysis. However, Magura et al. suspected that one possible confounding influence on the results of these studies was the relatively inaccurate urinalysis method (thin layer chromatography) used in these studies. A low rate of detection would perhaps have produced spurious correlations between the self-report and the urinalysis results. To test this they conducted a study comparing self-reported drug use and urinalysis results using the more sensitive EMIT system as well as the usual thin layer chromatography procedure.

As suspected, the number of detected drug-positive samples was much higher when analysed by EMIT than by thin layer chromatography. In one of the studies, the latter method detected only 27% of the samples identified as drug positive by EMIT (Magura et al., 1987). However, a fall in correspondence between self-report and the urinalysis data was not observed as expected when the more sensitive EMIT method was used (15% of self-reported opioid use was detected by thin layer chromatography: kappa = 0.17, p≤.01; and 34% by EMIT: kappa = 0.23, p≤.01). Despite this continued match, it was still the case that some subjects who had not admitted their drug use were found to be drug positive through urinalysis (12% of opioid-negative self-reports were positive by EMIT and 3% by thin layer chromatography). Magura et al. (1987) concluded that self-report reveals as much drug use as does urinalysis, but that both methods together reveal more than either method when used alone.

Under certain conditions, then, a majority of methadone maintenance patients will give accurate accounts about their drug use. However, these conditions are not to be found in traditional methadone maintenance treatment programs. Magura et al. (1988) point out that there are no non-controversial ways of resolving the problems associated with the use of urinalysis in methadone maintenance programs. One alternative they propose is the abandonment of scheduled urinalysis, pointing out that many clinical staff believe that if the treatment environment was oriented towards developing more cooperative relationships with patients, then the patients would be able to be honest about their drug use without fearing punishment and, in the end, would also be more amenable to change.

OPTIONS FOR THE USE OF URINALYSIS IN METHADONE TREATMENT

Given that research to date on urinalysis provides no clear guidelines for its optimal implementation in methadone maintenance treatment, we set out below a number of possible options for its use and the implications involved with each of them.

Routine Urinalysis

Although there is no evidence to support the view that urinalysis controls or reduces the illicit drug use of methadone maintenance patients, this is not the only reason for its traditional place in methadone maintenance programs. Urinalysis is also thought to be worthwhile as a clinical aid in guiding treatment and as an objective source of data for program evaluation and research. These benefits have to be weighed against the substantial personal and economic costs involved in frequent, routine testing.

If urinalysis continues to be employed in methadone

maintenance programs, then there are a number of measures that can be taken to reduce costs and to ensure that the results obtained are the best possible indicator of patients' drug use. Having different schedules for patients at different stages of treatment, which is a common practice in many methadone maintenance clinics, is one way to reduce the overall frequency of tests and therefore the cost involved. New patients could be monitored frequently in the first few weeks of treatment and the frequency of tests could be reduced as they become stabilised.

Wells and McKay (1989) have suggested that testing stabilised patients who have responded well to treatment more than once a month may be excessive considering the cost involved. There is perhaps no reason why such patients need to be tested at all except for program evaluation; behavioural signs of relapse could be used as an indication of when testing is needed for clinical purposes. While this proposal does not remove the negative aspects associated with the use of urinalysis (like the humiliation and lack of trust involved), it does allow for the development of trust and the possibility of graduating beyond a treatment practice that many patients dislike.

Two important conditions must be met if urinalysis is used to monitor patients' drug use. Every sample should be randomly taken at a time unknown to the patient concerned and should be observed, or the temperature of the sample taken, to ensure that it is not tampered with in any way. If these two conditions are not met, then testing is a waste of time and money.

Infrequent Urinalysis

This option involves the abandonment of regular testing and would retain infrequent, random tests unmatched to individual patients for the purposes of program evaluation. It does not preclude the option of on-the-spot testing for any patient showing signs of intoxication or any other indications of relapse to chronic illicit drug use. This option would save a substantial amount of money and may have positive benefits on staff–patient relationships.

Adopting Other Methods to Monitor Drug Use

If urinalysis were abandoned altogether as a means of monitoring drug use, then other means might be employed to assess programs and make clinical decisions. A number of authors have suggested this option (Goldstein & Judson, 1974; Gottheil et al., 1976; Magura & Lipton, 1988). Goldstein and Judson (1974) proposed that if equivalent treatment success rates could be achieved for the same or less expense by emphasising other aspects of treatment, then there is no justifiable reason to continue using urinalysis. Gottheil et al. (1976) suggested using the substantial money spent on urinalysis for expanding counselling services. Finally, Magura and Liptor (1988) reiterated this proposal when they argued that if urinalysis no longer became a part of methadone maintenance treatment, then better staff–patient ratios and a different conception of methadone maintenance programs would have to be developed. However, if treatment delivery remains contingent upon abstinence from illicit drug use, then the reliance on self-report that these measures would ultimately depend upon would not be possible. Put simply, no patient is going to be honest about their drug use if there is a possibility that they will be dropped from treatment for doing so.

One possibility for meeting the needs of program evaluation if urinalysis were abandoned entirely would be to use independent interviewers. As the evidence reviewed earlier suggests (pp. 131–32), such interviewers would reveal as much drug use as urinalysis and, in the case of the less sensitive urinalysis methods, probably more. It should be noted that the recent introduction of low-threshold methadone maintenance programs in the Netherlands has meant that there are now programs that do not use urinalysis (Wells & McKay, 1989). When assessments of these programs become available they may provide more information about the consequences of not using urinalysis.

Hair Analysis

Another way of monitoring drug use, and and one that has received media attention, is hair analysis (Magura et al., 1992). Traces of drugs taken by the subject can be extracted and identified from hair within a few days of any given use episode and one strand of hair will contain a living record of the subject's recent drug use history. This history may be as long or as short as the length of any given person's hair (5 cm = approximately four months growth). Hair analysis may also provide information on the amount as well as the pattern of consumption. The method of hair analysis that has been most researched to date is radioimmunoassay of hair.

Clearly, hair analysis has the potential to be useful for both clinical and research purposes and it avoids many of the shortcomings of urinalysis. The taking of a sample does not involve the unpleasant features that are associated with the taking of a supervised urine sample. Hair retains traces of drugs used for much longer than they are present in urine, and ways in which the subject might interfere with a sample are not apparent, although the effect of hair treatments and dyes is not as yet known. As well as the usual uses of urinalysis as a measure of drug use both during and after treatment, hair analysis, unlike urinalysis, would be useful for establishing the history and extent of drug use at assessment for treatment. The one important qualification to this list of obvious advantages is that hair analysis is, at the time of writing, prohibitively expensive.

Magura et al. (1992) also caution about the possibility that new technology such as hair analysis might lead to an over-enthusiastic spate of drug surveillance within drug treatment programs. According to them, and referring as much to urinalysis as any other form of drug testing:

> ...for patients who otherwise are 'doing well' (e.g. complying with therapy, employed), continuous testing to identify minimal illicit drug use or periodic 'slips' might actually do more harm than good if the clinician is (or feels) obligated to make a strong punitive response. It is important not to allow drug testing to become an end in itself during drug abuse treatment, but to consider carefully the rationale and value of any planned testing protocol for the program, the clinicians, and the individual patients (p. 66).

CONCLUSION

t is difficult to draw any definite conclusions on the basis of the research that has been done and the opinions that have been published for and against the use of urinalysis in methadone maintenance treatment. Surprisingly, the issue has largely been ignored by researchers and as a result it remains difficult to weigh the relative costs and benefits of the procedure. We have, therefore, tried to suggest what the possible options are for the use of urinalysis and what the implications of each of these options might be.

The substantial cost involved in urinalysis is good reason for its use to be reassessed and to ensure that when it is used the samples taken have a good chance of providing a true indication of patients' drug use. The observation made by Wells and McKay (1989) that urinalysis results are at times ignored by treatment staff, and the procedure is only employed because it has become an entrenched feature of methadone maintenance treatment, is a matter for concern. Staff time and public money could be saved if such a practice is widespread. There is perhaps a need to ensure that when

urinalysis is used to monitor drug use, staff understand the many
factors involved in carrying out the procedure in a worthwhile
fashion, including the cost involved.

Finally, the option of abandoning urinalysis altogether is not
far-fetched. The little research that has been done suggests that
scaling down its involvement in methadone maintenance treatment
would not necessarily lead to widespread illicit drug use among
patients and that it may change the atmosphere of clinics from one
imbued with control and surveillance to something more along
therapeutic lines. It has to be kept in mind that no matter what
method is used to monitor illicit drug use in methadone
maintenance programs, the reduction or elimination of drug use is
only one way in which a beneficial treatment outcome might be
measured. Improvements in health, social and psychological
functioning, and reductions in involvement with crime are also
important.

SUMMARY

rinalysis is used in methadone maintenance treatment to
monitor patients' illicit drug use and to ensure that they are
ingesting the methadone prescribed to them. The advantages of
urinalysis are that it provides an objective means of monitoring
drug use that can be used for program evaluation, making clinical
decisions about patients, and monitoring methadone ingestion, and
as evidence in court. Urinalysis is also thought to reduce illicit drug
use. The disadvantages of urinalysis are that the procedure
communicates to patients from the outset that they cannot be
trusted; it is humiliating for both patients and staff to either be
observed urinating or to observe the act of urination; it is a
relatively inaccurate measure of drug use; and it is expensive.

Unless samples are taken every day, urinalysis is not a reliable
method of monitoring drug use. Because daily testing is
prohibitively expensive, tests are usually done less frequently but on
a random basis to try to retain a reasonable chance of detecting
illicit drug use while at the same time keeping costs down. Testing
less than daily without adopting a random schedule allows patients
safe periods for illicit drug use and is probably a waste of time.
Random schedules can be devised in a number of ways. The most
efficient is when patients neither know the day they will be tested
nor the period of time around which the schedule is conducted. To

ensure that samples are not interfered with, the act of urination must be observed.

Research that has examined the ability of urinalysis to reduce illicit drug use has found that it is not reliably effective. Attempts to increase the effectiveness of urinalysis results by contingency management have not demonstrated any enhanced impact over usual procedures, although they have not been well-executed and the results remain ambiguous. Few patients seem to respond to such interventions and any benefit that might be involved is offset by losing substantial numbers of patients from treatment. By way of contrast, research has consistently demonstrated that under certain conditions methadone patients will be truthful about their drug use. These conditions do not prevail in methadone clinics and no research has been done, or attempts described, about how treatment might be changed to allow patients to feel that it is safe to be honest with staff about their drug use.

COUNSELLING AND PSYCHOTHERAPY

INTRODUCTION

he role and importance of counselling has become one of the more controversial issues associated with methadone maintenance treatment. On the one hand, the randomised controlled trials of methadone maintenance reviewed in Chapter 2 included high levels of assistance to the patients beyond the provision of methadone (Dole et al., 1969; Gunne & Grönbladh, 1981; Newman & Whitehill, 1979). On the other hand, low intervention programs (that is, programs with low-level or minimal counselling and other ancillary services) have been advocated as a way of making methadone maintenance available to more people due to the lower cost involved. This chapter attempts to clarify the role that counselling plays in methadone maintenance treatment by examining the accumulated evidence with regard to the contribution of counselling to patient outcome. Research on the related issue of the effectiveness and appropriateness of psychotherapy is also reviewed, along with recent evidence on the characteristics of effective therapists and counsellors.

COUNSELLING

Introduction

ounselling, along with other ancillary services, was originally conceived of as assisting the rehabilitative goals of methadone maintenance treatment. Put simply, it was thought that the provision of methadone would stabilise patients physically and psychologically, while counselling would address the adjustment problems which often accrue after long-term illicit heroin use. The early practitioners of methadone maintenance treatment rejected the view that dependent individuals have pre-existing psychological problems of some sort, arguing strongly that most of their patients' problems were a result of having to maintain a heroin habit, or were due to the socio-economic conditions that they had grown up in (e.g., Dole & Nyswander, 1967; Newman, 1974). The form of counselling that the opioid dependent were thought to require, therefore, was focused on the practicalities of organising their lives, including assistance with housing, job-seeking, and sorting out their legal problems and family relationships. However, the exact constituents of counselling as delivered in methadone maintenance programs are sometimes unclear. The next section considers the nature of the activities that fall under the rubric of counselling.

What Does Counselling Involve?

Although occasional articles have been published over the past three decades describing particular models of methadone maintenance treatment (for example, Kaufman & Blaine, 1974), until recently very little has been known about the day-to-day activities of methadone maintenance programs, what services they deliver, and how those services affect their patients. Counselling is in some ways exemplary in this regard. Fortunately, Ball and Ross's (1991) in-depth account of six methadone maintenance clinics in three cities in the north-east of the USA has provided for the first time a detailed account of what counsellors actually do on a day-to-day basis in methadone maintenance programs. A recent report by the General Accounting Office (1990) has also provided information about counselling services offered in 24 public methadone maintenance programs across the USA, and Calsyn et al. (1990) have published the results of a 1984 national survey of the staffing patterns of USA methadone maintenance units that provides some insight into the services being offered to patients. The recent book-length account of the findings of the Treatment Outcome

Prospective Study (TOPS) has also provided some information on counselling services delivered in the 17 methadone maintenance units that participated in the study (Hubbard et al., 1989).

In Australia, comparable information has been provided by a recent report on 17 public methadone maintenance clinics in New South Wales (Australian Social Issues Research, 1991) and a national survey of treatment practices conducted by the National Drug and Alcohol Research Centre (Baillie et al., 1991). We were unable to find any other published accounts detailing actual counselling practices in methadone maintenance units, though there have been occasional didactic articles addressed to drug counsellors about psychotherapeutic approaches to the treatment of drug dependence (for example, Khantzian, 1985a; Zweben, 1986, 1991).

Counsellors were found to make up 67% of the staff employed at the six methadone maintenance programs surveyed by Ball and Ross (1991), and about half of the staff in the Calsyn et al. (1990) nationwide USA survey. The high proportion of staff being employed as 'counsellors' is a situation which is probably unique to the USA, reflecting Federal regulations that have stipulated a counsellor to patient ratio of 50 to 1. (See General Accounting Office (1990) report for a discussion of this issue.) By contrast, in Australia the professionals most commonly employed in methadone maintenance programs are nurses rather than counsellors (Australian Social Issues Research, 1991). This situation reflects government policy and regulations in Australia that stipulate that at least one nurse must be present when the methadone dose is administered. Finally, unlike the Ball and Ross (1991) study which found one-third of the counsellors to be ex-addicts, it is unusual for ex-addicts to be employed in methadone maintenance programs in Australia.

What does a counsellor in a methadone maintenance clinic do? Ball and Ross (1991) found that most of what counsellors do can be described by 10 activities: case management; liaising with other social service agencies; assessing new applicants; one-to-one counselling; brief contacts; group therapy; family and couples therapy; assessment of psychological problems; vocational counselling; and education. Case management refers to the ongoing documentation and care of the clients that make up a counsellor's case-load. This involves keeping records, representing the client at case meetings, and disciplining the client for misbehaviour and drug-positive urinalysis results. Ball and Ross (1991) emphasised the importance of the 'brief contact' — a term that refers to the brief communications between a counsellor and their client when they meet in the hallway, or when the client drops in to ask a question. Though all of the above listed activities were offered at one or other of the participating methadone maintenance programs, by far the majority of the counselling activity was taken up by brief contacts, one-to-one counselling and group work, in that order.

Nearly all patients in the six programs had regular (on average fortnightly) one-to-one counselling sessions, a pattern that was also found in the study conducted by the General Accounting Office (1990). The topics dealt with in these sessions ranged from current problems related to work, health and the law, and to case management issues such as clinic attendance and ongoing drug use. One important topic early in treatment was helping the patient to understand and comply with the program rules. The general focus, both in terms of time spent on the issue and in terms of the overall goal of treatment, was on what Ball and Ross described as rehabilitation. The way in which counsellors 'rehabilitated' their clients varied considerably, with the approach being determined by training and/or program philosophy and goals, as well as the individual needs of their clients. Whereas some counsellors took a more active approach in terms of giving advice and focusing on behaviour modification, other counsellors took a more traditional counselling approach and focused on their clients' psychological problems rather than their drug use alone.

Group sessions accounted for much less of the face-to-face contact between patients and counsellors and tended to be topic-oriented rather than generally therapeutic. This result is consistent with that from the TOPS study where 78% of the patients surveyed received mostly individual counselling and only 7% reported any group therapy (Hubbard et al., 1989). Ball and Ross (1991) found that groups were usually convened for special purposes, such as dealing with cocaine or alcohol problems, and were attended by individuals with those problems. Other interventions, such as family therapy, were offered to only a few patients, as was psychological assessment, both being based on the needs of the patient. Vocational guidance and education, though available throughout the study period, were only taken advantage of by a minority of patients.

One important role that methadone maintenance programs fulfil for their patients is crisis intervention. Ball and Ross (1991) found that counsellors were not the only staff members who were involved in this activity, although in some programs at least one counsellor was always available on a roster basis. Medical, nursing and administrative staff also helped patients with urgent problems.

These crises involved a range of problems from serious trauma through to less serious matters. Ball and Ross cite the following examples:

> ...suicide attempts, acute depression, auto accident, arrest, fear of gang violence, rape, assault, bereavement, loss of place to live, discharge from program, recognition of HIV positivity, end of welfare payments for family, and so forth (p. 142).

The average case-load for each counsellor was 41 patients with a range of 28 to 63 patients; by contrast, the General Accounting Office found a range from one counsellor for every 15 clients, to one for every 96. Time spent on the various activities described above for the Ball and Ross study was 39% in face-to-face counselling, 31% on case management and administrative work, 12% at staff meetings, and 18% on other activities like urine sample collection and answering the telephone.

In Australia, there is no mandated or recommended counsellor–patient ratio, nor is counselling necessarily seen as part of the methadone maintenance clinic's activities. Nonetheless, according to the National Methadone Guidelines, such services should be available for patients who need them, either at the clinic or by referral if necessary (Commonwealth Department of Community Services and Health, 1991). The survey of public methadone maintenance clinics in New South Wales found that few clinics had staff qualified in psychology or social work (seven out of 17) and that there was considerable variability in the type and number of services offered (Australian Social Issues Research, 1991). Some of the clinics felt, and it was the policy in some districts, that the clinic should provide a point of contact where patients' problems could be assessed, and from where they could be referred elsewhere if they were found to need specialist treatment. If referrals are to be successful, however, special effort is necessary to ensure that the patient being referred arrives at their destination and is welcome when they arrive there — methadone maintenance patients are often not welcome in other sectors of the health care system. One way that has been suggested to ensure more successful referrals is for a member of the referring clinic to accompany the patient to the place of referral and to personally introduce their patient to the specialist concerned (Australian Social Issues Research, 1991).

At clinics that had staff with specialised training (for example, family therapy) and the staff numbers to allow time for it, more specialist services were offered, although the availability of these services appeared to depend more upon the individual interests of staff rather than clinic policy.

A small number of clinics did have much more comprehensive programs with different levels through which patients would graduate. In these programs a commitment to counselling was an expected part of this course. Overall, it would appear that much of the counselling offered in Australia is focused around what Ball and Ross refer to as case management and crisis intervention. Counselling offered over and above case management depends upon a variety factors that include clinic policy, staff–patient ratios and individual staff interests and training. In the recent national survey of treatment practices in Australia, it was found that 45% of patients in methadone maintenance clinics received regular counselling, with a range from 39% in New South Wales to 100% in the Australian Capital Territory and Western Australia (Baillie et al., 1991).

Is Counselling Necessary?

The answer to this question is not clearly known. Commenting on the area, Newman and Peyser (1991) have recently argued that there is a pervasive belief that ancillary services are the most important components of effective methadone maintenance treatment (see for example, Burgess et al., 1990; Renner, 1984), even though there is little research evidence to support this proposition. They contrast this belief with what they see as a reluctance to acknowledge the potency of methadone in bringing about the changes that have been associated with maintenance therapy. The evidence presented in this book that addresses the efficacy of methadone, the dose of methadone and the duration of methadone, argues for the central role of the drug substitution in bringing about reductions in drug use. Similarly the results of the study by Yancovitz et al. (1991) on interim methadone maintenance dosing have shown the potential of methadone maintenance devoid of ancillary services to reduce illicit opiate use (see Chapter 2).

The results of this New York trial by Yancovitz et al. of interim maintenance are interesting, but because of the brief study period (one month), further studies would be desirable. Such further study is unlikely to be promoted in the USA where interim maintenance is considered to be unacceptable by both the advocates and critics of methadone maintenance (Dole, 1991). Advocates fear that the higher intervention methadone maintenance model will be replaced by low intervention (low cost) treatment, and the critics of methadone maintenance fear the spread of a treatment modality they find unpalatable in a form which emphasises even more strongly the provision of methadone. Unfortunately, the study by

Yancovitz et al. (1991) does not tell us whether counselling and other related ancillary services are necessary for the full effectiveness of methadone maintenance to be realised; it merely tells us that interim maintenance reduces the heroin use (Dole, 1991).*

It must, however, be acknowledged that there is as yet no conclusive evidence that methadone maintenance without ancillary services (such as counselling) would be as effective as methadone maintenance with more intensive ancillary services. Yet, Newman and Peyser's point remains valid: it is reasonable to assume that the replacement of heroin with an adequate daily dose of methadone would have a substantial impact on the life of a person whose day-to-day activities are dominated by the pursuit of heroin and the money necessary to buy it.

There seems to have been a reluctance to answer the pertinent question with regard to the role of counselling in methadone maintenance treatment. This question is: is counselling necessary for effective treatment and, if so, for which patients is it necessary? Methadone maintenance programs that offer methadone without counselling or other ancillary services have existed for some time in a number of countries (notably the Netherlands, Hong Kong and Australia), but no evaluations have yet been published to indicate whether they are as effective as full service methadone maintenance programs or if they are especially suited to any specific type of heroin user (Newman & Peyser, 1991; Yancovitz et al., 1991). The few studies that have attempted to answer questions about the role of counselling have often been thwarted in their attempt to do so, and there remains no clear evidence one way or the other.

The first attempt to address the issue was reported by Ramer et al. (1971) who set out to test high dose methadone maintenance with and without ancillary services. The study was quickly abandoned in response to the requests of unit staff who felt that it was unethical to deny patients the benefit of counselling services, especially when they were experiencing crises in their lives. However, the study did provide some pertinent information. One important finding that arose was that patients with psychiatric diagnoses had the worst outcome of the patients participating in the study. In a subsequent comparative observational (non-randomised)

---

* The recent report from the General Accounting Office (1990) cites a study by Childress and her colleagues which found that interim maintenance was no more effective than being on a waiting list. Until the details of this study are available to allow for an assessment of relevant methodological variables (e.g., doses of methadone used), conclusions will have to be restricted to the best available evidence in this case the study by Yancovitz et al. (1991).

study that attempted to examine the issue, Longwell et al. (1978) compared the urinalysis results of two groups of patients in a methadone maintenance program in Arizona: those seeing a counsellor, and those who were not seeing a counsellor. They found that patients who received no counselling had significantly more opiate-positive urinalysis results compared to those who did. This result is consistent with the view that counselling has a positive effect on illicit drug use; yet it is difficult to be confident that the apparent difference is attributable to counselling, since the patients in the Longwell et al. (1978) study were not randomly allocated to receive counselling or not, and no statistical procedures were used to assess whether those patients in the counselling groups differed in any way from those in the non-counselling group. It may have been the case, for example, that the subjects in the non-counselling group were heavier heroin users to start with.

The second related reservation has to do with the time subjects had spent in methadone maintenance. To be eligible for the study, the subject had to have spent three months or more in treatment. There is no evidence to suggest that the authors checked to see if there were differences in time spent in methadone maintenance between the two groups, a factor that has been shown to have a positive effect on outcome (see Chapter 9). With these reservations in mind, the Longwell et al. (1978) study must be considered consistent with the view that counselling is important, but that it does not provide conclusive evidence.

The question of whether counselling is a necessary part of methadone maintenance treatment was also addressed by the Ball and Ross (1991) study. They note that both the staff and patients at the methadone maintenance units that participated in their study viewed counselling as the most important component of the rehabilitative aspect of methadone maintenance treatment. Ball and Ross provided some evidence that programs providing 'a high level of treatment services to patients' were associated with less heroin use, less cocaine use, less injecting drug use and less criminal behaviour among their patients. They reported that a high level of treatment services included: (a) patients being regularly seen in individual counselling sessions; (b) the overall adequacy of the counselling services; (c) a high rate of attendance for medication; (d) as well as a number of other variables that related to the program director and to a long-term maintenance and rehabilitation policy. The Ball and Ross (1991) finding is consistent with the recent report of Joe et al. (1991) from their re-analysis of the TOPS data. Joe et al. (1991) found an increase in retention as measured survival rate for more intense 'psychological' services.

The survival rate increased by 13% for each unit of a six-category measure of frequency of contact which went from none through to daily. For a full description of the Treatment Outcome Prospective Study (Joe et al., 1991) see Chapter 3. These two findings suggest that more intense counselling services lead to a better outcome — reduced drug use, injecting, and crime — and retention for methadone maintenance treatment, respectively.

However, definitive research as to whether counselling is necessary for effective methadone maintenance treatment has still not been carried out. Such research would necessarily involve a randomised controlled trial wherein patients would be provided with equivalent treatment except for counselling services. In such a study patients would receive equivalent and effective doses of methadone (in excess of 50–60 mg, on average), a condition not often met in interim/low intervention programs. They should also preferably be treated by the same staff to control for variables such as staff attitudes to patients. Patients in the no-counselling condition would still receive crisis intervention assistance but no regular individual counselling sessions. A study satisfying these minimum criteria has yet to be done and we can only reiterate Hall's (1983) conclusion that until such a study (or some reasonable approximation to it) has been done, this controversial issue will remain unresolved. It must, however, be acknowledged that in the meantime counselling involving case management and crisis management should be provided in methadone maintenance programs.

Counsellor Training

It has been commonplace in the USA to employ 'ex-addict' counsellors in methadone maintenance programs, presumably in the belief that ex-addicts have advantages in this role because of their own experience of being opioid dependent (Siassi et al. 1977b). However, as Hall (1983) has remarked, there is no reason to assume that an individual's experience of addiction is a ready-made qualification for helping others with their drug dependence. Still, as some claim, it may be the case that ex-addict counsellors are perceived by patients to be more approachable than their 'straight' counterparts, but there is no evidence that this has any significant effect on outcome.

Two findings in the literature suggest that ex-addict counsellors may not be as effective as ordinary counsellors. Siassi et al. (1977b) compared the performance of ex-addict and other counsellors and found that non-addict counsellors performed better on a range of indicators. McLellan et al. (1988), in a study comparing four counsellors, found that the three trained non-addict counsellors were more effective than their ex-addict counterpart.

In contrast, Longwell et al. (1978), in the study discussed earlier, found no difference in the effectiveness of ex-addict and non-addict counsellors. Aiken et al. (1984a), in an investigation to determine whether professional and non-professional counsellors (ex-addict and non-addict) fulfilled different roles in a range of drug treatment programs across the USA, found that there was little difference in what the various types of counsellors did, or in how they went about it, and few differences in counsellors' or clients' attitudes and expectations concerning each other or treatment. The only exception was that ex-addict counsellors were perceived by clients as being more accessible and better able to understand their clients' lives and problems (LoSciuto et al., 1984). Aiken and her colleagues (1984b) went on to compare the outcome of clients of paraprofessional (ex-addict and non-addict) and professional counsellors and found no differences on a range of outcomes.

The more pertinent question to be answered in relation to the studies reviewed above is whether trained counsellors, no matter what their drug use history, are more effective than untrained counsellors. Moreover, for this question to be answered, it will be necessary to clarify the meaning of the word 'training'. Does it mean that the counsellor concerned has been trained as a general counsellor in a postgraduate course for this purpose? Does it mean that the counsellor concerned has attended training courses while working in a methadone maintenance unit and has developed expertise in this fashion? The fact that there is no clear definition of the role and the goals of counselling in methadone maintenance programs makes this task even more difficult. There is a clear need to define the task of counselling and, on the evidence to date, there is no reason to believe that a person without training would be an effective counsellor. One is left wondering what other patient population would be left to the untrained health care worker to meet their needs.

PSYCHOTHERAPY

According to Kleber (1984) psychotherapy can be distinguished from counselling by the fact that it attempts to influence mental processes which are believed to underlie maladaptive behaviour. In the case of psychodynamic psychotherapy, these mental processes are assumed to consist of unconscious conflicts. For cognitive-behavioural therapy the underlying cognitive processes are believed to be maladaptive negative behaviours, thoughts and emotions. Another way of making the distinction is that suggested by Woody et al. (1983), according to whom counselling focuses on external matters that are often resolved by specific and direct assistance of some sort, whereas psychotherapy is concerned with the internal psychological processes of the client. In other words, counselling mainly consists of 'practical problem solving' (Hubbard et al., 1989) or as Kleber (1984) suggested, counselling involves adopting a common sense approach that focuses on support and help.

In this section we examine the more recent research on the use of psychotherapy as an adjunct to methadone maintenance treatment. Early (mainly psychoanalytic) case reports from the pre-methadone maintenance period are not reviewed, except to say that it has long been believed that opioid-dependent individuals are not amenable to psychotherapy.

The New Haven Psychotherapy Study

Rounsaville and his colleagues (1983; 1986c) conducted a well-designed, randomised controlled trial that compared six months of weekly interpersonal psychotherapy (IPT) with a low-contact control condition consisting of a brief monthly appointment with a psychiatrist. Interpersonal psychotherapy is an individual therapy in which the focus of discussion is primarily upon interpersonal, or relationship, issues. According to Rounsaville et al. (1983): 'Short-term IPT is based on the concept that psychiatric disorders, including depression and opiate addiction, are intimately associated with disturbances in interpersonal functioning, which may be associated with the genesis and perpetuation of the disorder' (p. 630).

In the trial conducted by Rounsaville, 72 subjects who had a current psychiatric disorder were assessed on a range of outcomes and psychiatric indicators at the commencement of the study, at four week intervals until the end of the treatment period, and followed two and a half years later. All subjects also had to attend a 90-minute session of group therapy once a week as part of their methadone maintenance program.

Rounsaville et al. (1983) found no indication of an advantage for short-term IPT on any of the assessed outcomes in comparison to the low-contact control condition. In fact, they found support for the long-held clinical wisdom that opioid-dependent individuals will not attend for psychotherapy (Woody et al., 1986), in that patients in the IPT condition were more likely to drop out of the study than were patients in the control condition. Rounsaville et al. (1983) point out that the lack of any demonstrable benefit for IPT, and indeed for psychotherapy, in this study is inconsistent with previous research that has shown IPT to be of benefit to depressed patients. It also conflicts with the findings of Stanton, Todd and Associates (1982) and Woody et al. (1983, 1987) which indicate that some methadone maintenance patients may benefit from psychotherapy. Rounsaville et al. suggest that there may be no discernible benefit for additional psychotherapy in a high intervention methadone maintenance program that offers both counselling on demand and compulsory group therapy on a weekly basis. Substantial attrition from the study may also have made it difficult to demonstrate an effect, although Rounsaville et al. point out that the subjects who left IPT did not generally leave the methadone maintenance program, suggesting they had lost interest in IPT rather than methadone maintenance treatment.

The VA-Penn Psychotherapy Study

The Philadelphia Veterans Administration Medical Center–University of Pennsylvania (VA-Penn) psychotherapy study was conducted by Woody et al. (1983, 1987) in an attempt to determine whether psychotherapy could be a useful adjunct to the high intervention, low dose methadone maintenance treatment being delivered at the medical center to male war veterans. Taking four and a half years to complete, this study remains the largest and most successfully conducted study of psychotherapy with opioid-dependent clients reported to date. In this study, 110 methadone-maintained, male war veterans were randomly assigned to one of three conditions: supportive-expressive psychotherapy (SE — a psychodynamic psychotherapy) plus drug counselling (DC); cognitive behavioural psychotherapy (CB) plus DC; and DC without additional psychotherapy. Sessions with psychotherapists and counsellors were scheduled weekly and the study period was for six months.

When assessed at seven months from the commencement of psychotherapy (that is, at one month after the psychotherapy was ceased) the patients who had received psychotherapy in addition to DC made both more and larger improvements than those who received only DC. Statistically significant differences between pre- and post-study assessment scores were observed in 12 of the outcome measures for the SE group, nine for the CB group and seven for the DC group. The SE group made strong gains in the areas of psychiatric symptoms and employment. In terms of drug use, all three groups improved but the SE and DC groups improved more than the CB group. When illicit opiate use was examined, the SE and CB groups had significantly less use than the DC group, even though the DC patients were maintained on higher doses of methadone than the SE and CB groups whose doses declined over the study period. Finally, DC patients were prescribed more ancillary psychotropic medication than the psychotherapy patients; in fact, the number of prescriptions written for the DC patients increased over the study period, whereas they decreased for the psychotherapy patients. Overall, the psychotherapy patients needed less methadone and ancillary medication, and made greater gains in a number of areas, than the DC patients. The two psychotherapy groups only differed significantly in a few areas: SE patients made greater improvements on measures for psychological functioning and employment, while CB patients had significantly less legal problems.

Woody and his colleagues reported the results of the 12-month follow-up assessments in 1987. They found that, in general, scores for the three treatment groups (SE, CB and DC) remained improved when compared with baseline measures. However, significant differences between the two sets of scores were found on 10 measures for the SE group, on 12 for the CB group, but on only two for the DC only group.

When the scores were looked at in more detail, it was evident that the majority of gains observed at seven months were maintained in the SE group, with further improvement being seen in employment, legal status, and psychiatric functioning. For the CB group, most of the gains were still evident at 12 months and further improvements had occurred in drug and alcohol problems and psychiatric condition. The DC only group maintained improvement in drug use and employment but the previous gains made in psychiatric functioning declined. Legal status in the DC only group had become significantly worse in the period between 7- and 12-month follow-up. When the records for patients still in methadone maintenance were scrutinised at 12 months it was found that, like at seven months, patients who had the benefit of psychotherapy seemed to require a lower dose of methadone, and fewer psychotropic medications, while maintaining low levels of illicit drug use.

In a further study of cognitive-behavioural psychotherapy at the Veterans Administration methadone program in Philadelphia, subjects who were randomly assigned to cognitive behavioural therapy did better on a range of outcomes measured one month after the completion of treatment than did subjects who received drug counselling (McLellan et al. 1986). The addition of a procedure to extinguish conditioned responses to drug-related stimuli (for example, preparing drugs to inject) to cognitive-behavioural psychotherapy did not lead to a better outcome, and the authors concluded that this procedure was therefore unsuitable for patients who were being maintained on methadone, or being treated on an outpatient basis. Woody and his colleagues (1990) are currently carrying out a further study in methadone maintenance units based in the community to assess the effectiveness of adding SE psychotherapy to methadone maintenance treatment.

Woody et al. (1983) argued that the addition of psychotherapy to a traditional methadone maintenance treatment service was successful because the therapy entailed a special kind of relationship — a therapeutic alliance — as well as special knowledge about how to manage that relationship. They observed that although many of the drug counsellors develop very good relationships with their clients, they had difficulty managing the relationship at times, especially when dealing with the more disturbed clients. In order to examine this possibility they went on to analyse the data taking into account the severity of psychiatric problems found among the patients participating in the study.

Psychiatric Severity and Response to Psychotherapy

Methadone maintenance patients suffer from high levels of psychiatric disorders, especially depressive disorders, and the severity with which they suffer from these disorders is predictive of treatment outcome (Chapter 13). Woody et al. (1984) examined the seven-month follow-up data collected in the VA-Penn study to determine if the addition of psychotherapy had made any difference to the relationship between psychiatric severity and outcome. A composite psychiatric severity score was calculated on the basis of the ASI psychiatric severity score and the other psychological assessment scales administered at the commencement of the study. Psychiatric severity scores for each patient were then categorised into low, medium and high severity groups and the data re-analysed by treatment group.

Significant improvements were found for low severity patients in all three groups and the addition of psychotherapy of either kind (SE or CB) offered no advantage. However, in the group of patients with medium severity scores, positive change occurred in all three therapy conditions, but the psychotherapy groups showed more changes on psychological assessment scores. Significant differences were observed between the psychotherapy and DC conditions, the majority of them showing an advantage for psychotherapy. The medium severity DC patients were also maintained on significantly higher methadone doses and required more psychotropic medication than the patients who received additional psychotherapy.

A clear benefit for receiving psychotherapy was also apparent for the high severity group. Both the CB and SE groups had improved at seven-month follow-up on most outcome measures and had made large gains on measures for employment, legal status and psychiatric functioning. By comparison, high psychiatric severity patients who received DC only changed little on any of the assessment measures, except for drug use, which showed a significant improvement. When the three groups were compared with each other, it was found that the DC group was poorer on nine out of 10 significant outcome measures. DC patients also required higher mean methadone doses and more psychotropic medicine than the psychotherapy patients. High severity patients, when compared as a group to the other two severity categories, had higher mean doses of methadone, a higher proportion of drug positive urine results, and were prescribed more psychotropic medicine. The low and medium severity groups did not differ on these measures.

As Woody et al. (1984) point out, three main points emerge from these data. First, patients in the high severity category had poorer pre-treatment functioning in all of the measures assessed than did medium or low severity patients. This is consistent with previous findings. The most common diagnosis in the high severity group was a depressive disorder. Secondly, high severity patients did not respond in any of the three conditions as well as patients with less severe psychiatric problems. High severity patients gained little from DC by itself. Thirdly, psychotherapy, when added to traditional methadone maintenance, made a difference to the relationship between psychiatric severity and treatment outcome. In this study, high severity patients improved in many areas of functioning and, in comparison with the DC patients, were able to do so on lower doses of methadone and with less psychotropic medication while taking fewer illicit drugs.

One difficulty with the interpretation of the main findings of the study had been that patients overall in the DC condition had less exposure to a counsellor or therapist than had patients in the psychotherapy conditions. This may have led to a treatment effect for the SE and CB conditions simply due to more attention. However, when this matter was examined by level of psychiatric severity, it was found that there were no significant differences in exposure to therapist/counsellor in the medium and high severity groups, suggesting that the observed effect was from therapy type rather than quantity of treatment *per se*. Woody et al. (1984) concluded that psychotherapy was a useful addition to methadone maintenance for patients with severe psychiatric symptoms.

Antisocial Personality and Response to Psychotherapy

Woody et al. (1985b) also used the seven-month follow-up data to examine the traditional belief that individuals with a diagnosis of antisocial personality (ASP) disorder do not respond well to psychological treatments. The subjects were divided into four categories:

(a) those whose only diagnosis was opioid dependence;

(b) those who had a diagnosis of depression in addition to opioid dependence;

(c) those who were depressed, opioid-dependent and diagnosed as having ASP disorder; and

(d) those who were opioid-dependent and had a diagnosis of ASP but no depressive disorder.

Patients without depressive or ASP disorder, and those who were depressed, responded well to treatment. The group with ASP disorder and depression also responded to treatment but not as well as the former groups. By contrast, the group with ASP disorder and no depression did not respond on most of the outcomes assessed, although they did improve in their drug use and legal status. In comparison to the other three groups, who did benefit from psychotherapy when compared to DC only patients, the ASP only group did not.

Woody et al. (1985b) concluded that psychotherapy, as has long been believed, does not benefit patients with a diagnosis of ASP disorder without a concurrent diagnosis of depression. One defining characteristic of ASP disorder for some diagnostic instruments (e.g. Research Diagnostic Criteria, see Gerstley et al., 1990) is the inability to form meaningful and enduring relationships with other people. Given that such a relationship is a precondition for effective psychotherapy, it is not surprising that it was found to be of no benefit in individuals with ASP. However, antisocial behaviour itself is common to the patient population, and by itself is not a contraindicator for psychotherapy. Woody et al. argue that an additional diagnosis of depression indicates that the individual concerned is capable of an emotional response and is therefore amenable to psychological treatment. Patients with ASP disorder are amenable to methadone maintenance, however, as is indicated by the observed reduction in drug use and crime.

Other Specific Interventions

A number of specific psychotherapeutic interventions that might be
added to counselling procedures to bring about behaviour change
have been studied with methadone maintenance patients. Many
have been relatively brief approaches that have met with limited
success. They are largely unreplicated, and it is not possible to be
fully confident of their likely impact. For example, Houston and
Milby (1983) attempted to assess the impact of aversion therapy
with methadone maintenance patients. They used electric shocks
paired with patients' imaginings of drug seeking behaviour, and
(perhaps not surprisingly) found no discernible effect on drug use.
In a similarly disappointing and limited study, Goldberg et al.
(1976) reported four case studies of methadone maintenance
patients who were taught 'alpha conditioning' (a relaxation
technique using biofeedback), and although the patients reported
that the technique induced a pleasant mental state, the authors
found no evidence for effects on traditional treatment outcomes like
extent of drug use. Another study using biofeedback techniques to
facilitate relaxation found that it reduced measures of anxiety in a
small group of methadone maintenance patients; however, the high
drop-out rate suggested that the primary difficulty might be getting
methadone maintenance patients to participate in sessions at all
(Kuna et al., 1976).

In another behaviourally-oriented study of reducing injecting
heroin use among methadone maintenance patients, Snowden
(1978) found a decline in heroin use in response to covert
desensitisation (sessions of imagined negative consequences to
injecting heroin) for methadone maintenance patients who were
assessed as having an internal locus of control. The finding, in the
absence of other research, has to be considered suggestive at best,
given that the experiment lasted for only seven weeks, that the
subjects were paid to attend sessions, and that the same
researcher/therapist conducted all sessions in all three conditions,
and therefore could not be considered a disinterested evaluator of
success.

More recently, and reflecting developments in the alcohol
dependence treatment field, new psychological interventions have
been applied to methadone maintenance patients. Specifically,
motivational interviewing has been subjected to some study.
Motivational interviewing is an approach to drug problems that is
based on the reflective listening style of counselling developed by
Carl Rogers (Rogers, 1957; Miller & Rollnick, 1991). Saunders and
his colleagues (Saunders & Wilkinson, 1990; Saunders et al., 1991)
have compared the effect of a two-session motivational interviewing

intervention to a two-session educational intervention at the commencement of methadone maintenance. They found few important differences between the two groups at six-month follow-up, but did find that the motivational interviewing subjects complied better with treatment. The most important contribution that motivational interviewing may make to methadone maintenance treatment might be in improving the general relationship between patients and unit staff as well as counsellors. Future research will clarify this issue. The therapeutic style associated with motivational interviewing is discussed in more detail later in this chapter.

In an investigation of a more global change to methadone maintenance treatment, patients surveyed in an Oregon methadone maintenance unit which had developed a 'psychoeducational' approach to ancillary service delivery were found to dislike group activities and life education classes; they preferred individual counselling in the methadone program (Stark & Campbell, 1991). This finding suggests that individual counselling is a form of ancillary intervention that methadone maintenance patients most like, and that a needs analysis approach, in which patients are surveyed to find out what kinds of interventions they need and prefer, is probably a useful step in developing a patient-centred set of services.

Clearly a group format for the counselling of methadone maintenance patients is an attractive option as an intervention because it is cost efficient. However, it does appear that the research evidence and clinical lore agree that methadone maintenance patients do not like to participate in group therapy. Although this may be the case for unstructured therapeutic sessions, recent evidence suggests that special purpose self-help groups may be more attractive if they are presented in the right way. For example, groups for pregnant women and HIV positive patients and patients with AIDS have been reported as having some success in attracting patients into treatment (see Chapters 11 and 12).

There have, however, been very few studies of group therapy with methadone maintenance patients. An early study by Willet (1973) compared two types of group therapy (psychoanalytic and T-group) to methadone alone. It failed to find any significant differences in drug use or interpersonal functioning. Unfortunately, a substantial drop-out rate from all three conditions resulted in a very small sample size that rendered the study uninterpretable. Abrahams (1979), in a later study, compared a cognitive-behavioural group to a non-directive group over a 10-week period on a range of outcomes. The cognitive-behavioural intervention incorporated an extensive package of skills training which included relaxation, assertion training and how to deal with problem situations. The control group met once a week for the same amount of time and participated in unstructured group discussions with a therapist present. The cognitive-behavioural intervention showed significant improvements on measures for anxiety, depression, and assertiveness. There was no advantage for the cognitive-behavioural group on drug use as measured by urinalysis. This study suggests that the value of group therapy, if patients will comply, may be found in meeting the psychiatric needs of methadone maintenance patients.

Family Therapy

The term 'family therapy' covers a range of interventions that have been developed over the past three decades, all of which have a common theoretical rationale that assumes that behavioural and psychological problems are a function of disordered or maladaptive interpersonal relationships within the family. Each family is understood from a systems theory perspective as a system with rules that govern its functioning (Hazelrigg et al., 1987). Although a family therapist will usually conduct sessions with members of the family and the client together, this is not necessarily a defining feature of the interventions that family therapy covers; some interventions may only involve the individual while others may involve other people in the client's life (e.g. co-workers, drug treatment agency staff, etc.) (Durrant, 1989; Hazelrigg et al., 1987). Family therapy has attracted the interest of counsellors and therapists who work with drug-dependent individuals, including methadone maintenance unit staff. In a national survey of drug and alcohol treatment agencies conducted in the 1970s in the USA, methadone maintenance units expressed the most interest in family therapy (Coleman & Davis, 1978).

Durrant (1989) suggests that there are seven definable types of family therapy practised in Australia, which differ from each other as much as any of them do from other types of psychotherapy and counselling. According to Hazelrigg et al. (1987), however, family therapies can be classified into two broad types: those that are 'pragmatic', in that they are focused on symptom removal and behaviour change; and those that are 'aesthetic', and have the broader goal of transforming the family system and achieving a holistic integration of the self. Only the pragmatic types of family therapy (structural, strategic, behavioural) have been evaluated using traditional research methods, and these types will be considered here.

Only two controlled studies have looked at the effectiveness of family therapy with an opioid-dependent clientele. The first of these was conducted in the USA (Stanton et al., 1982), while the second, which was intended to be a replication of the USA study, was carried out recently in the Netherlands (Romijn et al., 1990). Both assessed structural family therapy as described by Stanton and his co-workers. This is a goal-directed intervention which requires the client and his or her family of origin (parents and siblings) to be present in the therapy sessions (Stanton et al., 1982). The therapist takes an active role and tries to influence the ways in which family members communicate with each other about the client's drug use. Therapy is time-limited, intense, and focused on the client's drug problems. An important component is that the client's parents have to take an active role in managing their child's treatment.

The Stanton et al. (1982) study was a collaboration between the Philadelphia Child Guidance Clinic and the Drug Dependence Treatment Center of the Philadelphia Veterans Administration Hospital. The subjects were all males applying for methadone maintenance who satisfied the eligibility criteria, the most important of which was that they were in more than weekly contact with their parents or parent surrogates. The eligibility criteria were in fact changed a third of the way through the study — subjects had to be living with their parents or parent surrogates. They and their families were randomly allocated to one of three conditions or to a control group if they satisfied the eligibility criteria and there was no therapist available at their time of entry to the program.

This resulted in four conditions being compared:

(a) *paid family therapy* that involved 10 therapy sessions in which all members of the family were paid a fee to attend, with the fee increasing if the subject was drug free for that week (extra money was paid for withdrawing from methadone);

(b) *unpaid family therapy*, which was the same as the paid condition, except that no money was paid for attendance, or for reduced drug use;

(c) *paid family movie condition*, which consisted of an equivalent number of sessions of family movie watching for which family members were paid in the same manner as the paid family therapy condition (for attendance and reduction in drug use); and

(d) *methadone maintenance control condition*, which consisted of subjects who were in methadone maintenance.

Subjects in the movie group and the methadone maintenance control condition had access to a counsellor on demand, whereas in the two family therapy conditions the family therapist assumed the role of drug counsellor and took control of the treatment, including the dispensing of methadone and take-home doses.

As Hall (1983) has remarked, this study is unique in the literature for the sophistication of its design in that it includes what is known as a non-specific control group (i.e. a group that received the same amount of exposure to certain basic conditions of therapy but is not exposed to the therapy itself). Borkovec (1990) provides a lucid discussion of the issue of control groups in psychotherapy research. The methadone control condition provided baseline data for what could be expected of a matched group of patients receiving methadone maintenance treatment as usual. The family movie group (non-specific control) provided a control for both payment and the simple effect of the family getting together once a week for 10 weeks. The unpaid family therapy group controlled for what might happen when a financial incentive for attendance and reduced drug use was not employed. To summarise, Stanton et al. compared a sample of male veteran methadone maintenance patients who were exposed to paid family therapy, unpaid family therapy, paid family movie plus counselling, and counselling.

Stanton et al. assessed each of the four groups of subjects on two measures: the percentage of days spent drug free in various drug classes (legal opioids, illegal opioids, other illicit drugs, marijuana and alcohol) and time spent in work or school. Outcome was also measured by the percentage of subjects in each group who were categorised as having a poor, medium or good outcome. Data was collected at six and 12 months after treatment. Differences were found in the direction expected for a family therapy effect for the drug classes other than alcohol (i.e. those who were exposed to family therapy had less drug use). No effect was found for employment or schooling. The differences in favour of family therapy were, however, only statistically significant for illicit drug use other than opiates, while the findings for the two classes of opioids were marginally significant (p<0.06).

The way in which the data are presented and analysed (one-way analysis of variance — no error term or F-ratios tabled) makes it difficult to know how to evaluate these data. The authors went on to carry out further analyses (analysis of covariance) to remove unwanted variation introduced by client characteristics which did result in statistically significant results for each of the outcomes favouring family therapy. As presented, these data suggest that family therapy contributes to a better outcome when combined with methadone maintenance than does drug counselling, but the data remain difficult to interpret.

In a further analysis, the data from the four conditions were combined into two comparable groups — family therapy (paid and unpaid) and a control group (methadone maintenance control and family movie) — and then analysed according to whether subjects were found to have a poor, medium or good outcome. The allocation of poor, medium and good outcome categories was determined by combining all the outcome measures. Significant differences in favour of family therapy were found for legal opiates, illegal opiates, other illegal drugs and marijuana. No advantage for family therapy was found for alcohol consumption or employment. However, when the mortality rates for the two groups were examined, it was found that 10% of the control subjects had died in the period to follow-up compared with 2% of the family therapy subjects — a difference that was significant. Further follow-ups to five years after the completion of therapy were planned. Todd (1984) reports that the positive effects for family therapy had persisted at two to three years after finishing treatment, but he presents no data to support this claim. We have been unable to find any other reports of further follow-ups for this study.

Taken overall, the Stanton et al. study was a well designed test of the use of family therapy in a methadone program. Patients who had the benefit of family therapy seem to have been able to reduce both their need for methadone and their use of illicit drugs. However, it has to be acknowledged that the eligibility criteria for the study meant that a defined sub-group of patients in the VA methadone program were compared with one another under a range of therapy conditions. Obviously, if a patient does not have contact with his or her family, or refuses to allow family members to become involved in the treatment process, then they are not suitable for family therapy. Further, structural family therapy is an intense and directive intervention that requires considerable interpersonal and observational skills of the therapist that can only be acquired through specialist training. It would seem then that if such a therapist was available and willing to go to the considerable effort of engaging a patient's family in treatment, and if the client was suitable for a family intervention, then family therapy may prove useful as an adjunct to traditional methadone maintenance treatment. It is impossible to say with any confidence on the basis of this single study, given the inadequate data presentation and analysis, whether such an intervention will or will not benefit a patient.

There has been one attempt to replicate the Stanton et al. study. Romijn et al. (1990) compared family therapy without methadone maintenance with low dose (20 mg) methadone maintenance plus drug counselling using two groups of subjects who were retrospectively matched on a range of client variables (age, sex, drug use etc.). Using the same outcome criteria as in the original study, the two groups were compared on follow-up measures taken 18 months after the commencement of treatment. In addition to the outcomes used by Stanton et al., crime and extent of drug culture involvement were assessed. The two groups differed significantly on only one measure — crime — and this favoured the methadone maintenance group.

This study differs obviously from the USA study in a number of ways. First, it compares family therapy alone to methadone maintenance, whereas the original Stanton et al. study compared family therapy to drug counselling among methadone maintenance patients. Secondly, the USA study randomly allocated subjects to each of the conditions, an allocation procedure that is superior to matched controls, especially when it is taken into account that the family therapy and the methadone maintenance subjects in the Dutch study came from different geographical locations. Thirdly, a number of aspects of the study are not clear. No detail is given about the length of the family therapy, or about the average tenure of the patients in the methadone maintenance condition. No detail is given about the methadone maintenance program, making it difficult to assess the effectiveness of such a program. In this regard, doses of methadone as low as 20 mg have been consistently shown to be associated with treatment failure (see Chapter 6).

For all of the above reasons, it has to be concluded that the null result of the Dutch study does not overturn the promise for family therapy as part of a methadone maintenance program shown in the Philadelphia study. Of relevance also are two recent meta-analyses of family therapy that reviewed controlled studies of the effectiveness of family therapy for a range of disorders (which did not include drug dependence), both of which have independently found family therapy to be moderately effective when compared to no-treatment control groups (Hazelrigg et al., 1987; Markus et al., 1990). It is reasonable to assume that if family therapy is effective in other areas, (for example, behaviour disorders in adolescents) then it may be effective in cases of drug dependence that are suitable for the intervention.

The extent to which this is desirable in methadone maintenance programs would have to be established: how many patients have sufficient contact with their family of origin and are willing to allow them to become involved in treatment? If there is a need, then further studies will need to establish whether such patients would benefit from family therapy if it was made available to them. The extent to which methadone maintenance program staff are willing to be trained in family therapy, or to which family therapists are willing to participate in methadone maintenance treatment, would also have to be established. Finally, the difficulties in getting methadone maintenance patients to attend family therapy sessions should not be underestimated. For example, Todd (1984) reports that paying patients did influence attendance at sessions in the Stanton et al. (1982) study. While all of the subjects and their families attended a minimum of four sessions in the paid family therapy condition, only 52% did so when they were not paid to attend.

Mandatory Psychotherapy?

Desmond and Maddux (1983) compared mandatory versus optional psychotherapy (described as supportive therapy and relationship therapy) over a one-year period and found no significant differences on a range of outcomes between the two groups. The pattern of results favoured the optional group, which is not surprising given that it is difficult to imagine how mandatory psychotherapy could be effective. Both groups received drug counselling as well as psychotherapy from the same counsellor, one for each group. It is unfortunate that the two groups were not compared to a third control group receiving drug counselling alone. The simple conclusion to be drawn from this study is that *mandatory* psychotherapy, if this needed to be demonstrated, should not be used as an adjunct to methadone maintenance. As Kaufman and Blaine (1974) have remarked, in methadone maintenance units where counselling or psychotherapy is mandatory, patients think of counselling sessions as a game they have to play to keep up their supply of methadone.

THERAPIST EFFECTS

Do Therapists Differ in Their Impact on Patients?

An important finding arising out of the analysis of the results of the VA-Penn psychotherapy project was that there were significant differences in the effectiveness of different therapists within each of the types of therapy compared (Luborsky et al., 1985). This finding confirms what is common knowledge among clinicians — that some therapists are better than others, no matter what style of therapy they subscribe to. This finding, which has since been replicated, has important implications for both treatment practices and future research on counselling, psychotherapy and (as will be seen) methadone maintenance treatment in general.

Most psychotherapy and counselling research has, until recently, compared the relative effectiveness of different types of interventions (for example, psychodynamic versus behavioural) and in doing so has assumed that one therapist is equivalent to another. Indeed, as Luborsky et al. (1986) point out, in the more than 500 studies that had been reported in the period to 1980 on psychotherapy, few examined whether there were differences between therapists within the various modalities that were being assessed. Luborsky et al. (1986) re-examined the data for four psychotherapy outcome studies (which included the seven-month follow-up data from the VA-Penn psychotherapy project) and found that differences between therapists were significantly related to patient outcome in all four. Importantly, therapist effects were found to be as, if not more, important than the contribution of therapy type to outcome. These findings have serious implications for the interpretation of research comparing different interventions that does not routinely control for therapist effects, that is, the therapist's as opposed to the therapy's influence on outcome.

Crits-Christoph et al. (1990) discuss in detail the implications of therapist effects for psychotherapy and counselling research. They argue that therapists are often treated in statistical analyses as if they were a fixed form of treatment, like a therapeutic drug, when they should be treated as if they were a random selection from the population of therapists who practise the particular form of therapy being investigated. In cases where the therapist is treated as a fixed form of treatment, the proper conclusion to be drawn is that the therapy concerned is effective as practised by the participating therapists. If there are no differences between therapists then this advice can be ignored. Crits-Christoph re-examined the data from eight psychotherapy studies to see how often this might occur. They found therapist effects in six out of eight of the studies. The largest therapist effect for any outcome measure in these studies meant that 55% of the variability in outcome seen in the patients was due to differences between therapists.

In order to determine the implications of therapist effects for study findings, Crits-Christoph et al. conducted a large series of simulated psychotherapy studies on computer using data generated randomly. Each of these 'studies' compared three treatment groups and varied both the number of therapists in each condition and the amount of variation in treatment effect contributed by differences between therapists. For each possible study, they then generated 2 000 analyses of variance using the randomly generated data. They found that neither the number of treatments, nor the number of therapists for each treatment would affect the results, but that the number of clients being treated by each therapist and the size of therapist effects would. In a study where there were 15 clients assigned to each therapist and where 25% of the variation seen in outcome was due to differences between therapists, one would expect a false positive result approximately 50% of the time. That is, one out of every two studies showing one intervention to be superior to another would be incorrect if differences between therapists were not investigated, and statistically controlled for if found.

The implications of this finding extend to studies of methadone maintenance treatment (Crits-Christoph et al., 1990). Recent research (for example, Ball and Ross, 1991) has found that methadone maintenance units differ in their effectiveness. This suggests that methadone maintenance units should be treated as random factors in treatment outcome studies that compare different modalities, unless it can be demonstrated that the variation in unit effect is zero. However, for the purposes of treatment practice, the most important implication of these findings is that an examination of therapist characteristics and their relationship to client improvement may lead to more effective therapies in general.

Characteristics of Effective Therapists

In addition to studies discussed in the previous section, there are two studies from the VA-Penn group, and findings from the alcohol treatment literature, which suggest that the therapist is an important factor in interventions with people with drug problems. In their investigation of the VA-Penn psychotherapy project data for therapist effects, Luborsky et al. (1985) found a number of aspects of both therapist and therapeutic style to be associated with improved outcomes when random samples of the therapy and counselling sessions were analysed. These findings can be summarised by four main points:

- therapists who were able to develop a warm, supportive relationship as a basis for working together (a therapeutic alliance) had better outcomes;
- components of sessions in all three modalities — supportive–expressive psychotherapy (SE), cognitive behavioural psychotherapy (CB), and drug counselling (DC) — that were coded as being part of SE or CB protocols from audio tapes of the sessions were associated with better outcomes, while DC techniques were not;
- the extent to which the psychotherapy sessions were consistent with the protocol for each of the therapies was related to better

outcome, and this was true for comparisons between clients for individual therapists (that is, those clients who received 'purer' SE or CB therapy did better);

- the extent to which therapists were judged to be well adjusted, skilled and interested in helping their patients was positively associated with a better outcome (although these were not statistically significant, perhaps as Luborsky et al. suggest, because of the small sample size of nine therapists).

Luborsky et al. (1985) interpreted these findings to mean that both personal characteristics of the therapist (adjustment, skill, interest in work, ability to establish a therapeutic alliance) and the psychotherapeutic techniques themselves (SE and CB) contributed to a better outcome. The latter point was highlighted by the finding that drug counsellors whose sessions were coded with more CB and SE components had clients who improved more. However, the data suggest that differences between therapists rather than modalities, are the more powerful influence on client response. Luborsky et al. suggest that the most important characteristic in this regard is the ability to develop a therapeutic alliance.

In a further study from the VA-Penn group, McLellan et al. (1988) retrospectively examined the differences in outcome for four drug counsellors who were appointed to a large number of clients in a virtually random fashion after the sudden resignation of two counsellors on the VA methadone maintenance program in Philadelphia. They found consistent differences across a range of outcomes between the counsellors. While two counsellors were moderately effective, the third was very effective and the fourth was not effective at all. The most effective counsellor was able to bring his clients to a point over a six-month period where their drug use and unemployment were significantly reduced when compared with the six months prior to the change in counsellor, while at the same time reducing their use of both methadone and ancillary psychotropic prescriptions. By contrast, the clients of the least effective counsellor showed increased levels of unemployment, drug use and criminal activity, and needed more methadone and ancillary medication.

When the differences between counsellors were examined, it was found that the most effective counsellor had postgraduate qualifications in psychology, while the least effective counsellor was an ex-addict with no tertiary education; the two moderately effective counsellors also had tertiary education. The three more effective counsellors kept well organised case notes, saw their patients frequently, were consistent in the application of program rules, and often referred their patients to other members of staff within the methadone maintenance unit and to outside agencies for specialist help. The least effective counsellor did not keep adequate case management notes, saw clients relatively infrequently, was inconsistent in responding to rule infractions, and seemed not to refer clients for specialist help. McLellan et al. (1988) claimed that when the case notes were examined in detail for some indication of session content, it became clear that the most effective counsellor was able to help clients anticipate their problems and assist them in developing ways of dealing with them before they arose. This was the quality that most clearly distinguished this counsellor from the moderately effective ones who were similarly qualified. They went on to argue that the techniques reflected in the case notes were consistent with those features of psychotherapy that were found to be effective in comparison with DC in the psychotherapy project.

The findings discussed in this section suggest that two important qualities contribute to the effectiveness of a counsellor: the ability to establish a warm, supportive relationship with the client relatively quickly, and having specialist knowledge about how to manage that relationship once it has developed (Woody et al., 1984; Zweben, 1991). The findings of the VA-Penn psychotherapy project overall suggest the latter is of most relevance when dealing with more disturbed clients. This also seems to be true of therapeutic relationships with 'difficult' methadone maintenance patients. Case management duties, which often involve dealing with rule infractions, conflict with the need to establish an alliance with clients. This is especially true of 'difficult' patients who persistently break program rules. Zweben (1991) remarks that such rules are based on the notion that the behaviour of patients can be controlled through having rules and enforcing them. This, she argues, is in conflict with: 'the understanding on the part of most addiction treatment professionals that one person is essentially powerless to control the drug use of another'. (p. 178). (See also Miller & Rollnick (1991) for an extended discussion of this issue.) In dealing with ongoing illicit drug use, Zweben suggests that counsellors who use 'power tactics' when patients refuse to comply are merely demonstrating their lack of clinical skills. This point of view is consistent with that of Miller and Brown (1991) who take the VA-Penn group's argument one step further and suggest that not only is establishing a therapeutic alliance important to a positive treatment response, but that confronting clients about their drug use contributes to a negative one.

The point has been made on a number of occasions that the importance of establishing supportive relationships when counselling clients with drug problems is simply a specific application of what has been found to be more generally true for counselling and psychotherapy (for example, Luborsky et al., 1985; Miller and Brown, 1991; Miller & Rollnick, 1991; Saunders et al., 1991). Miller and his colleagues have been especially emphatic on this point, arguing that the traditional approach of confronting clients about their drug use in an attempt to get through to them works against everything that has been learned about how to change human behaviour. Miller and Brown (1991) interpret the Luborsky et al. (1985) findings as showing that counselling that consists solely of case management is ineffective. On this interpretation, this aspect of methadone maintenance treatment is conducive to a confrontational and directive style (see also Zweben, 1991). In a study of clients with alcohol problems, Miller and Sovereign (1989) found that the more therapists confronted clients, the less likely they were to reduce their drinking, and the more the therapist was empathic and supported the client, the more likely it was that they would reduce their drinking. Miller and Rollnick (1991) argue, on the basis of results like these, that the therapist is largely responsible for the extent to which the client resists therapy and, therefore, for the failure of therapy to the extent that it is the result of client resistance.

CONCLUSION

In concluding, it seems appropriate to reiterate the final statements from Hall (1983) in her review of the role of ancillary services in methadone maintenance treatment. There is a need to establish whether or not counselling is essential to effective methadone treatment, and for which patients this is true. There has been a reluctance to research this issue, possibly because it challenges cherished beliefs about the relative roles of methadone and counselling in treatment outcome, and about what it is possible to achieve with the opioid-dependent population. The need to research this issue should be seen as a priority in the area of methadone maintenance treatment.

The evidence reviewed in this book suggests that methadone maintenance treatment is effective only with adequate doses of methadone and for the period that the person remains in treatment. The conclusion to be drawn from this evidence is that counselling is not a stand-alone treatment for opioid-dependence, and that methadone maintenance treatment should not aspire to a goal of total abstinence in the belief that counselling makes such a goal possible.

However, it has to be acknowledged that the model of methadone maintenance treatment that the evidence supports as being effective is the Dole and Nyswander model — high-dose, maintenance-oriented treatment with high quality ancillary services to assist patients to recover (Chapter 2). The fears of the advocates of this model — that low intervention methadone maintenance is motivated by a desire to cut costs rather than the needs of the patient population — have some basis. The same motivation has been responsible for similar moves with other patient populations, such as the chronically mentally ill. However, this fear has to be tempered by the fact that it is unlikely all methadone maintenance patients need such a high level of intervention in their lives. The evidence we have reviewed shows that there are patients who need more assistance than others to get their lives in order, and counselling should be made available to them. On the other hand, it is hard to see why stabilised patients with no substantial life problems should need (or be required to routinely see) a counsellor at all. This is consistent with the main message of this book — that methadone maintenance patients are like any other treatment population. They have different needs and differ in their response to different components of treatment and therefore should have their treatment individualised for them.

Another issue arising from the literature reviewed in this chapter is that there is a clear need to develop protocols for counselling and training programs that are based on techniques shown to be useful elsewhere. Replacing confrontation with a client-centred style would be a step in this direction. Perhaps the most interesting findings reviewed in this chapter are those that suggest that not all counsellors are equally effective in bringing about change for their clients. Finding out more about the characteristics of effective counsellors is an obvious research need. As Luborsky et al. (1986) have remarked, it will be interesting to see to what extent these characteristics are teachable techniques, or are part of the effective counsellor's personality.

SUMMARY

The traditional role of counselling in methadone maintenance treatment has been to help patients resolve problems associated with their opioid dependence. Widespread poly-drug use, high rates of some psychiatric disorders, and changing social conditions suggest that there is a need to redefine this role.

Counselling in methadone maintenance programs, which consists predominantly of case management and assisting with crisis situations, takes place mainly in individual counselling and by way of brief unscheduled meetings. More serious problems (for example, psychiatric disorders) are not usually dealt with by case counsellors unless they are qualified to do so. Referral both within and outside the methadone maintenance unit is sometimes used to provide these services.

The style of counselling any patient receives depends in part on unit policy and in part on the beliefs of his or her counsellor. There is no well worked out model of drug counselling as part of methadone maintenance treatment.

There is no evidence to suggest that counselling is a necessary part of methadone maintenance treatment for all patients, although this issue has never been adequately researched. It does have to be acknowledged that the model of methadone maintenance treatment that has been shown to be effective has always included counselling as part of its service delivery. This remains the case even though methadone maintenance without counselling is not uncommon throughout the world.

There is limited evidence that methadone maintenance units with better quality counselling services have more success than units with lesser quality services. There is no evidence to suggest that ex-addict counsellors are more effective than other counsellors; if anything, the evidence suggests that they may be less effective. There is a need to define the word 'training' with regard to counselling in methadone maintenance programs. There is no evidence to suggest that an in-service trained person without formal counselling qualifications is any less effective than a person with formal counselling qualifications.

Studies of specific techniques, such as relaxation training, with methadone maintenance patients have failed to find any impact on the traditional outcomes of level of illicit drug use or criminal activity. The use of newer techniques (e.g. motivational interviewing) may prove to be useful in establishing a working relationship with patients and increasing their compliance with treatment, but require further research before they can be accepted as a necessary or integral part of treatment.

Psychotherapy (cognitive-behavioural or psychodynamic) might be a useful adjunct to methadone maintenance treatment for patients with psychiatric disorders which are amenable to such treatment, for example, depression. However, more research is needed to confirm this finding, which comes from one study. There is, however, no reason to believe that psychotherapy is a treatment for opioid dependence, or that it is indicated for methadone maintenance patients without psychiatric problems.

Patients with a diagnosis of ASP do not appear to be amenable to psychotherapy unless they have a concurrent diagnosis of depression. Such patients are suitable for methadone maintenance treatment. Family therapy may be useful for methadone maintenance patients who qualify for family treatment and are willing to participate in it. The limited evidence from one study for family therapy is positive. Further research is needed to establish its usefulness. Mandatory psychotherapy or counselling is unlikely to be of benefit to methadone maintenance patients and may have a negative impact on patient attitudes to treatment in general.

It has been established that some psychotherapists and counsellors are more effective than others. Differences between therapists (therapist effects) may be more important than differences between therapies, i.e. differences in clients' responses to therapy may be more an effect of therapist characteristics than the relative effectiveness of particular therapies. The discovery that therapist effects exist has important implications for designing studies that compare different therapies.

The ability to establish a relationship with clients based on trust, known as a therapeutic alliance, is an important contributor to a positive outcome from therapy. As well, certain components of both psychodynamic and cognitive-behavioural therapy have been found to be associated with a better outcome, and the use of these components by therapists contributes in part to the differences seen in therapist effectiveness.

Evidence arising out of studies of differences between therapists suggests that counselling in methadone maintenance programs should be based on sound general counselling principles (reflective listening, establishing empathic alliance etc.) rather than the traditional drug counselling method of confrontation.

DURATION OF METHADONE MAINTENANCE

INTRODUCTION

Any consideration of the appropriate duration of a treatment has to take into account three factors: the characteristics of the patient; the characteristics of the treatment; and the effect the treatment has on the patient. For a condition of long duration, such as opioid dependence, and a drug-based intervention such as methadone maintenance, a dose-response relationship is to be expected. In the case of methadone maintenance, a dose-response relationship could be manifested in a number of different ways: the effectiveness of methadone maintenance could be expected to increase with increasing methadone dose; the overall treatment could be expected to be more effective the more intensely it is applied (across the range of interventions at its disposal); and the treatment could be expected to be more effective the longer it lasts. It is with the latter dose-response relationship that this chapter is concerned.

As we have explained earlier, the original conception of methadone maintenance treatment was a medical one. The practitioners responsible for its initiation in New York in the early

1960s explained their successes by suggesting that opioid dependence was a metabolic disease (Dole & Nyswander, 1967) and any social or psychological problems that patients might have were considered to be a result of their drug use. It followed from this disease model that the duration of methadone maintenance was indefinite and that its success or otherwise was to be assessed on the basis of the remission of heroin use and the secondary problems associated with that use in methadone-maintained individuals. As methadone maintenance was rapidly adopted in other parts of the USA, and then in other countries, different models of treatment were developed on the basis of less medical notions about the genesis and maintenance of opioid dependence.

These two broad types of methadone maintenance — medical and non-medical — have been identified and described by a number of authors (Cole & James, 1975; Graff & Ball, 1976; Hubbard et al., 1989; Rosenbaum, 1985). Focusing on the duration of methadone maintenance considered to be desirable according to the two models, they can conveniently be referred to for the purposes of this chapter as long-term maintenance (LTM) and short-term maintenance (STM). Cole and James (1975) refer to LTM and STM as adaptive and change-oriented modes of methadone maintenance, while Graff and Ball (1976) refer to them as metabolic and psychotherapeutic models of treatment. Rosenbaum (1985) identifies two types of LTM (medical and libertarian) and describes STM programs as being reformist in orientation. Finally, Hubbard et al. (1989) prefer the terms 'methadone maintenance' and 'methadone-to-abstinence' to describe these two types of methadone maintenance programs. Although all of these authors were describing the situation in the USA, the results of a recent Australian survey of nationwide practices in drug and alcohol treatment agencies suggests that these two models of methadone maintenance, as reflected in stated treatment goals, are relevant for Australia as well (Baillie et al., 1991).

DURATION OF METHADONE MAINTENANCE AND TREATMENT OUTCOME

In this section we examine research that has investigated the relationship between length of time spent in methadone maintenance and post-treatment outcome. This literature has been reviewed previously by Hargreaves (1983). The definitive test of shorter or longer periods of methadone maintenance would be a randomised controlled trial in which patients were randomly allocated to different time periods of methadone maintenance and then assessed at treatment completion (Hargreaves, 1983). No such experiments have been done. In the absence of rigorous experimental results, the effect of treatment duration on outcome has to be assessed on the basis of a range of observational outcome studies, most of which use a pre-post design. Some of these studies use statistical techniques to control for the influence of extraneous variables on the relationship between time in methadone maintenance and post-methadone maintenance outcome and can therefore be interpreted with more confidence. Others, however, merely report correlations between duration and outcome and, in such cases, it is unclear whether it is the duration that is correlated with outcome or some other variable or variables like patient characteristics.

One common threat to the validity of the findings of such studies is selective attrition, or the biased loss of a proportion of the original study sample (Hall, 1983). In such cases an apparent significant correlation between duration and outcome is found, because those patients with more serious problems drop out of treatment over time and the performance of the remaining sample appears to improve, when in actual fact the reported averages (e.g. for heroin use) are diminishing due to changes in the composition of the group rather than to the impact of treatment.

It has been a consistent finding that length of time spent in methadone maintenance is a predictor of post-methadone maintenance outcome. The finding that the longer a patient spends in methadone maintenance, the more likely they are to benefit, has been reported in a number of studies (Cushman, 1981; Dole & Joseph, 1978; Hubbard et al., 1989; McGlothlin & Anglin, 1981a; Simpson, 1979, 1981; Simpson & Sells, 1982; Stimmel et al., 1978). However, there have been two studies where this relationship has not been found (Cushman, 1978b; Judson et al., 1980). This section examines this evidence as a whole to assess whether it is reasonable to conclude that the longer an individual spends in methadone maintenance, the more likely they are to have a better outcome.

New York Studies

Dole and Joseph (1978) conducted a study of the long-term outcomes of 1 544 patients admitted to methadone maintenance in the period 1966 to 1967 and in 1970 in New York. They found that for the 846 patients who had been discharged or had left methadone maintenance, a favourable outcome in terms of relapse to heroin use and criminal activity was associated with having spent a longer time in methadone maintenance. Cushman (1978b) in another New

York study of a group of patients who had detoxified from methadone maintenance with staff assent (i.e. 'completed' methadone maintenance) did not find a relationship between time spent in methadone maintenance and a successful outcome (see pp. 177–78). In a later paper, however, Cushman (1981) used data from the same clinic which included all patients who left methadone maintenance (including those who were expelled, who absconded and who were jailed as well as those who completed treatment), as well as patients who left methadone maintenance from two other New York programs. In this study, a relationship was observed between time spent in methadone maintenance and outcome, with patients staying longer than three years doing significantly better than those who stayed for less than three years.

Stimmel et al. (1978), in another study of methadone maintenance programs in New York, followed up patients admitted to methadone maintenance during the period March 1969 to February 1976 who had left by May 1977. They found a positive association between time spent in methadone maintenance and illicit opioid use at follow-up. Eighty-six per cent of patients who had spent less than 12 months in methadone maintenance had relapsed compared with 79% who had one to two years of maintenance, 67% who had two to three years of maintenance, and 60% of those who had more than three years of methadone maintenance. An examination of these data shows that the odds of a patient being heroin-free become more likely after at least two years of methadone maintenance.

McGlothlin and Anglin (1981)

In a retrospective study that has already been discussed briefly in Chapter 6, McGlothlin and Anglin (1981a) compared the outcome of patients from three methadone programs in California at an average of 6.6 years after entry to methadone maintenance. Two of the programs followed a high dose, long retention policy, while the third program followed a low dose, two-year maximum duration policy in combination with a strict policy regarding expulsion for program rule violations. Overall the patients in the two high dose, long retention programs were doing better at follow-up.

Of special interest was the difference in treatment duration among those who did and did not become dependent again. Of the patients who had left methadone maintenance, those who had not become dependent averaged 32 months of methadone maintenance compared to 18 months for those who became dependent. An examination of the numbers of patients graduating, absconding and expelled are revealing (Hargreaves, 1983). The two LTM programs graduated 12% and 18% of their patients, compared to 2% being graduated from the STM program. For patients who absconded (i.e. stopped attending) the figures were 10% and 16% for the LTM programs and 29% for the STM program. Expulsions accounted for 18% and 22% for the LTM program and 44% for the STM program. These figures suggest that the STM program was associated with less success in terms of patients graduating from the program, more failure in terms of keeping their patients in methadone maintenance, and less capacity to change patients' behaviour without expelling them. However, in interpreting this study, it has to be acknowledged that different dose levels and policies concerning expulsion are confounding variables in the apparent relationship between duration and outcome.

Drug Abuse Reporting Program

Some of the most widely cited results supporting the relationship between length of time spent in methadone maintenance and positive treatment outcome are those arising out of the Drug Abuse Reporting Program (DARP) study discussed in detail in Chapter 3 (Simpson, 1979, 1981; Simpson & Sells, 1982). For the three major treatment modalities concerned — methadone maintenance, therapeutic community and outpatient drug-free — the outcome of patients was better as length of time spent in treatment increased. This relationship was evident after three-months stay and was linear (Simpson & Sells, 1982). The association between time in treatment and outcome was consistently found among various sub-samples of the follow-up group, whether single or composite outcome measures were used, whether different post-methadone maintenance time periods were examined, after statistical procedures were employed to control for background and baseline differences between clients, and when post-DARP treatment was examined in the same way (Simpson, 1979, 1981; Simpson & Sells, 1982). Patients who stayed in treatment for periods longer than three months did significantly better than the comparison group who attended detoxification or did not begin the form of treatment for which they applied, although for methadone maintenance it was concluded that at least one year of maintenance was necessary in order for any effect to be detected (Simpson, 1979; Simpson & Sells, 1982). One caveat on this general result was that time spent in methadone maintenance was not predictive of the use of non-opioid illicit drugs.

The finding in the DARP study of a linear relationship between duration of methadone maintenance and outcome that commences after a period of 3 months has led Simpson (1979) to suggest that there may be no specifiable optimum duration for methadone maintenance. For the overall DARP sample, the linear relationship observed extended from 3 months to 2 years at follow-up, the time at which the data became inadequate (Simpson & Sells, 1982). As we concluded in Chapter 2, the retrospective nature of the data collection procedure casts some doubt over these findings. Furthermore, as Hargreaves (1983) has pointed out, it is difficult to know what these findings mean, especially when it is acknowledged that the correlation between time spent in treatment and outcome reported by Simpson (1982) accounts for only 4% of the variation seen in outcome.

Treatment Outcome Prospective Study

The TOPS study was a second large-scale, multi-site treatment outcome study carried out in the USA (see Chapter 3 for a detailed discussion of this study.) The analysis of the data in the TOPS study made use of statistical procedures to test various hypotheses about the relationship between a wide range of variables and the outcomes observed. Outcome for patients at follow-up was compared with a comparison group of patients who had left treatment within the first week. These analyses revealed that overall for the three modalities that showed an effect of treatment in the study (methadone maintenance, therapeutic communities, outpatient drug-free), the best predictor of a positive outcome was the length of time spent in treatment. This finding remained consistent for each of the modalities examined separately, for each of the three annual cohorts followed, for different groups of patients, and for different programs participating in the study. According to the authors:

> The multiple confirmation of findings, combined with the reasoned rejection of alternative explanations, is compelling evidence that retention of at least six months in treatment is responsible for the changes in behavior observed after treatment (Hubbard et al., 1989, p. 166).

However, an examination of the findings for time in treatment by outcome (see Table 3, Chapter 3) reveals that, for methadone maintenance, a statistically significant reduction in heroin use was only observed after spending more than a year in methadone maintenance, and that significant reductions in criminality were only observed in those patients who had remained continuously in methadone maintenance during the follow-up period (i.e. they were still in methadone maintenance at the time of interview). Consistent with the DARP findings is a lack of relationship between time spent in methadone maintenance and the use of non-opioid illicit drugs. Also consistent with the DARP results is an effect of time in treatment, which apparently continues beyond the time limit for follow-up used in the study. As will be discussed later in this chapter, it is difficult to consider such effects as proper *post*-treatment effects when overall they really amount to a comparison of being in methadone maintenance with not being in methadone maintenance. Such evidence supports the view that there are no demonstrated *post*-treatment effects as such for methadone maintenance for the majority of patients.

Bell, Hall and Byth (1992)

In a recent Australian study of the influence of methadone maintenance on the level of criminal activity as indicated by the rate of recorded convictions before and after entry to methadone maintenance treatment in Western Sydney, it was found that increasing duration of methadone maintenance was associated with a decreasing risk of being convicted for property or drug offences (Bell et al., 1992). As in the TOPS study, the use of statistical procedures to control for the influence of other important variables on the observed relationship between time spent in methadone maintenance and criminal activity increases the confidence with which it can be accepted that duration of methadone maintenance predicts the outcome reported.

Ball and Ross (1991)

Ball and Ross (1991) in their analysis of the data from the Three Cities Study (discussed in detail in Chapter 2) used statistical procedures to control for patient and treatment characteristics in their analysis of the follow-up data. Once the other relevant characteristics were controlled for, time spent in methadone maintenance was not found to be related to levels of heroin use or crime reported at one-year follow-up. Duration of methadone maintenance did predict, however, length of time since the last injecting drug use episode. According to Ball and Ross, the sample that this analysis was conducted on consisted of patients who had spent at least 15 months in methadone maintenance at the time of the follow-up interviews (i.e. patients had been in methadone maintenance for at least three months at the commencement of the study period). They argue that treatment would have had its chance to be effective by the time that the patients entered the study and that improvement after that time would be slight and remain undetected. While this evidence is consistent with Ball and Ross's conclusion that methadone maintenance is effective as a maintenance treatment (i.e. while patients remain in methadone maintenance), it may the case that the reason for not detecting a difference was that selective attrition had taken place and that the remaining sample of patients consisted of the more well-adjusted patients, a possibility discussed in detail later in this chapter (see pp. 178–79).

Two Contrary Findings

As has already been mentioned, there have been two published reports of length of time in methadone maintenance not being statistically associated with any positive post-methadone maintenance outcome. Cushman (1978b) reported that for a group of patients who had completed methadone maintenance (i.e. detoxified with the assent of staff) the average time spent in methadone maintenance for successful patients (defined as not relapsing to heroin use) was not significantly different from the average stay for those patients who had relapsed to heroin use. The average stay for successful patients (60% of sample) was 4.3 (±1.5) years and for relapsed patients 3.7 (±0.14) years. Two aspects of this study make it a special case when considering its status as evidence against the studies discussed above that did find a relationship between time spent in methadone maintenance and outcome. First of all, the group itself is unusual in that it is a group of patients who have successfully completed methadone maintenance. Secondly, the success rate (60% had not relapsed) for this group is very high when compared with the usual rates for patients assessed post-methadone maintenance. The probable reason for this is that reason for leaving treatment is a strong predictor of post-methadone maintenance behaviour (see pp. 183–85). As common sense would suggest, those patients who respond well during methadone maintenance do better when assessed afterwards. Finally, as is the case in the other report discussed immediately below, the finding that there is no statistically significant effect does not prove the hypothesis that there is no effect (the null hypothesis), especially given the small sample size that was interviewed at follow up (n = 68).

The second finding of there being no statistically significant effect was reported by Judson et al. (1980). A random sample of all admissions to a Californian methadone program during its first 28 months of admission was followed up five years after entry to methadone maintenance. For a sample of 112 subjects who had been off methadone maintenance for at least one year, no significant differences were found between the average time spent in methadone maintenance for successful and unsuccessful patients on a range of outcomes. The requirement that patients not have been in methadone maintenance for at least one year is unusual and it is not clear what effect this selection criterion would have had on the sample.

Given the weight of the evidence in favour of there being a relationship between time spent in methadone maintenance and post-treatment behaviour and the qualifying factors discussed above for the contrary studies, it has to be concluded that these two studies do not provide evidence that there is no relationship between duration and outcome. Even if there were no difficulties with these studies, it is still the case, as mentioned above, that due to the probabilistic nature of statistical analysis, it is to be occasionally expected that errors will occur, suggesting there is no effect even though in reality there is one.

Predicting Outcome from Duration: Alternative Explanations

One common criticism of research concerning the effectiveness of treatments for drug problems is that most studies do not allow one to conclude whether the outcomes observed are the result of treatment or not. As we have already noted, because a substantial proportion of patients drop out, it may be the case that those patients who are, for example, more highly motivated remain in treatment longer and do better (selective attrition). If this were the case, the apparent benefit of treatment could be partly due to motivation rather than the effects of the treatment they are receiving. Randomised controlled trials that demonstrate treatment effects control for patient factors by random assignment, so that any difference in patient outcome can be attributed to treatment. However, in the case of observational studies of the relationship between duration and outcome this has to be demonstrated.

It could be the case, therefore, that as patients drop out of methadone maintenance over time, the more well-adjusted patients, who tend to use less drugs overall, stay longer in treatment and are found to be doing better at post-treatment follow-up. According to this argument, the association found in the studies reviewed above between post-treatment functioning and length of time spent in treatment could be primarily a result of systematic differences between those who stay for longer and those who stay for shorter periods rather than an effect of more or less treatment. As suggested at the beginning of this section, the only definitive way to demonstrate that it is length of time in methadone maintenance that has influenced outcome would be to do an experiment in which patients were randomly assigned to differing durations of methadone maintenance and to compare outcomes between the groups. Such an experiment is unimaginable for both ethical and practical considerations. The next best alternative is to use the strategy adopted by Bell et al. (1992) and the TOPS researchers (Hubbard et al., 1989) where patient characteristics are measured extensively at entry to treatment and then controlled for in statistical analyses to demonstrate that even when these characteristics are taken into account, time in treatment still influences outcome.

It has to be kept in mind that even if the observed correlation between longer stays in treatment and better outcome is confounded to a certain extent by patient characteristics, this does not mean that treatment does not work. It simply means that it works better — and is more acceptable — for some individuals than for others. In the next two sections we look at evidence which places important qualifications on any simple statement that longer stays in treatment lead to better outcomes.

Reasons for Leaving Treatment

Patients leave methadone maintenance treatment for a variety of reasons: because both patient and staff agree that methadone maintenance is no longer needed; because the patient feels that he or she no longer needs methadone maintenance but staff do not agree; because the patient has infringed some program rule and is expelled; because the patient fails to appear for treatment; or because the patient is jailed. Patients who complete methadone maintenance (detoxify with staff assent) are more likely to be successful than patients who leave for other reasons (Cushman, 1978a, 1981; Des Jarlais et al., 1981; Dole & Joseph, 1978; Milby, 1988; Simpson & Sells, 1982; Stimmel et al., 1978).

Stimmel et al. (1978) calculated relative risks for post-treatment relapse to opioid use for those completing methadone maintenance and those who left for other reasons, and found that those who did not complete treatment were almost five times (relative risk = 4.7) more likely to relapse than those who completed treatment. However, it has to be acknowledged that those who completed treatment would no doubt have stayed longer in treatment and that it could be the case that a longer duration may account for the results (Hargreaves, 1983). In the data analysis performed by Stimmel et al., a shorter duration of methadone maintenance did significantly increase the risk of relapse associated with reason for leaving for methadone maintenance, but it is not clear from the report, as Hargreaves (1983) points out, what would happen if the procedure had been reversed and risk was calculated first for duration and then for what extra contribution reason for leaving methadone maintenance would make. However, it is plausible to conclude that patients who leave methadone maintenance for reasons other than completing treatment are at risk of relapse. It is likely that patients who improve during treatment are more likely to do well when they leave compared with patients who show little improvement and then leave against the advice of staff. In accordance with this view, and as might be expected, an association has also been observed between positive behaviour change during methadone maintenance and success after leaving treatment (Dole & Joseph, 1978; McGlothlin & Anglin, 1981a; Simpson & Sells, 1982). As making such changes in behaviour are a prerequisite of completing methadone treatment, presumably this predictor is not independent of reason for leaving treatment.

Milby (1988), after reviewing this literature, concluded that reason for leaving treatment was the most important predictor of successful detoxification from methadone maintenance. Given the strong association between longer periods of methadone maintenance and completing treatment, it is likely that completing treatment is more important than the length of time spent, but it is difficult on the basis of the available evidence to untangle relative contributions of these two factors. The finding that change during treatment and reason for leaving treatment are strong predictors of post-methadone maintenance outcome, suggests that not only do the patients who do better stay in treatment longer (as in selective attrition) but that behaviour change during that time is also important.

Time-Limited Methadone Maintenance

Three studies have looked at the effect on patients of instituting an arbitrary maximum time limit for methadone maintenance (Anglin et al., 1989; McGlothlin & Anglin, 1981b; Rosenbaum et al., 1988). McGlothlin and Anglin (1981b — see Chapter 3 for a more detailed account of this study) examined the effect of the closure of an methadone maintenance program on its patients and compared outcome at two-year follow-up with patients from a similar program that continued operating during the follow-up period. In comparison to the patients who remained in methadone maintenance, the patients who had to leave treatment were substantially worse off. Anglin et al. (1989) report a similar study conducted after the closure of the San Diego County methadone program in 1978. In this case, they found few differences between the San Diego patients and a comparison group. However, this failure to detect an effect of removing methadone maintenance treatment must be considered along with the fact that the majority of the San Diego patients entered private methadone maintenance programs.

In a similar study, Rosenbaum and her colleagues (1988) examined the impact on patients of the adoption of a two-year limit for public methadone maintenance in Alemada County, California. After two years of publicly-funded methadone maintenance, patients had to detoxify or begin paying US$200 a month if they wanted to stay on methadone. The sample (n = 143) consisted of nearly half the patients on public methadone maintenance in Alemada who were affected by the new policy at the time of its introduction. Each of the patients was interviewed at this time and at six-month intervals thereafter for two and a half years. The data discussed in this report are qualitative. (The term 'qualitative' refers to a form of data collection in which subjects are interviewed in an unstructured way in order to give the subject an opportunity to influence the content of the information that is collected. It is usually contrasted with quantitative data collection which relies on structured data collection procedures for the purposes of hypothesis testing.)

Rosenbaum et al. found that the patients they interviewed fell into three broad groups and that each of these groups responded to the two-year limit in different ways. They described these three groups of patients as being 'model', 'stabilised' and 'marginal'. Model patients (6% of sample) tended to have some history of employment, a minimal involvement in crime, did not use illicit drugs during treatment and had found work while on methadone maintenance. These patients used the advent of the two-year limit to get off methadone maintenance.

At the other end of the spectrum, marginal patients (25% of sample) were described as having long histories of opioid dependence and criminal activity, little or no past employment, being poorly educated, poly-drug using, and as having entered methadone maintenance as a last resort rather than out of a desire to rehabilitate. While in methadone maintenance they used a lot of heroin and other illicit drugs, regularly missed appointments, and tended to be abusive to program staff. Because these patients had not really abandoned their pre-methadone maintenance lifestyle, the imposition of the two-year limit meant for them simply an intensification of their illicit drug use and the lifestyle associated with it.

The majority of the patients (69%) were in the stabilised group. These patients responded to methadone maintenance and became stabilised, although their backgrounds were similar to the marginal patients. Many of this group had mental health problems. They continued to use heroin occasionally after entry to methadone maintenance, but this tapered off over time. Methadone maintenance stabilised their lives and they responded in a positive fashion as their drug use and criminal activity diminished. The introduction of the two-year limit was catastrophic for this group as a whole with many becoming dependent on heroin again. The results of this study, as the authors point out, expose the irony involved in arbitrarily limiting the duration of methadone maintenance. The population that methadone maintenance is most suitable for — the stabilised group — is the one most disadvantaged by the policy.

Overall, the findings from studies of time-limited methadone maintenance suggest that imposing arbitrary time limits on the availability of methadone maintenance, either for financial purposes or in the belief that a limit will foster rehabilitation, does not contribute to a positive treatment outcome for the patients most in need of it. They also, in combination with the findings concerning reason for leaving treatment, suggest that methadone maintenance treatment should be a *maintenance* until such time as the patient is ready to try and live without methadone.

Conclusion: Duration and Outcome

The balance of the evidence reviewed in this section suggests that length of time spent in methadone maintenance is related in some way to post-methadone maintenance behaviour. However, what remains unclear is whether this effect is accounted for by definable lengths of stay or whether it is due to the positive results found for patients who have remained continuously in methadone maintenance from the time of initial assessment to the time of final follow-up. The evidence from the DARP and the TOPS suggests that 'longer is better'. The results of the studies overall suggest that more than two to three years of methadone maintenance is necessary before significant behaviour change is observed. However, arbitrarily limiting the duration of methadone maintenance to such time periods has been found to have negative consequences for the patients most in need of it.

When the evidence reviewed in Chapters 2 and 3 is taken into account, we have to qualify these statements by adding that the evidence overall suggests that methadone maintenance works as a *maintenance* intervention. Significant differences have been observed for methadone maintenance between subjects in and out of treatment, between pre-treatment and during treatment behaviour and between during treatment behaviour and post-treatment behaviour when treatment is either removed or the patient leaves for reasons other than completion.

PATIENT CHARACTERISTICS AND TREATMENT OUTCOME

While the overall picture that emerges from the studies reviewed above suggests that longer stays in methadone maintenance are better than shorter stays, it is still the case that some patients do well after relatively brief stays in methadone maintenance. This section attempts to delineate which patients do well after a short period of methadone maintenance and which patients need longer term methadone maintenance. We also consider how the conclusion reached in the last section might have to be modified in light of this evidence about patient characteristics. Each of the patient characteristics that have been found to be predictive of outcome are examined below. (See McLellan (1983) for another review of this literature.)

AGE: Although age is predictive of retention in methadone maintenance, with older patients tending to stay longer, it does not seem to be related in any uncomplicated fashion to post-treatment outcome (McLellan, 1983).

CRIMINAL HISTORY: One of the most consistent predictors of post-treatment behaviour reported in the literature is the extent of pre-treatment criminal involvement. The more extensive a patient's pre-treatment criminal involvement, the less likely they are to have a positive post-methadone maintenance outcome (e.g. Bell et al., 1992; Dole & Joseph, 1978; Hubbard et al., 1989; Judson & Goldstein, 1982; McGlothlin & Anglin, 1981a, 1981b; McLellan, 1983; Simpson & Sells, 1982). In the DARP study, level of pre-treatment criminal activity was the best predictor of post-treatment outcome on a range of outcome measures. This relationship was observed for up to six years after initial entry to methadone maintenance (Simpson et al., 1982), but was not evident when a sub-sample was followed up at 12 years (Simpson et al., 1986). In both the TOPS and a recent Australian study, level of pre-treatment criminal activity was the strongest predictor of criminal activity after entry to methadone maintenance (Hubbard et al., 1989; Bell et al., 1992). This evidence suggests that patients who have an extensive criminal history will not do well if they leave methadone maintenance. For these patients, however, being in methadone maintenance is associated with significant reductions in illicit drug use and criminal activity (e.g. Ball & Ross, 1991 — see Chapter 3).

OPIOID USE HISTORY: The duration and intensity of pre-treatment opioid use has been shown to predict outcome in studies that have measured it (Ball & Ross, 1991; Dole & Joseph, 1978; Hubbard et al., 1989; McLellan, 1983; Simpson & Sells, 1982). The evidence suggests that patients who have a long history of heavy opioid use will not do well if they leave methadone maintenance, though they do significantly reduce their illicit opioid use while in methadone maintenance.

PSYCHOLOGICAL ADJUSTMENT: McLellan (1983) concluded that descriptive measures of personality variables or psychopathological symptoms had not been predictive of retention or post-treatment outcome, but that studies which had used quantitative measures of psychopathology were suggestive of a relationship between more severe symptomatology and lower retention rates (see Chapters 8 and 13). Joe et al. (1991), in a recent report on the TOPS data, also found such a relationship between more severe 'mental health problems' and poor retention, although more symptoms of depression were associated with better retention.

EMPLOYMENT STATUS: Being employed is a predictor of a positive post-methadone maintenance outcome (Cushman, 1978b, 1981; Dole & Joseph, 1978; McGlothlin & Anglin, 1981a; McLellan, 1983). The best predictor of post-treatment employment in the DARP and TOPS studies was having been employed before methadone maintenance (Hubbard et al., 1989; Simpson & Sells, 1982). Being employed also predicts retention in methadone maintenance (Szapocznik & Ladner, 1977). Again, as Cushman (1981) remarks, being employed is often one of the criteria to be met for completing methadone maintenance, so this predictor may not be independent of reason for leaving treatment (see pp. 179–80).

LIVING WITH FAMILY/PARTNER: Stimmel et al. (1978) found that patients completing treatment were more likely to be living with family than patients who left methadone maintenance for other reasons. Szapocznik and Ladner (1977), in an early review of research that examined predictors of retention in methadone maintenance, found that marital status was associated with retention in treatment. Hubbard et al. (1989) also report a relationship between length of stay in methadone maintenance and being married. These results are consistent with common sense in suggesting that those patients with more social support would do better in methadone maintenance (McLellan, 1983).

LEVEL OF ALCOHOL USE: High levels of alcohol use have been found to be negatively associated with retention (Szapocznik & Ladner, 1977), overall treatment outcome (Judson & Goldstein, 1982), and to predict post-methadone maintenance level of alcohol use (Hubbard et al., 1989).

POLY-DRUG USE: Patients who use only opioids tend to stay in methadone maintenance longer (Hubbard et al., 1989). As already mentioned in the discussion of the relationship between duration of methadone maintenance and outcome, time in methadone maintenance does not have a significant effect on the use of non-opioid illicit drugs, and poly-drug use is predictive of shorter stays (Joe et al., 1991; Szapocznik & Ladner, 1977).

It is clear from the evidence reviewed in this section that patients who have a long history of opioid dependence and criminal activity will do poorly if they leave methadone maintenance prematurely. This should be seen in the light of the more general point that patients who leave methadone maintenance for reasons other than completing treatment with staff assent have a high risk of relapsing. As common sense would dictate, patients who have less severe drug and legal problems, who have some form of social support, who have few or no psychological problems, and who are more likely to find work, are more likely to reach a point after a relatively short period of methadone maintenance where they have a reasonable chance of capitalising on the positive behaviour changes they have made while in methadone maintenance. In the next section we consider ways in which methadone maintenance programs might maximise retention rates for the patients with more serious problems who need longer periods of methadone maintenance before they will improve.

CHARACTERISTICS OF METHADONE PROGRAMS AND RETENTION IN TREATMENT

It is clear from the evidence reviewed in the previous section that a substantial proportion of patients leave methadone maintenance before they have any likelihood of even short-term success in recovering from their dependence. Ironically, these are the patients most in need of methadone maintenance in that they have more severe drug and drug-related problems. This section examines ways in which treatment factors have been found to affect patient retention in methadone maintenance in order to identify ways in which retention rates might be improved.

Although there has been a great deal of interest on the part of researchers in the influence of patient characteristics on retention rates and outcome for methadone maintenance, interest in how the various aspects of methadone maintenance treatment affect retention and outcome has been comparatively recent. While clear conclusions can be made about the major variables of methadone maintenance treatment such as dose and duration, understanding of the context within which methadone maintenance is delivered, and the dynamics of the treatment process itself, is limited to the findings of a few very recent studies.

Methadone Dose

For a full discussion of the importance of methadone dose levels in methadone maintenance treatment see Chapter 6. For the purposes of this chapter, it can be noted that methadone dose is an important predictor of retention in methadone maintenance (e.g. Caplehorn & Bell, 1991; Joe et al., 1991). Patients who are maintained on higher doses of methadone stay in treatment longer. Patients who are maintained on low doses of methadone as a consequence of the clinic following a low dose policy, rather than dose being determined on an individual basis, tend to drop out of treatment. The tendency over the last two decades to prescribe lower doses of methadone in methadone maintenance programs is not supported by the research literature.

Program Policy

A number of aspects of the treatment policy adopted by a program have been found to affect retention and outcome from methadone maintenance. An inflexible policy with regard to dose has been found to be associated with losing patients from methadone maintenance (Brown et al., 1982–83). The adoption of a short- or long-term maintenance policy is obviously going to affect the duration of treatment and therefore retention rates. However, as already outlined earlier (see pp. 173–74), the available evidence suggests that adopting a STM policy is associated with poorer retention, more discharges and fewer treatment completions independent of the commitment to a shorter period of methadone maintenance (McGlothlin & Anglin, 1981a — see also pp. 191–92). A policy of expelling patients for illicit drug use, while at the same time not providing adequate doses of methadone, seems to be an important part of the poor results of the STM model. Ball and Ross (1991) found that methadone maintenance programs that have a policy of LTM combined with an emphasis on service provision rather than good administrative functioning (i.e. meeting the needs of patients rather than an emphasis on keeping to the rules) are more successful at reducing drug use and criminality among their patients (see also D'Amanda, 1983).

Ancillary Services

The term 'ancillary services' refers to services provided by methadone maintenance programs other than the dispensing of methadone. They may include the provision of services such as medical treatment, counselling and job training, or referral to them. The important issue of counselling is dealt with in detail in Chapter 8. Like other aspects of the treatment characteristics of methadone maintenance programs, there has been little research on the role of ancillary services in retention and outcome until recently. However, both Ball and Ross (1991) and Joe et al. (1991) in their recently published reports found the provision of medical services to be an important component of methadone maintenance treatment. In the study reported by Ball and Ross, those programs that provided better medical services had lower rates of drug use and crime among their patients. Joe et al. found that if patients requested medical assistance at the time of assessment and received medical treatment for those problems during the first three months of methadone maintenance, then their survivorship in the program was increased by 22%. Ball and Ross also claimed that programs which provided better quality and more frequent counselling services had lower rates of drug use and crime among their patients (though this interpretation of their data is questionable — see Chapter 8), while Joe et al. found that provision of counselling and financial services both significantly increased retention. Although these findings suggest that ancillary services probably play an important role in retaining patients in treatment, it has yet to be established how they relate to other components of treatment (e.g. methadone dose and clinic policies).

Conclusion: Treatment Characteristics and Retention

It is perhaps because of the moral dimensions of illicit drug use that patient characteristics were thought for such a long time to be the important determinants of outcome and retention in methadone maintenance. There was in this regard an underlying attribution that patients were wholly responsible for treatment failure. While it is almost certainly the case that there are a small minority of individuals who do not respond to any interventions (Rosenbaum et al.'s (1988) marginal patients), it is clear from the evidence that methadone maintenance programs do differ in important ways, and that the ways in which they differ relate to their success in assisting their patients. Although we are only beginning to understand what these important variables are, it is clear that treatment characteristics do affect retention and outcome and that, therefore, the responsibility for successful treatment does not lie only with the patients.

MODELS OF TREATMENT AND DURATION OF METHADONE MAINTENANCE

As outlined earlier in this chapter, there are two basic treatment models for methadone maintenance: one that emphasises successfully maintaining individuals until they are ready to do without methadone (the LTM model), and another that emphasises the goal of a drug-free life after a relatively short period of methadone maintenance (the STM model). Given the clear message of the research to date, it is surprising that the STM model slowly gained ascendancy during the seventies and eighties. For example, a two-year review became part of Federal regulations in the USA in the early 1970s. It arose not out of research or clinical practice, but out of political pressure that was brought to bear as a result of a concern that methadone maintenance patients were being sentenced to a life of methadone dependence — a view that was shared by proponents of the STM model and 'radicals' who saw methadone maintenance as a form of social control (Attewell & Gerstein, 1979; Newman, 1977).

The influence of the STM model was, until very recently, evident in Australia in the *National Methadone Guidelines* (Commonwealth Department of Community Services and Health, 1988)* in which it was also recommended that patients maintained on methadone have their status reviewed after two years, suggesting, if only by implication, that two years is an appropriate maximum duration of methadone maintenance for most patients. Given that there is little evidence for the STM model, this is indeed surprising. Two important reasons for the undue influence of the STM model are the association of the LTM model with Dole and Nyswander's disease model of opioid dependence, and the substitution of the debate about whether methadone maintenance intensifies and prolongs dependence for debates about methadone dose and treatment duration. The STM model has also been advocated at times as a solution to the problem of meeting the needs of patients when there are more applicants for methadone maintenance than available places.

The Argument for LTM

In a series of articles published in the late seventies and early eighties, Dole and his colleagues presented data in support of the

---

* This has been changed for the current *National Methadone Guidelines* (Commonwealth Department of Community Services and Health, 1991)

illicit opioid use that occurred when patients left methadone maintenance, it was inadvisable for many patients to leave methadone maintenance treatment (Des Jarlais et al., 1981; Dole & Joseph, 1977; 1978). In response to various government agencies that sought to place a limit on the length of methadone maintenance, they conducted a series of follow-up studies of patients who completed, left or were discharged from methadone maintenance. They argued that these studies were not assessments of the outcome of methadone *maintenance* treatment, because, according to their view, such an assessment must be of performance during methadone maintenance (Des Jarlais et al., 1981).

The first of these studies (Dole & Joseph, 1977) compared a random sample of 202 patients who entered methadone maintenance in New York in 1972, and who had left methadone maintenance at follow-up in 1974, with a sample of 143 who began methadone maintenance in the same year and were still in treatment at follow-up. Most of the patients who had left methadone maintenance had done so against the advice of program staff. The outcomes compared were illicit opioid use and death. Overall, 68% of the group who left treatment had some illicit opioid use, although it is not clear how this was estimated. In comparison, 7% of the group who remained in treatment fell into this category as measured by urinalysis. No differences were found in the overall number of deaths between the two groups, but the attributed cause of death differed, with more of the post-methadone maintenance deaths being attributed to a drug-related cause.

Although this study does provide impressive evidence for the reduction of illicit opioid use during methadone maintenance, the comparisons between the two groups are hard to interpret. The authors have not provided information on type of discharge or on the differences between the two groups in terms of important variables that would predict post-methadone maintenance performance (Hargreaves, 1983). If most of the patients had been expelled from methadone maintenance for drug use, then the results would be expected. However, the findings of this study are consistent with the stronger findings listed below and lend some weight to Dole et al.'s arguments.

In a second study, Dole and Joseph (1978) compared patients who remained in methadone maintenance with those who did not. The subjects consisted of two cohorts: the first cohort comprised all the patients admitted to methadone maintenance during 1966 to 1967; the second consisted of a stratified random sample drawn from the approximately 17 000 first-admission patients that entered methadone maintenance during 1972. This amounted to 1 544 subjects, 92% (1 413) of whom were followed up. Of these, 567 had remained in treatment continuously and 846 had left or been expelled one or more times. The results of this study generally support the conclusion of the previous study in that being in methadone maintenance effectively suppressed illicit opioid use (10%), and most patients who left treatment relapsed (70%).

In a third report from this group, Des Jarlais et al. (1981) presented data from a sample of 956 patients who entered methadone maintenance during 1965 to 1966 and 1972 and who subsequently left or were discharged at least once. Information was acquired through interviews (528 people) and agency records (357 people). Ninety-three per cent of the original sample was followed up in this way. Seventy-two per cent of the group relapsed to opioid use after discharge. The authors provide impressive figures for pre-, during and post-methadone maintenance opioid use. Daily use went from 96% to 2% to 54% for each of these categories respectively.

Overall, these three studies provide evidence in support of Dole and his colleagues' argument that long-term methadone maintenance is an effective intervention for the population that it was originally introduced to treat — long-term heroin users with an extensive history of criminal activity. The authors acknowledged that a few patients remained abstinent after a short period of methadone maintenance, but that these were relatively stable patients with short histories of opioid dependence and crime (Dole & Joseph, 1978).

As Dole and his colleagues argued in all three of these papers, there has been no large-scale study which has shown that a relatively short period of methadone maintenance produces any significant or enduring period of abstinence in a chronically opioid-dependent and criminally active population. The evidence reviewed in this book in Chapters 2 and 3 is consistent with this argument. It is also consistent with the evidence in this chapter concerned with reason for leaving treatment predicting post-methadone maintenance behaviour, with the findings of the studies of time-limited methadone maintenance, and other studies that have followed up patients who left treatment before completion (for the latter see e.g. Ball & Ross, 1991; Perkins & Bloch, 1971). The combined weight of this evidence has led a number of authors besides Dole and his colleagues to justifiably conclude that detoxification from methadone maintenance and a drug-free life is not a realistic goal for all patients (Ball & Ross, 1991; Cushman, 1981; Hubbard et al., 1989; McGlothlin & Anglin, 1981b; McLellan, 1983; Rosenbaum et al., 1988; Stimmel et al., 1978).

The LTM Model and the Disease Explanation

While we acknowledge that the research evidence favours the LTM model, we do not accept that this necessarily means that we have to accept the explanation of opioid dependence as being a metabolic disease. Newman (1991), for example, has recently argued that the only plausible explanation for the success of methadone maintenance is that opioid dependence is a metabolic disease. There is, however, no necessary connection between the LTM model and the metabolic disease hypothesis. In fact, we see no reason at this time to make any assumptions about the aetiology of opioid dependence in order to explain the success of dispensing methadone in reducing opioid use and drug-related crime. The most parsimonious explanation is that methadone maintenance works because it provides in a controlled fashion an opioid substance that is acceptable to patients as an alternative to illegally obtained opioids such as heroin.

While we understand that in the American context there may be advantages in proposing the disease model, we feel that it is disadvantageous in countries like Australia for the LTM model to depend so heavily on disease theories of dependence for which there is little evidence. Another major disadvantage of employing these notions is that by telling patients they have a disease for which they will need to take methadone indefinitely, proponents of the disease hypothesis induce in patients the belief that they will never be able to recover from their dependence, thus creating a self-fulfilling prophecy (D'Amanda, 1983). Patients in methadone maintenance programs have been found to internalise program staff's ideas about treatment and the nature of dependence and to begin to view their prospects, and their drug use, from that perspective (Brown et al., 1975; Rosenbaum, 1985).

STM: Setting Up Patients for Failure

It has been argued by some authors that the STM model is not only at variance with the research evidence, but that it is positively harmful to patients. For example, Rosenbaum (1985), in a study of the way in which methadone maintenance clinics control their patients, reports that patients who attended STM clinics had been told by treatment staff that they should be able to overcome their drug problems and lead a drug-free life. To this end they were encouraged to detoxify after relatively short periods of methadone maintenance. As the evidence surveyed in this review suggests, many, if not most, of these patients acting on such advice will quickly relapse to heroin use. Rosenbaum (1985) argued that the cycle of detoxification, failure and return to methadone maintenance quickly erodes patients' sense of self-worth and self-efficacy, thereby generating more harm than good.

There would seem to be something counter-productive about the STM model. The package of low methadone doses, punitive illicit drug-use policy and expectations of a quick cure seem designed to place patients in a situation in which it is impossible to succeed. Such a combination is not effective either as a form of maintenance, or as a method of achieving abstinence.

TAILORING TREATMENT TO THE INDIVIDUAL

The evidence reviewed in this paper suggests that there are discernible characteristics of patients and methadone maintenance programs that influence outcome both during and after methadone maintenance. It would make sense to titrate treatment in some way on the basis of this information according to the severity of the problems of the patient concerned (Gerstein & Harwood, 1990). At the beginning of this chapter, three dose-response relationships were mentioned: methadone dose, duration of methadone maintenance, and the intensity with which ancillary services are applied. In this section, we would like to suggest what methadone maintenance treatment might be like if it were based on what we know about these three dose-response relationships.

While the LTM and STM models have tended to come in ideological packages complete with beliefs about aetiology (e.g. STM = low dose + short duration + high intervention + psychogenic model of opioid dependence), the model we suggest relies on a menu approach to treatment planning similar to that suggested by Hubbard et al. (1989). Using such an approach means that patients are involved in deciding what may be the best program for them. The clinician presents the patient with a menu of available treatment options and helps him or her to come to a decision about what might be best for them. This procedure reduces the need to communicate to patients beliefs about disease or the desirability of abstinence in the short term, and the implications for success or otherwise inherent in these notions. In this way, different treatment lengths and dosage regimes could be explained to patients along with their potential advantages and disadvantages.

If the three major variables of methadone maintenance treatment (dose, duration, level of intervention) are viewed as being independent of one another, then each of them may be individualised to meet each patient's needs. This avoids the assumption that there is one 'correct' treatment plan (e.g. low dose, short-term, intensive counselling) for each patient no matter what their needs or level of commitment to a drug-free life may be. It also avoids the view that has developed with regard to 'streaming' within methadone maintenance that there is a necessary connection between the three variables for some courses. For example, low intervention methadone maintenance has been widely considered as also being necessarily a low dose (20 to 30 mg) course. While there may be reasons why this has developed (e.g. concern about clinical safety), we would predict that this would be unsuccessful because of the inadequate dosage employed, if dosage is determined for the group as a whole rather than tailored to individual need.

As an alternative, treatment matching on the basis of considering dose, duration and counselling as being independent can be demonstrated using a few examples. On the basis of the evidence discussed in this review, it is clear that a patient with a long history of criminal involvement and heavy heroin use would usually be inappropriate for a low dose, short-term treatment course. If there is little evidence of psychopathology and no interest in counselling, there would seem to be little reason to suggest it at all. So for this patient a high dose, long-term, low intervention regimen might be most appropriate. If at some time during the course of their tenure the patient begins to show signs of significant behaviour change, then a change in treatment plan would of course be possible if the patient so wished. However, there is no logical reason why such a patient should be encouraged to detoxify once they have stabilised on methadone. At the other end of the spectrum, a patient who has a relatively short history of heroin use, little past criminal activity, reasonable social support and some history of being employed may be suitable for a low dose, short-term, high intervention program, with a goal of achieving abstinence. However, the evidence indicates that such patients would be in a minority.

SUMMARY

here are two broad models of methadone maintenance. One model is primarily medically based and views opioid dependence as a metabolic disease, and the goal of treatment as successful maintenance on methadone. The other model is non-medical, views opioid dependence as a behavioural disorder that may be psychogenic, conditioned, or a form of criminal activity; it views the goal of treatment as a drug-free life. According to the latter model, a brief period of methadone maintenance is seen as a useful intervention on the way to abstinence. Various authors have developed typologies to describe these models. This review examines these treatment models from the perspective of their viability as indicated by research findings.

Research to date suggests that there is an association between longer stays in methadone maintenance and a positive post-methadone maintenance outcome as measured by reduced illicit opioid use and criminal activity. This evidence suggests that periods of at least two to three years of continuous methadone maintenance are more likely to be beneficial for a majority of patients than are briefer periods. However, the evidence does not allow the specification of an optimum duration for methadone maintenance. The evidence indicates that longer stays are better than shorter stays, and that being in methadone maintenance is better than not being in methadone maintenance. Limiting the duration of methadone maintenance arbitrarily, for financial or philosophical reasons, has serious negative consequences for a majority of patients.

The research on patients' characteristics provides some clues as to which patients fare poorly if they leave methadone maintenance prematurely. The following patient characteristics have been found to be associated with drug use and/or criminal activity after leaving methadone maintenance:
- a longer and heavier history of opioid use;
- a longer and more extensive criminal history;
- leaving methadone maintenance against staff advice;
- exhibiting little behaviour change during methadone maintenance;
- not living with family or partner;
- not finding employment before, during or after methadone maintenance.

On the other hand, patients with less severe drug problems, who have little history of criminal activity, who have reasonable social support, and who become employed have some chance of success if they complete methadone maintenance. Overall, the evidence on patient characteristics suggests that patients should not be encouraged to leave methadone maintenance before they show reliable signs of rehabilitation (employment, stable social adjustment, no illicit drug use, etc.).

The scant research that has been done on the contribution of treatment program characteristics to patient outcome suggests that some forms of methadone maintenance are more successful than others. Programs that prescribe higher methadone doses, that have a flexible policy regarding dosage, a non-punitive approach to illicit drug use, and that provide adequate medical and counselling services are more likely to meet the needs of their patients than programs that do not.

Even though there is very little research to support it, the short-term model of methadone maintenance has had a strong influence on government policy and treatment practice over the last two decades. This is surprising given that there is no evidence that short periods of methadone maintenance will result in abstinence for the majority of patients. On the contrary, there is sufficient evidence to conclude that a majority of patients substantially reduce their drug use and criminal activity while they are on methadone maintenance programs that meet their needs. It has to be concluded that of the two major treatment models, the evidence favours the medical, long-term maintenance model. However, the research also suggests that there are problems with this model as well.

The three major treatment variables of methadone maintenance treatment — dose, duration and level of intervention — have tended to come in ideological packages along with notions concerning the origins of opioid dependence. A model based on the research to date would view these three variables as independent, and would titrate them according to the needs and characteristics of the patients. An appropriate model for methadone maintenance would then be patient-centred; it would not, on the basis of treatment philosophy, restrict the range of availability of methadone, time of treatment, or ancillary services.

The original program devised by Dole and Nyswander (1965) for methadone maintenance was a drug replacement regime. A return to this basic model is suggested by the evidence reviewed above. The optimum duration for methadone maintenance is, therefore, for as long as the patient finds it necessary to continue taking a daily dose of methadone. Given the chronic, relapsing nature of opioid dependence, there is no reason to expect that this would be for a short period of time while heroin remains relatively freely available in our society.

THE END OF TREATMENT

INTRODUCTION

In the previous chapter on the duration of methadone maintenance treatment, it was concluded that the available evidence suggests that, for most people, methadone maintenance is only effective while they remain in treatment. We also concluded that for those who leave methadone maintenance, their reason for leaving treatment was an important predictor of how they would fare afterwards. In this chapter, we examine the research on different methods of withdrawing patients from methadone at the end of treatment. Treatment may have come to an end through a decision to leave with staff support, a decision to leave against staff advice, or because it is no longer possible for the unit to keep the patient on the program.

Understandably, most patients who leave methadone maintenance in the hope that they are ready to lead an opioid-free existence are apprehensive. They are afraid of the withdrawal symptoms they may experience and of relapsing to heroin use. The immediate post-methadone maintenance period is a difficult time and systematic programs that are effective and acceptable to patients are just being developed. It is in this last area, rather than in the development of new detoxification techniques, that future improvements in methadone maintenance programs are likely to be made. However, as has been seen in the previous chapters, these improvements will only be of value if programs can ensure that patients stay in treatment long enough for the beginnings of a new lifestyle to have developed.

THE METHADONE WITHDRAWAL SYNDROME

Physical Aspects

As with other opioids, when a person who is dependent on methadone abruptly ceases taking the drug, they exhibit a set of signs and symptoms that are known as a withdrawal, or abstinence, syndrome. While the details of the physiological processes involved in the manifestation of this syndrome are not fully known, it is thought that regular exposure to exogenous opioids causes changes in neuronal functioning in the brain and that when exposure suddenly stops or dose is sharply reduced, a rebound-like effect occurs resulting in hyper-excitability. In short, it is thought that certain endogenous systems in the central nervous system adapt to chronic opioid use and that when this use ceases it takes some time for the body to readjust.

According to Jaffe (1985):

The *abrupt withdrawal of methadone* produces a syndrome that is qualitatively similar to that of morphine, but it develops more slowly and is more prolonged, although usually less intense. The addict has few or no symptoms until 24 to 48 hours after the last dose, and then complains of weakness, anxiety, anorexia, insomnia, abdominal discomfort, headaches, sweating, pain in muscles and bones, and hot and cold flashes. As with morphine withdrawal, there is nausea, vomiting, and an increase in body temperature, blood pressure, pulse, respiratory rate, and pupillary size. In general, after abrupt withdrawal, the primary or early abstinence syndrome reaches its maximal intensity by about the third day and may not begin to decrease until the third week, and apparent recovery may not occur until the sixth or seventh week (p. 544).

There is evidence that the first or primary phase of withdrawal is succeeded by a secondary and more prolonged abstinence syndrome in which both subjective symptoms of distress and physiological signs of abnormal functioning can be observed (Martin et al., 1973). The conventional wisdom about the comparative intensity and duration of the withdrawal syndromes for heroin and methadone has recently been questioned by Gossop and Strang (1991) who observed a more intense abstinence syndrome (of a similar duration) for methadone-dependent patients than they did for heroin-dependent patients during a 10-day inpatient methadone withdrawal program. However, the patients in the study were not solely dependent on heroin or methadone, and the extent to which the results of this study are applicable to patients in methadone maintenance is questionable, given what is known about the accumulation of methadone in body tissue during maintenance treatment (Kreek, 1979). The ideal way in which to resolve this issue would be to compare heroin- to methadone-maintained individuals with half of each group being detoxified with tapering doses of heroin and the other half being subjected to the same procedure with methadone. Such an experiment would also allow the investigation of the belief held by many heroin addicts that it is better to switch back to heroin at the end of methadone maintenance, because the withdrawal is shorter and easier to bear (Rosenbaum & Murphy, 1984).

The existence of a withdrawal syndrome, unpleasant as it may be, is not sufficient to explain the very high rates of relapse observed among opioid users after detoxification. Opioid-dependent individuals are capable of fully or partially detoxifying themselves and use a variety of methods to achieve this goal without professional assistance (Gossop et al., 1991). This is also the experience of detoxification programs that are quite successful as long as the goal of detoxification is seen as completing the withdrawal process. Such programs would, however, have to be seen as unsuccessful if there was the unrealistic expectation that the people who briefly pass through them will then go on to lead a drug-free life (Newman, 1983a).

Psychological Aspects

The distress associated with withdrawing from opioids is better tolerated by some individuals than others. A number of factors are thought to be associated with this. Andrews and Himmelsbach (1944) demonstrated that the greater the amount of opioid required to prevent withdrawal, the more intense the syndrome will be when withdrawal occurs. Similarly, it is widely believed that the longer the person has been dependent, the more intense the withdrawal syndrome will be (Kleber, 1981). However, contrary to these findings, Phillips et al., (1986) found that both the dose of methadone required to stabilise patients at the beginning of a detoxification program, and length of opioid dependence were not associated with the level of withdrawal distress. Instead, they found stronger associations between withdrawal symptoms and neuroticism (as assessed by the Eysenck Personality Questionnaire) and expectations about withdrawal distress.

Whitehead (1974) had earlier suggested that there may be a psychological component of the response to methadone during methadone maintenance treatment. In a series of case reports, he presented the clinical observation that some individuals who are being maintained on otherwise adequate doses of methadone would unexpectedly experience withdrawal, often in association with stressful periods in their lives. McLellan et al. (1986) have observed that conditioned withdrawal, which they also found to be common among methadone maintenance patients, may be elicited by negative emotional states (e.g. anger, depression). Complaints that the dose being dispensed is not enough to 'hold' the patient concerned (i.e. prevent withdrawal) are familiar to anyone who has worked in a methadone maintenance clinic. Whitehead called this phenomenon the methadone 'pseudowithdrawal' syndrome.

Related to the notion of pseudowithdrawal is a phenomenon known as the abstinence phobia or pathological detoxification fear. Hall (1979) described abstinence phobia in methadone maintenance patients who are attempting to slowly withdraw from methadone as an exaggerated anxious reaction to comparatively mild withdrawal symptoms. She notes that anxiety is a common symptom of the opioid withdrawal syndrome, but that in the cases she is describing extreme levels of anxiety are observed which evoke phobic-like responses such as avoidance (i.e. refusal to proceed with the detoxification). Hall suggests that this reaction is probably the result of previous experience of traumatic, sudden and involuntary withdrawal such as may occur in prison, or of observing others experience severe withdrawal symptoms, or of inaccurate information about the severity of methadone withdrawal that circulates within the heroin-using subculture.

Hall (1979) proposed that abstinence phobia might, like other phobias, be amenable to some form of intervention. Hall et al., (1984) tested this proposition by examining whether the addition of a cognitive behavioural intervention (relaxation training tied to anxiety as cue plus cognitive restructuring of withdrawal symptoms) assisted patients who wished to detoxify from methadone maintenance. When they compared two stratified random samples of methadone maintenance patients, they found no discernible influence for the intervention on reductions in methadone dose, detoxification rate or detoxification anxiety. However, the findings of the study did support the existence and importance of a phenomenon of detoxification anxiety. Patients who were assessed as being anxious about detoxifying at the beginning of the study showed only minimal changes in their maintenance dosage, and assessed levels of detoxification anxiety were found to increase as dose decreased. These findings suggest that anxiety is associated with detoxification which, to date, has not proven amenable to traditional anxiety treatments.

Milby and his colleagues have developed the concept of what they term detoxification fear and have devised an instrument for assessing it (Milby et al., 1986; 1987; Raczynski et al., 1988). Milby et al. (1986) make a distinction between mild anxiety in anticipation of an unpleasant experience and unrealistic fear which is out of proportion to the symptoms experienced in a dose reduction withdrawal procedure. They suggest that this fear may be realistic if it is based on experiences that have been very traumatic, such as unassisted detoxification in a prison or police station. In such cases, Milby et al. (1986) suggest that the appropriate paradigmatic psychiatric disorder would be post-traumatic stress syndrome rather than phobia.

Milby et al. (1986) used their instrument that had been devised to assess detoxification fear to survey methadone maintenance patients from three cities in the USA. They found 28% to be suffering from pathological levels of detoxification fear. They also found that significantly more women than men suffered from this fear. This finding is consistent with the observation of Rosenbaum and Murphy (1984), who suggested that women may experience the emotional dimensions of withdrawal more intensely than men do, and evidence that women in general are more likely to experience anxiety disorders than men (Robins et al., 1991b).

Raczynski et al. (1988) have also provided physiological evidence as an independent validation of some of the assumptions of this model of detoxification fear. They found that methadone maintenance patients exhibited greater reactivity to imagined detoxification situations than to neutral situations, and that patients assessed as having significant levels of detoxification fear experienced this increased reactivity to a greater extent than did others.

There is, in summary, enough evidence to suggest that there may be a subgroup of methadone maintenance patients who are anxious enough about detoxifying from methadone for this to be an impediment to completing withdrawal. The only intervention reported in the literature that has shown any success in alleviating anxiety in withdrawing opioid users is reported by Green and Gossop (1988). They based their intervention on the assumption that clear, accurate information may reduce the distress involved in withdrawal, just as in other areas of medicine where unpleasant interventions have to be employed. Green and Gossop compared the responses of opioid-dependent individuals randomly assigned to an information and no-information condition for a 21-day methadone detoxification program. The subjects who received the information were more likely to complete detoxification and experienced less subjective withdrawal distress during the period immediately after their methadone dose reached zero. The implications of this study are that accurate information may be useful in alleviating anxiety among withdrawing methadone maintenance patients. The extent to which this would also be true for patients with severe detoxification anxiety is not clear.

The findings reviewed in this section have to be kept in perspective. Alleviating anxiety about detoxification might contribute to greater completion rates which would be an important accomplishment. However, as Milby et al. (1986) note, reducing opioid dose to zero is necessary but not sufficient for living a drug-free life. In the next section, we examine the ways in which the withdrawal process can be made less distressing by employing diminishing doses of methadone and other drugs.

WITHDRAWAL REGIMENS

ntil recently, the only other treatment available besides opioid maintenance has traditionally been detoxification. In order to make detoxification a more humane process, there has been a constant search for medications and procedures that will alleviate the suffering involved, and a startling array have been tried over the years (see Kleber, 1981). The treatment of choice for detoxification regimens has for some time been a course of diminishing doses of methadone, so that the individuals detoxifying could do so with as little distress as possible. This has also been the procedure of choice for methadone maintenance patients when they are leaving treatment. Recent experimentation with other medications (e.g. clonidine) has shown promise, but, when the disadvantages associated with the use of these medications are taken into account, tapering off from methadone still remains the most effective and humane method for withdrawing opioid-dependent individuals, including methadone maintenance patients.

Methadone

There have been few studies that have examined the relative effectiveness of different methadone withdrawal regimens in detoxifying methadone maintenance patients. Mintz et el. (1975) randomly assigned patients to a withdrawal regimen (reduction in dose by 10% per week over two days for 14 weeks) or to continued methadone maintenance under double-blind conditions. Although the study was thwarted by nearly all the patients leaving the experiment by the end of the study period, one finding did emerge: under double-blind conditions, methadone maintenance patients whose dose was being reduced by 10% per week reported withdrawal symptoms, which because of the double-blind design were unlikely to be the result of patient expectation.

In a more successful study, Senay et al. (1977) found that under double-blind conditions a slow (3% per week) dose reduction withdrawal regimen was better than a faster (10%) regimen which was associated with higher drop-out rates, more heroin use and greater subjective distress. The inclusion of both blind and open methadone maintenance conditions in the study allowed the authors to estimate the influence of expectation on withdrawal symptoms. They found that in the blind methadone maintenance condition and the slow withdrawal condition (remembering that subjects did not know what conditions they were in) more withdrawal symptoms were observed than in the methadone maintenance condition in which patients knew their dose, suggesting that the uncertainty about whether their dose was being reduced or not induced withdrawal symptoms in the blind methadone maintenance condition. By contrast, both the blind methadone maintenance condition and the slow withdrawal condition exhibited less withdrawal symptoms than the fast withdrawal condition, demonstrating that rate of detoxification also played a part. This study is consistent with the result of Mintz et al. discussed in the previous paragraph in demonstrating that withdrawal phenomena are related to both rate of methadone reduction and to patient expectations about withdrawal symptoms.

Given that patient expectations appear to play a role in the withdrawal process, it may be possible to devise conditions in which these expectations assist in achieving detoxification from methadone. Paneptino et al. (1977) report on a procedure used in a methadone maintenance program for pregnant women and their partners in which the patients know their doses and have some control over their detoxification schedule. Using this procedure, they found that 63% of a group of patients who participated in this schedule successfully detoxified. An important part of the regimen was regular attendance at a group held for detoxifying methadone maintenance patients, in which issues of relevance to the patients were discussed. The evidence for both the open schedule and the usefulness of detoxification groups is plausible, but there are too many confounding factors to accept that the findings of this study can easily be interpreted for the general population of methadone maintenance patients. Pregnant women were over-represented in the sample (74%), which means presumably that at the time of detoxification all would have had young babies to take care of. The small number of men in the sample, in comparison to the usual methadone maintenance patient population where men usually outnumber women, were all partners of these women. The significance of the influence children may have on methadone maintenance patients may be considerable. Rosenbaum (1981; 1991) has found in two surveys that both opioid addicts out of treatment and methadone maintenance patients report that their children spur them on to make an extra effort to get over their problems.

The three studies reviewed immediately above (Mintz et al., 1975; Paneptino et al., 1977; Senay et al., 1977) raise the main issues that need to be addressed in a withdrawal regimen: the rate at which the methadone dose should be reduced and whether this relates to maintenance dose level; whether the reductions in dose should be blind or open; and whether group or individual counselling is an important part of the process. (Counselling is dealt with later. See pp. 208–09). Clinical opinion is consistent with these findings in suggesting that withdrawing patients from methadone maintenance should be done in a slow, gradual fashion (Kleber, 1977). For example, Lowinson et al., (1976) recommend dose reductions of 10 mg per fortnight until a daily dose of 40 mg is reached; thereafter the patient should be split-dosed and further reductions made at 5 mg per fortnight until the daily dose reaches 10 mg. When 10 mg is reached, they recommend reductions of 2 to 3 mg per week according to individual response. Cushman (1981) suggests reductions of 5 mg per week until the daily dose reaches 20 mg, when the reduction rate should be halved to 2.5 mg per week.

Two conclusions emerge from these recommendations: that the process should be gradual and that there is a point where the tapering of the dose is slowed down. In this regard, it is widely believed that many patients begin to experience difficulties with the withdrawal procedure when the dose reaches around 20 mg

(Goldstein, 1971; Lowinson et al., 1976). If a patient does begin to experience withdrawal symptoms, it is better to readjust the methadone dose rather than offer ancillary medications, such as the benzodiazepines, which are often abused by methadone maintenance patients.

A recent study by Strang and Gossop (1990) contributes to the available knowledge on the effects of different withdrawal regimens on the symptoms experienced by patients during withdrawal. They compared linear to inverse exponential dose reduction schedules in a rapid 10-day methadone detoxification program. All patients were initially stabilised on a dose of methadone over three days, which was individualised to their needs before being slowly reduced to zero over the next 10 days. In the linear reduction schedule, the dose was reduced at a rate of 10% of the starting dose per day, that is, if the stabilising dose was 50 mg it would be reduced daily by 5 mg. In the inverse exponential reduction schedule, the stabilising dose was reduced daily by 20% of the previous day's dose, that is, 50 mg then 40 mg, then 32 mg, etc. Using the latter schedule, there is a more rapid reduction in dose at the beginning of the schedule which tapers off to a slower reduction near the end of the 10-day period

Strang and Gossop (1990) found that patients in the inverse exponential reduction condition who required high doses (>50 mg) of methadone to stabilise them experienced a more intense withdrawal syndrome during the early part of the withdrawal period than their counterparts in the linear reduction group without any shortening in the total length of time the withdrawal syndrome was experienced. In contrast, patients who were stabilised on low doses (<50 mg) of methadone before being withdrawn suffered a shorter withdrawal syndrome in the inverse exponential condition without showing any increase in drop-out rate, or in the intensity of the withdrawal syndrome. This may mean that patients who are maintained on lower doses of methadone can be tapered from methadone more quickly, although, as we will see below, there may be more disadvantages than advantages in hastening the methadone withdrawal process.

There is no evidence to suggest that either blind or open dose reduction schedules are more effective in assisting patients to complete their detoxification. As Kleber (1977) points out, when patients know their dose reduction schedule they are encouraged to participate in the procedure, and to take some responsibility for each dose reduction decision, but their knowledge may lead to anxiety when the dose gets close to zero. Blind withdrawal lessens this anxiety, and is for this reason preferred by some patients.

Letting patients know that both options are available, and the relative advantages and disadvantages of each, is probably the best way of maximising participation, while allowing for individual differences in anxiety before and during the detoxification process.

There is probably no optimum method for tapering methadone dosage that is applicable to all patients. Cushman and Dole (1973) conducted a prospective study with 48 methadone maintenance patients who were detoxifying from methadone with the assent of program staff because they were considered to be rehabilitated. All patients were blind to the dose reduction schedule. It was found that the patients could be categorised into four distinct groups according to their response to being detoxified:

- a small number of patients who, even though they did not experience withdrawal symptoms, became anxious about their dose before it reached 30 mg and asked for methadone maintenance to be reinstated;
- a small number of patients whose dose went below 30 mg and asked for methadone maintenance to be reinstated, because they could not tolerate the withdrawal symptoms;
- about one half of the overall majority of patients who successfully detoxified but who re-entered methadone maintenance because of relapse to drug use or an inability to tolerate the protracted withdrawal syndrome they were experiencing;
- the other half of the detoxified group who were successful in getting off methadone maintenance and leading an opioid-free life.

Cushman and Dole (1973) note that 93% of the patients overall experienced a withdrawal syndrome, and that secondary withdrawal was sufficiently intense to make 25% of the study group return to methadone maintenance after being detoxified. According to the authors, the implication of these findings is that both program staff and patients have to realise that a withdrawal syndrome of some sort is inevitable when a patient leaves methadone maintenance, regardless of the degree of rehabilitation achieved during treatment.

Clonidine

Clonidine is a non-opioid medication (alpha adrenergic blocking agent) that has been mainly used in the treatment of hypertension. In the mid-seventies, it was discovered that clonidine reduced the signs of withdrawal in rats and it was then trialled towards the end of the decade for the detoxification of opioid-dependent humans. In a series of experiments it was found to effectively suppress the opioid withdrawal syndrome. With methadone maintenance patients, it was found that administration of clonidine for the duration of the primary withdrawal period (10 days) reduced both the observable signs and subjective distress of the study participants (see Ginzburg, 1983).

When clonidine was compared with tapered methadone withdrawal, it was usually been found to be equally effective in reducing the signs and symptoms of the abstinence syndrome. The two regimens differed, however, in the times during withdrawal when patients experienced difficulty. For clonidine, the first few days seemed to be difficult, while for methadone tapering, the end of the tapering regimen as the dose neared zero seemed to be the time at which many patients suffered the most (Ginzburg, 1983; Gossop, 1988). Given that the methadone withdrawal regimen is the preferred treatment for detoxifying opioid-dependent individuals, the apparent equal efficacy of clonidine was an important finding (Gossop, 1988). For methadone maintenance patients, there would also appear to be an advantage in the use of clonidine. Using a reducing dose regimen, it may take many months before the patient becomes completely detoxified from methadone. According to its advocates, using clonidine can shorten this period to 10 days. In one study, when used in combination with the narcotic antagonist naltrexone, it was found that the detoxification period could be halved to five days (Charney et al., 1986). The purpose in achieving this rapid detoxification is to initiate maintenance with an opioid antagonist like naltrexone, a treatment that would effectively block the effects of any opioids taken by the patient.

Marked problems have, however, been found to be associated with the use of clonidine. These were serious enough for the two authors who have reviewed the literature on the use of clonidine in opioid detoxification to conclude that there are serious disadvantages with the procedure when it is compared to a tapered methadone regimen (Ginzburg, 1983; Gossop, 1988). Clonidine has a number of undesirable effects when used at dose levels necessary to suppress withdrawal symptoms. The most serious of these effects are a lowering of systolic and diastolic blood pressures, and sedation. These untoward effects are serious enough to require the close medical supervision of patients who are being administered clonidine at levels necessary for opioid detoxification. Most of the trials of clonidine have accordingly been conducted with hospitalised subjects. When outpatient trials have been conducted, the delicate balance between administering an adequate dose to suppress withdrawal and one which will not result in too great a lowering of blood pressure and sedation has not really been achieved. Patients also often have difficulty sleeping when taking clonidine during withdrawal and, in some early studies, the procedure induced psychosis in a small number of patients (although this outcome is less likely if patients are screened for a history of psychiatric disorder).

Clonidine seems to be no more effective than methadone in managing the opioid withdrawal syndrome. As well as suppressing withdrawal symptoms, clonidine has a number of serious concurrent effects associated with its use. As Gossop (1988) has pointed out, although clonidine advocates claim that it is more effective than methadone tapering, the evidence does not really indicate this. Recent evidence confirms Gossop's view. In a randomised controlled trial comparing, among other things, clonidine to methadone tapering, San et al. (1990) found methadone to be more effective at eliminating withdrawal signs and symptoms than clonidine.

There would seem little reason to recommend the use of clonidine for methadone maintenance patients tapering from methadone at the end of treatment. Although becoming detoxified from methadone is required in order to complete the recovery process, it does not mean that it is a desirable goal in its own right. Many patients now in methadone maintenance would probably successfully detoxify rapidly using clonidine if this was done in a hospitalised setting. However, we know from the evidence reviewed in the previous chapter on the duration of methadone maintenance that most patients would quickly relapse to heroin use after leaving hospital. Rawson et al. (1984) compared the outcome of methadone maintenance patients detoxified over 10 days using clonidine, who either did or did not then go on to naltrexone maintenance. They found that most of the clonidine only subjects relapsed because of urges to use heroin rather than because they experienced withdrawal symptoms. This finding emphasises that, just as in the case of illicit opioids, successful detoxification from methadone is a relatively easy goal to achieve under controlled conditions, but that this has very little meaning in terms of recovery from opioid dependence. This result is fully consistent with what we know from other substance dependence disorders (alcohol, nicotine).

Milby (1988), in a comprehensive review of research on detoxifying from methadone maintenance, concluded that improved detoxification rates observed over the 15-year period since the advent of methadone maintenance treatment were due primarily to the use of new medications like clonidine. This interpretation of the evidence is questionable for a number of reasons. First, the rates for successful detoxification with methadone improved nearly as much on earlier rates as did those for studies using clonidine. Secondly, many of the early studies of methadone tapering were descriptive studies of the fates of large numbers of patients leaving methadone maintenance programs under uncontrolled conditions. The extent to which these are comparable to highly controlled studies of short periods of clonidine withdrawal that were conducted on inpatients is questionable. Thirdly, there is the confounding variable of the duration of detoxification, which Milby acknowledges. The improved rates shown for the later clonidine studies may be the result of the different durations of detoxification involved. That is, if the clonidine study periods were as long as the methadone tapering study periods, the same failure rate might be observed simply because there is a constant drop-out rate found in all detoxification studies no matter what medication is used. If this were the case, the apparent superiority of clonidine would be due to the different study periods rather than to the different characteristics of the two medications being employed. Finally, as Gossop (1988) has pointed out, many of the studies using clonidine have used special selection criteria that make it more likely that the procedure will achieve high rates of successful detoxification. Taking these factors into account, it is difficult to share Milby's enthusiasm for medications like clonidine.

It is likely that new approaches to managing the opioid withdrawal syndrome will become available in the near future (e.g. Hartmann et al. (1991) describe positive results in a clinical trial comparing acetorphan, an enkephalinase inhibitor, and clonidine). However, the evidence reviewed in this book suggests that successful recovery has more to do with changes that will have occurred while the patient was in treatment. Leaving methadone maintenance is best seen as a period of transition and, as such, is probably best left to the slow pace of methadone tapering. The person concerned is not only being weaned off methadone, but sloughing off the identity of being a methadone maintenance patient which is related to its predecessor, the opioid addict. It cannot be expected that these changes will occur in a matter of days after years of dependence.

Adjunctive Counselling

There is a clinical consensus that withdrawal from methadone maintenance is a difficult time for most patients and that additional support is needed during this period (Cushman, 1981; Kleber, 1977; Lowinson et al., 1976; Resnick, 1983). Milby (1988) concluded that some form of psychotherapy or counselling probably assists the withdrawal process, but, given the paucity of studies in this area, was unable to state that the research strongly indicated this. Similarly, there was no evidence that either group or individual counselling is better in this regard (Kleber, 1977). As already mentioned earlier in this chapter, some methadone maintenance programs do form 'detox' groups for patients who are ready to leave treatment (Kleber, 1977; Panepinto et al., 1977). Such groups allow individuals going through the same experience to get together and encourage and support one another.

In their survey of staff and patient attitudes to withdrawing from methadone maintenance, Gold et al. (1988) found that three-quarters of the patients and nearly of all of the staff members surveyed thought that counselling and psychotherapy would contribute to successfully leaving methadone maintenance. Besides anxiety about withdrawal and difficulties due to withdrawal symptoms, many patients experience a sense of loss about leaving treatment, especially if they have been in methadone maintenance for a long period of time. The patients in the Gold et al. survey indicated that they would miss contact with clinic staff and the counselling provided within the program more than coming to the clinic itself or the contact this made possible with the other patients. In addition, there is the loss associated with giving up methadone itself (Rosenbaum & Murphy, 1984).

Although there is little research evidence on which to base such a conclusion, it is likely from the observations set out in the clinical literature that supportive counselling does contribute to successful weaning from methadone maintenance for most patients. In the next section, we look at the importance of paying attention to patients' motivation for wanting to leave methadone maintenance and the further role that counselling and self-help groups can play in the post-methadone period.

LIFE AFTER METHADONE

A number of factors have been identified as influencing a patient's readiness to attempt withdrawal from methadone maintenance. These include staff attitudes to methadone maintenance and withdrawal, the influence of significant others in the patient's life, and the gains that the patient has made during his or her time in treatment. A patient who has improved during methadone maintenance and who leaves with the blessing of program staff has a reasonable chance of success in leading an opioid free life (Milby, 1988).

Deciding to Withdraw

As we have noted previously (see Chapter 9), patients withdraw from methadone maintenance for a variety of reasons. There are three basic categories of patients who leave methadone maintenance: those that complete their course of methadone maintenance in the sense that they and their unit staff believe they will be able to leave without relapsing to heroin use; those that leave methadone maintenance against the advice of program staff; and those that leave involuntarily, usually because they have continued to use illicit drugs or broken program rules, or have been sentenced to prison. In the first and last categories the precursors to the exit from the program are reasonably clear. In the first case, a long period of not using the more serious illicit drugs and other signs of recovery will be evident to program staff. In the case of involuntary withdrawal from methadone maintenance, serious infraction of program rules or being sentenced by a court (which may have nothing to do with response to treatment given the delay between arrest and conviction) are usually the immediate precursors.

With the second category — leaving contrary to advice — a number of factors might precipitate a premature exit from treatment. Initially, patients who enter methadone maintenance may have unrealistic expectations about what is possible for them. Often they think that after many years of opioid dependence they will be able to get themselves together and get off methadone within a few months (Caplehorn & Bell, 1991; Stimmel et al., 1977). A patient who wishes to leave methadone maintenance after a short period may need to discuss their reasons for wanting to detoxify with program staff. Other pressures that methadone maintenance patients feel are the stigma associated with being a methadone maintenance patient and the burden of having to come into the clinic regularly. Some patients are coerced into leaving treatment by family or friends who do not understand the treatment or its goals. In all of these cases, staff can clarify with the patient the reasons why they feel they have to leave treatment at that particular point and assist, if necessary, in ensuring the patient is treated fairly (e.g. at other sites within the health care system) or in educating family and friends about what methadone maintenance is all about (Kleber, 1977; Lowinson et al., 1976).

The attitude of staff may also affect a patient's decision to leave treatment. Lowinson et al. (1976) suggest that the best course to take is to develop an attitude that is at the same time neutral (in the sense of not subscribing to any given duration of methadone maintenance as being the best) and patient-centred. If staff members appear either eager or pessimistic about leaving treatment they may thwart any attempts in the latter case, or they make the patient feel that they cannot live up to staff expectations in the former. (The issue of the way in which staff attitudes to the optimum duration of treatment may unduly influence patients is covered in more detail in Chapter 9.) Being patient-centred also means that if a patient decides after consultation that he or she wants to leave treatment at a time that staff feel is inappropriate, then staff should still offer their full encouragement and support once the process begins.

Aftercare

It is widely acknowledged that individuals who have left methadone maintenance need assistance and support for some time afterwards (e.g. Gold et al., 1988; Goldstein, 1972b; Lowinson et al., 1976). Former methadone maintenance patients may experience a protracted withdrawal syndrome and may also have to contend with a renewed desire to use heroin in response to environmental cues and emotional states that arise as they go into this new phase in their life. Rosenbaum (1991) provides descriptions of the lives of former patients who have been successful in making a new life for themselves and the methods they used to get there. As Kleber (1977) has noted, however, although aftercare is often recommended and offered to many former methadone maintenance patients, it is unusual for them to remain in contact with the program. Rosenbaum and Murphy (1984) note that patients who have graduated usually have very good relationships with program staff for some time before having left treatment and that this loss is considerable in terms of their social support network. Providing after-care that former methadone maintenance patients will take advantage of is an important aspect of methadone maintenance treatment that has not been adequately developed. In this section, we examine the types of aftercare that have been proposed and the results of the few studies that have investigated their effectiveness. A much more extensive discussion of aftercare possibilities is provided by Weddington (1990–91).

One suggestion for assisting in the transition from methadone maintenance to abstinence has been for the tapering process to take place while the patient resides in a therapeutic community (Sorensen et al., 1984a). Results of research examining this mode of getting off methadone maintenance suggest that it may be a useful form of aftercare, but that, as is true of the therapeutic community treatment generally, it is acceptable to few patients (Sorensen et al.,

1984b). Wermuth et al., (1987) describe an aftercare service that can be delivered by methadone maintenance units on an outpatient basis that involves individual counselling, group meetings, relapse prevention training and referral to Narcotics Anonymous. Wermuth et al. suggest that at least six months of aftercare is necessary to help patients get over what they call the post-methadone syndrome. Other suggestions for aftercare have included opioid antagonist maintenance and the integration of 12-step style programs into methadone maintenance programs (Weddington, 1990–91).

The best available evidence for the effectiveness of aftercare in enabling opioid-dependent individuals to make a new life for themselves is provided by a randomised controlled trial conducted in Hong Kong and the USA. This study compared a structured aftercare program with assistance on request which was provided by both study and former treatment personnel (McAuliffe, 1990; McAuliffe & Ch'ien, 1986). The aftercare program, which was trialled in this study, consisted of a combined recovery training and self-help group approach. Subjects had been treated in a range of treatment modalities (methadone maintenance, therapeutic communities, detoxification programs). Each recovery group met for three hours each week for a period of six months, or for longer if participants wished to continue. Half the time the group was led by a trained counsellor who conducted relapse prevention sessions, while the rest of the time was devoted to an unstructured self-help meeting led by one of the group participants. Group members were encouraged to attend extra-curricular social activities and to use the 'buddy' system if they felt themselves at risk of relapsing. The study found that, in comparison with the control condition, the intervention reduced the risk of relapse, self-reported crime and helped unemployed subjects find work. All of the subjects participating in the study were highly motivated individuals who wanted to lead a drug-free life. The important point of this study, as McAuliffe (1990) suggests, is that even such highly motivated subjects can be assisted by a structured aftercare intervention.

Although methadone maintenance patients rarely return to their former programs for assistance, it may be that patients would be more likely to return if specialised aftercare services were made available and presented as part of the treatment process. One possible impediment to providing aftercare services is their cost. However, two things should be kept in mind when the costs of such services are considered. The first is that every patient who is successful is one less patient who will return for another course of treatment (McAuliffe, 1990). The second is that it may be possible to offer such services within existing programs. Wermuth et al. (1987), for example, suggest appointing one member of staff as the aftercare specialist who will organise the aftercare program and keep up with developments in the area. Future research should clarify how important aftercare is to recovery and in what form it can be most effective.

CONCLUSION

Withdrawing from methadone is only one part of the process of leaving methadone maintenance. It is important to keep in mind that a patient who leaves methadone maintenance without being ready is highly likely to relapse, and that patients who leave early are unlikely to want to go through an aftercare program that may take some months to complete. The development of aftercare programs is important, but given the few patients who are ready to use them, it may be more important to look at ways of getting more patients to this point. This means, in the first instance, keeping patients in treatment long enough for change to take place and attaining this requires the adoption of treatment practices that have been shown through research to work.

SUMMARY

Methadone maintenance patients, like other people who are dependent on opioid drugs, will experience a characteristic withdrawal syndrome if the administration of methadone is ceased abruptly. Because of the relatively long elimination half-life of methadone and the fact that it accumulates in body tissue during maintenance treatment, the methadone withdrawal syndrome is more protracted than that of shorter acting opioids like morphine and heroin, but is also less intense.

The methadone withdrawal syndrome has a number of associated psychological phenomena that are important in the management of patients. It has been noted that during methadone maintenance many patients experience withdrawal symptoms, even though they are being maintained on an adequate dose. The most probable explanation for this phenomenon is that features of opioid withdrawal syndromes can be evoked by internal and external stimuli that have come to elicit these symptoms via conditioning processes.

As is probably the case with any incipient unpleasant experience, most methadone maintenance patients experience a mild anticipatory anxiety when faced with the prospect of withdrawing from methadone. Providing clear, accurate information about what is about to happen may be helpful in alleviating some of this anxiety. In some patients, however, this mild anxiety becomes a fear of phobic proportions and may make the prospect of leaving methadone maintenance difficult. At present, there is no intervention known to be effective in ameliorating this detoxification fear.

The most effective and humane procedure for withdrawing methadone maintenance patients from methadone at the end of treatment has been a slow course of diminishing doses of methadone. The limited research available suggests that the slower the course the better, although clinically the pace is best set individually in consultation with the patient. Tapering can occur in an open fashion in which the patient knows the details of the dose reduction schedule, or in a blind manner in which the patient does not know these details. Some patients prefer to be blind to dose reductions in order to reduce anxiety and prevent expectancy effects Informing patients about what is possible when withdrawing from methadone maintenance and allowing them to decide what is the best for them is the optimum method for allowing for differences between patients, and of maximising their participation in decisionmaking process, so that they are more likely to take responsibility for any course of withdrawal they embark upon.

Clonidine, although apparently comparable to methadone tapering in trials conducted in inpatient and residential settings, is ill-suited for use in methadone maintenance because there is no reason to believe that a more rapid withdrawal procedure would benefit patients. Leaving methadone maintenance after a long period of time is a complex process of disengagement for patients and detoxification is only one of the more important issues.

Supportive counselling is an important part of leaving methadone maintenance. There is a clinical consensus that this a particularly difficult time for patients and that the disengagement process should be seen as part of the treatment process, not the end of it.

The decision to leave methadone maintenance may have complex features associated with it. New patients often have unrealistic notions about detoxifying from methadone quickly and then leading a problem-free life. Some patients are pressured by family and friends who do not understand that recovery from opioid dependence takes time. Patients may also feel that there is a stigma associated with being on methadone. And finally, staff may, through their beliefs and attitudes about the desirability of either abstinence or maintenance, influence patients to either attempt or abandon withdrawal from methadone maintenance no matter what their state of readiness. A patient-centred approach to these issues is one where staff orient their attitudes about treatment to the patient rather than to their own beliefs about the desirability of this or that practice. A patient-centred approach also includes assisting patients to try to determine what is best for them and this, at times, involves educating family and friends and serving as an advocate for patients in instances of discrimination. A patient who leaves treatment before they are ready is at high risk of relapsing to opioid use with all the ensuing risks to health and welfare which that entails.

Most ex-methadone maintenance patients suffer what might be called a post-methadone syndrome. This consists of the mild symptoms of the protracted phase of the withdrawal syndrome and the issues involved in leading an opioid-free life without the regular counselling and contact with clinic staff that is part of methadone maintenance treatment. There has long been a clinical consensus that supportive counselling should be continued after the administration of methadone has ceased, but few patients have ever taken up this option. Recent developments in research on relapse prevention have led to the development of aftercare services, that is, structured programs which assist patients to disengage from methadone maintenance treatment. The research available suggests that well-motivated patients leaving treatment are more likely to be successful if they participate in an aftercare program. Such programs involve a mix of education, skills training and features derived from self-help groups like Narcotics Anonymous.

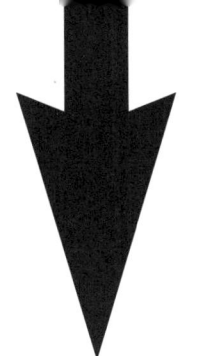

SECTION III
SPECIAL ISSUES

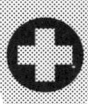

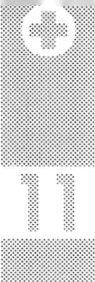

IMPLICATIONS OF THE HIV EPIDEMIC FOR METHADONE MAINTENANCE TREATMENT

INTRODUCTION

he advent of HIV has brought about a number of innovations in dealing with injecting drug use that would have been inconceivable little more than a decade ago. In Australia, for example, education campaigns to encourage safer sexual and drug use practices, along with the development of needle and syringe exchanges, are imaginative public health responses. The expansion of methadone maintenance programs has been another important part of the overall attempt to prevent an HIV epidemic among injecting drug users in Australia. It is arguably the case that because of these measures, Australia has not yet experienced the tragedy that has occurred among drug users in cities like New York and Edinburgh.

These new public health initiatives in the area of injecting drug use are part of a larger harm reduction approach to drug problems that was adopted as government policy in Australia in 1985. In this chapter, we examine the implications for methadone treatment of the adoption of these policies and the special problems that have arisen as a result of the appearance of HIV among patients attending methadone clinics. As will be seen below, although methadone maintenance is, in a sense, perhaps the prototypical harm reduction treatment, some of the basic tenets of the models of methadone treatment that have evolved have been challenged by this new set of circumstances. We examine suggestions that have been made about how these new dilemmas might be resolved and suggest some future directions that methadone treatment might move toward.

HARM REDUCTION

t is a common misconception that harm reduction policies are new on the drug treatment scene and that they have only been with us as long as HIV has been. A number of commentators have pointed out that interventions aimed at reducing the harm associated with drug use have always existed alongside other more abstinence-oriented treatment approaches (e.g. Berridge, 1990; Stimson & Lart, 1991). Methadone maintenance is the descendant of a long line of similar opiate maintenance programs that have existed in various forms throughout the world. For example, morphine maintenance was a common way of managing opioid dependence in the USA early this century (Courtwright, 1982), and heroin maintenance fulfilled a similar role in the United Kingdom for many years (Krivanek, 1988). All such programs have recognised that opioid dependence is not curable in the short term in many individuals and have adopted the humane and pragmatic alternative of providing such individuals with a regular supply of pure drugs as a way of minimising the harm caused by being dependent on a prohibited drug that is in plentiful supply.

More generally, the harm reduction approach acknowledges abstinence as a desirable goal of treatment, but also accepts that a reduction in the harm associated with drug use is also a worthwhile outcome of treatment in cases where total abstinence is unattainable. Focusing on the narrower concept of HIV risk reduction, the goals of interventions for injecting drug users can be conceived of as a hierarchy of desirable outcomes with abstinence from illicit drug use at the top followed by a number of less desirable outcomes (Stimson, 1990). Other viable outcomes include changing the mode of administration of the drug (e.g. oral methadone or replacing injected heroin with a smoked variety), abstaining from needle sharing, or, at the very least, if the person concerned continues to share, proper cleaning of injecting equipment before each new person uses it.

HIV AND THE CHANGING ROLE FOR DRUG TREATMENT

timson (1990; see also Stimson & Lart, 1991) has identified five broad changes that have come about as a result of HIV and the subsequent adoption of a public health-based policy on injecting drug use in the United Kingdom, an analysis that is just as pertinent for countries like Australia where similar harm reduction policies have been adopted. These are:

- a shift in the definition of what the problem is away from the drug user to the behaviours associated with drug use;
- a comparable shift in the definition of the drug user away from the notion that all drug users are irrational to one of the rational or 'health conscious drug user' who is capable of responsible drug use;
- a change in the focus of interventions with injecting drug users away from dependence to behaviours that promote health and reduce risk;
- a change in the nature of the relationship between drug treatment workers and their clients away from confrontation and control to a more 'user friendly' approach;
- a new need for drug treatment staff to be more multi-skilled (Stimson & Lart refer to the 'renaissance drug worker') than they have had to be in the past, so that they are able to deal with a range of new problems brought about by HIV.

In this chapter we will examine the implications of these changes for methadone clinics. While staff in the newer forms of harm reduction agencies, such as needle and syringe exchanges, feel quite comfortable with this new approach, staff in the more traditional treatment agencies, such as methadone maintenance clinics, have often felt confused about what the purpose of their interventions should be in this new policy environment.

THE ORIGINS OF CONTROL IN METHADONE CLINICS

s we have already mentioned, methadone maintenance was originally conceived as a harm reduction program that allowed for the provision of an acceptable and less harmful opioid substance to those who were dependent. The treatment attracted vitriolic criticism from critics who claimed that methadone maintenance was analogous to handing out alcohol to alcoholics, that it prolonged or created dependence in individuals who otherwise would not be so, and that it was a form of social control of individuals whose drug problems were a symptom of social disadvantage (Nelkin, 1973). Attewell and Gerstein (1979) have argued that critics of methadone in the USA were placated when the relevant regulatory body (Food & Drug Administration) ensured that their concerns were addressed in their published protocols for recommended treatment practices. Contrary to the original model of treatment developed by Dole and Nyswander (1965), these protocols established that a drug-free life was an appropriate goal of treatment and implicitly restricted other aspects of methadone maintenance like dosage levels. The eventual impact of these policy initiatives was that methadone programs eventually adopted standards and goals for treatment that had less to do with what had been demonstrated to be effective and more to do with making the treatment politically and socially acceptable.

Methadone programs were unable to live up to the enthusiastic claims made for them by their early proponents and were also set up to fail by the new ethos of methadone-to-abstinence that arose in methadone clinics and regulatory bodies during the 1970s. By the early 1980s in Australia, for example, methadone had fallen out of favour. It had not prevented epidemic heroin use and was still vilified by other drug and alcohol workers. Although the Australian Government had already considered expanding methadone programs as way of dealing with drug-related crime in the mid-1980s it was the advent of HIV that led to the rapid expansion soon afterwards. Along with this expansion came the rehabilitation of the image of methadone as the only effective way of dealing with injecting opioid use that was acceptable to large numbers of drug users. We suggest, and this is the point of this historical digression, that some of the role conflicts and confusions that can be observed today in methadone clinics are not entirely new and could usefully be viewed as a re-enactment of difficulties that have been encountered in the past for methadone treatment.

Deeper still, at the heart of the way in which drug problems have been articulated in countries like the USA and Australia, there is the ambivalence and confusion about whether dependence on illicit drugs is a medical or a legal problem. The re-appearance of opioid maintenance as a form of treatment in the USA was, in fact, a radical shift away from it being regarded solely as a criminal matter (for doctors as well as drug users — see Courtwright, 1982; Gerstein & Harwood, 1990). However this confusion remains and we would suggest that it lies at the heart of the methadone clinic, of the policies that constrain it, and of the procedures that are enacted in the name of clinical safety and control. HIV has brought about a crisis for methadone treatment in two ways. It has required that methadone clinics should be as effective and acceptable to drug users as possible; and it has brought into question the extent to which the policing and health care roles of methadone clinics can continue to be accommodated. In the next section, we look at the possible difficulties involved in adopting a harm reduction approach within methadone treatment and what additional measures might be adopted to increase its effectiveness.

REDUCING AND ELIMINATING RISK BEHAVIOURS

The conditions under which effective risk reduction counselling can take place pose two sets of problems for counsellors working in methadone units: one has to do with patients' injecting behaviour; the other with sexual behaviour.

Rule Enforcement and Counselling

In relation to injecting drug use, counsellors in methadone clinics often find themselves fulfilling two contradictory roles for their patients: policing and counselling (Attewell & Gerstein, 1979; Zweben, 1991). On the one hand they are expected to enforce the rules of the program, and on the other they are supposed to develop counselling relationships based on trust (Curet et al., 1985). As common sense dictates, if patients feel that talking with their counsellor about illicit drug use is going to have adverse consequences for future treatment, it is unlikely they will be honest about it. However, in order for a harm reduction approach (and the interventions described below) to work, the central focus of treatment has to be on the well-being of the client (Baker & Dixon, 1991). If the well-being of the client is the central concern of the counsellor, rather than some other concern such as making sure the program rules are not broken, then an appropriate response to ongoing drug use or needle sharing will not be to invoke the rules of the program, but to try to create the conditions under which the client will consider the risks associated with their behaviour and begin to do something about it.

Curet et al. (1985) have suggested one possible solution to the treatment versus control dilemma, if this is a problem due to the structure of the program concerned. They suggest that the law enforcement and counselling functions should be separated in such a way that a patient is guaranteed confidentiality with his or her counsellor, but is still subject to the rules of the program which would be enforced, if necessary, by staff other than the counsellor. This would allow the development of a therapeutic alliance between counsellor and patient without it being damaged by conflict over program rules. Another solution would be to abandon 'preaching treatment and practising control', as Attewell and Gerstein (1979) refer to it, and drop the control aspect of unit practice. If patients continue to take illicit drugs, then it is a reason to express concern, not to invoke the relevant sanctions dictated by program rules.

As we have noted before in Chapter 8, the use of rules and sanctions have failed at both a society and treatment level to control illicit drug use in the past. We agree with Zweben (1991) when she points out that one person is essentially powerless to control the drug use of another person. The use of rules and sanctions in methadone treatment mirrors the larger social context within which they operate. However, we do not believe that it is, or should be, the role of health care providers to act against the interests of their patients (e.g. see Blum 1984). Assisting those patients who continue to put themselves at risk requires the development of an alliance between patient and counsellor and this precondition for the possibility of a successful outcome can only be thwarted by a punitive approach to illicit drug use.

Sex Counselling

As we have seen in Chapter 4, an important part of HIV risk reduction for drug users, as it is for everyone else, is encouraging safer sexual behaviour. Injecting drug users are at increased risk for HIV infection and for other markers of unsafe sexual behaviour (e.g. other sexually transmitted diseases). As part of the new range of skills required of drug treatment workers as a result of HIV, being able to counsel patients about their sexual behaviour is an important task. However, drug treatment staff in the past have not had to deal with sexual matters in their relationships with their clients, are not trained in sex counselling, and may therefore feel uncomfortable in discussing such matters in counselling sessions (Macks, 1988). Nicolosi et al. (1991) have suggested that this inexperience in dealing with sexual behaviour in counselling may be reflected in the lack of success on the part of treatment programs in reducing the incidence of unsafe sex.

To enable full risk assessment, staff should have a good knowledge of human sexual behaviour and be able to speak frankly about sex without embarrassment (Macks, 1988). Kelly and St. Lawrence (1988) have suggested the following guidelines for HIV counselling concerning sexual behaviour. The counsellor's own definitions of what is normal sexual behaviour should not interfere with discussions with the client. At the same time, the counsellor should avoid embarrassing the client by being overly explicit before rapport has developed and should keep strict confidentiality concerning the client's sexual behaviour. The counsellor should abandon simplistic definitions of hetero- and homosexuality, understanding that because a person describes themselves as heterosexual or homosexual does not mean that they do not at times engage in sexual activity that contradicts the way in which they describe themselves. Finally, Macks (1988) has proposed that the counsellor should realise that what might appear to be a life or death issue to them — for example, in the use or non-use of condoms — might not appear that way to the client, and might not to the counsellor, if they found themselves in a similar situation. There is, therefore, a clear need for staff in methadone clinics who are involved in counselling to be trained in counselling about sexual behaviour.

Education

According to Turner et al. (1989) changing behaviour involves three basic steps: the person concerned has to perceive that there is a problem; they have to be motivated to do something about it; and they need the knowledge and the skills necessary to make the relevant changes in their behaviour. Education, or providing information, is the starting point for any program that wants to change behaviour. Information not only has the ability to influence behaviour, but also dispels inaccurate myths and helps in the fight against the discrimination of which HIV positive and AIDS patients have become victims. In order to be effective, the information has to be to the point and written in language that is understandable by the target audience.

Education by itself is effective for some people but is usually not enough to change most people's behaviour (Kelly & St. Lawrence, 1988). This does not mean, however, that it is unnecessary (Turner et al., 1989). AIDS education is important on entering a methadone program and as a first step in HIV counselling (Kelly & St. Lawrence, 1988). One of the reasons why education alone does not work effectively is because most injecting drug users do not perceive the risk to be a personal one (e.g. Magura et al., 1989b).

This is not uncommon when the risk is associated with well established, immediately gratifying behaviour that has long-term negative consequences (Kelly et al., 1989). One of the tasks of motivating clients is to assist them to see the risks involved as personal.

Education also serves the useful function of dispelling myths about HIV and AIDS. Sontag (1988) presents an interesting discussion of the subtle ways in which misinformation and the language used to describe HIV and AIDS can contribute to the mystification of the virus and its subsequent effects on the body. Although most injecting drug users are reasonably well informed about the major modes of HIV transmission, they are often unsure about many of the details (Magura et al., 1989b). An unpleasant aspect of being ignorant about HIV transmission can surface in the form of stigmatising other patients on methadone programs whose HIV or AIDS status has become known (Baker & Dixon, 1991). Education can help to reduce discrimination like this by helping other patients to see that they are in no way at risk by being on the same program as HIV positive patients or patients with AIDS.

The content of educational materials made available to patients should not be restricted by the treatment philosophy of the program. Patients should be advised that if they do inject, they should inject safely. Assuming that they will not inject is counter-productive in terms of the maintenance of the well-being of the patient.

Group Work and Self-Help Groups

Both self-help groups and group therapy have worked well for homosexual men. They have provided much needed support for those who have been infected with HIV and for changing high-risk behaviour for those who find it difficult to initiate and maintain safe sexual practices (Friedman et al., 1987; Kelly & St. Lawrence, 1988; Kelly et al., 1989; Kelly & Murphy, 1991). The willingness to participate in such groups has probably been made possible by the strong sense of community and heightened political awareness found in contemporary Western gay culture that has developed as a result of the liberation movements during the 1970s (Friedman et al., 1987). In general, injecting drug users lack any such sense of community and usually dislike participating in groups when in treatment (Magura et al., 1989b; 1991). At the time of writing, evidence from studies of group interventions among drug users have been found to be better than merely providing information alone, but the benefits have mainly been reflected in increased awareness about AIDS, changes in attitudes, and the acquisition of a variety of personal skills, rather than any definitive change in risk behaviours (see Sorensen, 1991; Magura et al., 1991).

One group intervention for reducing HIV risk-taking behaviour among methadone patients has been described by Magura et al. (1989b). According to the authors, self-help groups work effectively by increasing self-esteem through helping others; by encouraging individuals to protect their newly acquired self-esteem by adopting positive behaviour changes; by providing positive peer role models; by providing mutual reinforcement for positive behaviour changes; and by sharing information and skills that contribute to behaviour change.

Participants in the research project were paid to attend four group sessions conducted by group leaders who were not part of the staff of the participating methadone programs. The content of each of the four sessions was determined loosely by the group leader with a session each devoted to: an introductory discussion of group processes followed by AIDS education; injecting and needle sharing; sexual behaviour; and assessing what change had taken place followed by the possibility of the participants continuing the group. Most of the participants reported that their sole reason for attending the group was because of the payment involved. The money seemed to function as a face-saving reason for participating in the group which might be seen by other program patients and group members as a matter for scorn. The authors speculated that the well known reluctance of methadone patients for initially attending groups might be overcome by providing incentives for attendance such as take-home methadone. After attending a group for a while, the authors argue that the bonds that develop in the group and the capacity for self-revelation would function autonomously as a reward for attending. Without any other evidence to back up these conclusions, the study must remain suggestive at best. Clearly, if some way of encouraging group attendance were found, it might be a useful component of AIDS risk reduction and methadone treatment in general.

Specific Interventions

Baker, Heather, and Wodak (1991) describe a cognitive-behavioural intervention for reducing injecting and/or needle sharing and high risk sexual behaviour. The treatment developed for the purposes of research consists of six counselling sessions. Areas covered are: motivational interviewing (discussed below); the identification of high-risk situations and development of problem solving techniques; how to cope with craving using relaxation training and positive self-talk; the role of a series of mini-decisions in relapse and the way high-risk behaviours function as rewards; how to deal with relapse if it occurs; and a session in which the treatment is reviewed. Similar cognitive-behavioural interventions have been shown to be effective in reducing HIV risk behaviour among gay men and runaway adolescents but has yet to be shown to be effective among injecting drug users (Kelly & Murphy, 1991).

Baker and Dixon (1991) describe an intervention based on motivational interviewing techniques. Motivational interviewing necessitates a good working relationship in which the client trusts the counsellor and feels that he or she is concerned and wants to understand and be of help. A session of motivational interviewing tries to achieve three things: to assist the client to talk about his or her risk behaviours and their ambivalence about them; for the client to come to the point where he or she expresses concern about the risks being taken, that is, personalises the risk for HIV infection; and for the client to express a wish to change these behaviours.

As the two interventions above show — and what has been shown among gay men — is that in the absence of proven interventions that are acceptable to large numbers of injecting drug users, counsellors would be best recommended to use interventions that have been found to work in other areas. This could be done on the basis of what has been discovered by research concerning the dynamics of HIV risk-taking behaviour (see Chapter 4). For example, peer pressure as a contributing factor to both needle sharing and unsafe sex could be dealt with by assertiveness training. More recent research has shown that initiating behaviour change is only one dimension of the problem of eradicating risk behaviours, because significant proportions of injecting drug users who have made positive changes to their behaviour report episodes of relapse (Des Jarlais et al., 1991). Des Jarlais et al. (1991) suggest that more attention needs to be paid to the processes involved in maintaining behaviour change.

Needle Exchanges and Methadone Units

One final possible way in which methadone programs might contribute to reducing the risk for their patients is in the provision of sterile needles and syringes. Needle exchanges have been demonstrated to reduce the incidence of needle sharing among injecting drug users without increasing the likelihood of more people becoming injectors or the amount of drug use in the local area increasing (see Friedman & Des Jarlais, 1991). Wolk et al., (1990b) retrospectively studied the effect of a needle exchange being adjacent to a methadone unit. Using another unit as a comparison, they found that the presence of the needle exchange did not lead to an increase in drug use in the nearby methadone unit, a fear that had been held by staff at the time. Acknowledging that not all methadone patients will remain abstinent, and that some patients will take time to eliminate their drug use altogether, means that these patients remain at risk for sharing needles. Providing needles and syringes for these patients may be a realistic way in which to reduce their risk while they continue to inject. Letting patients know that if they are going to inject that they should do so safely may not only reduce this risk but also contribute to a less hostile and suspicious therapeutic relationship. The criticism that making sterile injecting equipment available to patients will give them mixed messages is misplaced and based on a naive understanding of the role of treatment for injecting drug users.

HIV AND METHADONE MAINTENANCE: CLINICAL ISSUES

As we have noted a number of times, the advent of epidemic HIV among injecting drug users has had a major impact on the goals of treatment for injecting drug use. As Brown and Beschner (1989) have succinctly remarked about the situation in the USA: 'The goal of an abstinent life is being overtaken with a concern with preserving life itself' (p. 144). Along with this, issues that have not been important previously in the clinical management of methadone patients have now become a part of the day-to-day activities of methadone units. Two of these issues are HIV testing and the management of HIV positive patients and patients with AIDS.

HIV Testing in Methadone Programs

A request to be tested for the presence of HIV antibodies is a good opportunity to counsel methadone patients about risk reduction. Testing for HIV has been shown to be effective in reducing HIV risk behaviour for some individuals (Higgins et al., 1990 cited in Friedman & Des Jarlais, 1991), and is thought to be an important component in more comprehensive risk reduction interventions among injecting drug users (Magura et al., 1991; Martin et al., 1990; Nicolosi et al., 1991). However, it is just as important to make sure that if HIV testing is carried out from a methadone unit, it is done with care and compassion.

Mersky (1989; see also World Health Organization, 1990) provides a good summary of the issues related to testing for HIV in drug treatment programs and, unless otherwise indicated, the following is based on the discussion and case presentations summarised there. All patients who enter methadone treatment should be counselled about their previous risk-taking behaviour and the possibility of being tested for HIV. Testing should be voluntary and a decision not to be tested should not have any consequences for treatment. Thought should be given to whether testing should be delayed until the patient is stabilised on methadone to avoid relapse and premature dropping out of treatment in response to positive test results which understandably usually cause acute emotional distress.

A drug treatment program that arranges for HIV testing on site should ensure that program staff are educated about HIV and AIDS and trained to provide pre- and post-test counselling (Howell & Niven, 1989). A patient who decides to be tested will need to be counselled both before the test and at the time he or she is informed of the results. The informed consent of the patient should be given. This means that the patient should understand the benefits of being tested, the meaning of the test results, the extent of the confidentiality of being tested and the results of the test, and that they have the right to decide not to be tested. Confidentiality of test results should be ensured and steps taken to eliminate them becoming known by accident (e.g. through the use of stickers on urine sample containers indicating that infection control procedures are necessary). In terms of the meaning of the test results, the meaning positive, negative and indeterminate test results should be explained. The delay between time of infection and presence of detectable antibodies to HIV should also be explained. Pre-test counselling should also include discussion of what different outcomes to the test would mean to the patient. Risk for suicide and relapse to drug use should be assessed in case the result is positive.

Post-test counselling includes informing the patient of his or her test results. If the patient's result is negative, the implications of the result should be explained. Discussion of possible retesting and the importance of continued safe sex and injecting should take place. As already stated, pre- and post-counselling are good opportunities to reinforce and encourage further risk reduction.

If the patient's results are positive more care should be taken. The meaning of the results should be explained, providing details about HIV and its relationship to AIDS. The possibility of telling previous sexual and needle sharing partners should also be addressed. Referral to appropriate medical services and a support group, if available, should be considered.

Understandably most people experience severe emotional

distress on being told of a positive test result. They do not differ in this regard from people who are told they are suffering from other life threatening illnesses (Kelly & St. Lawrence, 1988). Patients' partners, friends and family may also be distressed. The patient should be told that their distress reaction is usual for someone in their situation. Some patients find it difficult to absorb any other information due to shock. In such cases, the counsellor should avoid going into lengthy explanations and instead try to encourage the client to ask questions as a means of bringing them back into the immediate relationship. Some patients may experience a delayed distress reaction after they leave the unit, so a suggestion that they return or telephone if they feel the need may be appropriate. Reactions to a positive test result may continue and usually include symptoms like anxiety, anger, depression, somatization and denial. Follow-up counselling should include interventions to deal with the reactions of the client as they arise, e.g. ongoing anxiety can be dealt with using the usual techniques of relaxation and stress management training (Kelly & St. Lawrence, 1988). Stress prevention training, for example, has been shown to be helpful among a group of individuals after they had been informed of a positive HIV test result (Perry et al., 1991).

Although there is some evidence that homosexual men reduce their risk-taking behaviour in response to an HIV positive test result (Kelly & St. Lawrence, 1988), there is some American evidence that this may not be the case for some seropositive methadone patients (Abdul-Quader et al., 1987; Magura et al., 1990). One important aspect of post-test counselling for seropositive patients, therefore, is the need to discuss risk-taking behaviour, including sharing injection equipment, sexual relationships and pregnancy.

HIV Positive Patients and Patients with AIDS

In terms of the day-to-day functioning of a methadone unit, HIV positive patients and patients with AIDS should not be treated any differently from other methadone patients. However, it should be recognised that these patients experience many problems that other patients do not. The reactions mentioned above concerning notification of positive test results tend to remain a problem for these patients. HIV positive patients who are just beginning to experience symptoms of HIV-related illnesses have been observed to experience the most distress of this group due to the uncertainty of their situation — no longer being well and still not having been diagnosed as having AIDS (Kelly & St. Lawrence, 1988).

Other psychological problems may complicate treatment (Batki et al., 1988). Anger may be focused at unit staff directly or indirectly through refusing to comply with program rules and the limits set by staff about things such as drug use. Depression, which is not uncommon among injecting drug users, may become a serious problem. This may be compounded by a sense of isolation that results from the stigma associated with HIV and AIDS. Often these patients may feel ostracised by both the society at large and the drug subculture, feelings that are often in accord with reality. These problems, and the fact of illness itself in the case of AIDS, often means that patients have very little reason to abandon their drug use.

There are serious consequences to expelling a seropositive patient or patient with AIDS from treatment. AIDS patients who inject are at risk for injection-related infections caused by lack of care in cleaning equipment and the skin around injection sites; they may also lose the daily contact with the health care system that they have in attending a methadone unit (Sorensen et al., 1989a). There may be beneficial aspects specifically associated with methadone treatment for this group, e.g. injecting heroin use has been found to be associated with immunological abnormalities that clear up after a period of successful methadone maintenance treatment. Novick et al. (1989) argue that methadone maintenance may even delay the progression of HIV to AIDS, an argument that is supported by some studies (e.g. Weber, et al., 1990). The effects of methadone and other opioids on the immunological functioning of HIV-positive drug users and drug users with AIDS is just beginning to be researched. More studies are needed before this issue is clearly understood (Sobel, 1991). However, it should be kept in mind that such people are far better off in a methadone program where they are receiving medical care than they would be otherwise. The risks associated with injecting, with the use of impure 'street' drugs, and the associated legal, financial and social stresses far outweigh any immunosuppression that may be associated with the use of oral methadone, something which has yet to be demonstrated. Releasing such patients from a treatment known to reduce injecting and needle sharing also has serious public health consequences. It may be necessary, for all these reasons, to be more flexible with this group of patients concerning continued illicit drug use.

HIV and Methadone Clinic Staff

It is also important to note that staff who treat the growing numbers of people infected with HIV are known to experience considerable levels of stress (Kelly & St. Lawrence, 1988). Methadone programs are no different in this regard. Experience in the USA suggests that methadone program staff often experience difficulties in dealing with this group of patients who are even more demanding than the usual patients seen in methadone clinics. A related difficulty is that some staff have difficulty accepting the change away from an abstinence orientation to a harm reduction model of treatment. Implicit in this acceptance is a recognition of the limitations of the effectiveness of drug treatment in general, which some staff find disheartening (Sorensen, 1989b).

Issues of death and bereavement increase these stresses and are not unlike those experienced by staff dealing with other terminally ill populations (Kelly & St. Lawrence, 1988; Sorensen et al., 1989a; 1989b). Programs to assist staff and procedures within clinics to deal with these issues need to be developed to help staff come to terms with these issues and to prevent burn-out. Education programs may help staff to adjust to the changing nature of methadone treatment (move to harm reduction) and ways in which to deal with the problems associated with dealing with difficult patient populations and terminal illness could be adapted from materials developed for health care workers who deal with comparable populations.

SUMMARY

The advent of a HIV epidemic among injecting drug users and the adoption of drug treatment policies which are primarily focused on the reduction of the harm associated with drug use has brought about a number of changes in the practices of drug treatment agencies. Stimson (1990) has identified five such changes: (a) the problem being addressed is seen as the drug use behaviours rather than the person using the drugs; (b) the drug user is seen as rational rather than irrational and therefore capable of health conscious drug use; (c) the focus of treatment is no longer on drug dependence but on the reduction of the harm associated with certain drug use practices; (d) the relationship tends to be more cooperative and user friendly than confrontational; (e) drug treatment workers need to be multi-skilled because they have to deal with new issues like HIV infection and sexuality.

Methadone maintenance is essentially a harm reduction intervention for opioid dependence in that it involves a change in the route of administration from injecting heroin to orally ingesting methadone. However, over the past three decades, methadone treatment has been subjected to a variety of regulations and controls as a way of placating critics of drug substitution therapy. For this reason, and because heroin use is both a medical and criminal matter, an ethos has developed within methadone clinics that results in a confusing mix of treatment and control. The contradiction between control and treatment is inherent in the role of methadone unit staff who are involved in counselling patients. On the one hand they are expected to develop relationships based on trust, and on the other they are expected to enforce program rules concerning illicit drug use. In order to engage patients in effective HIV risk reduction counselling, it is necessary to create the conditions under which patients will feel free to talk about their drug use without fear of punishment.

Counselling patients about their sexual behaviour is not part of the traditional work of drug counsellors and may present some problems for counsellors who do not feel comfortable with this new aspect of their role. The dissemination of educational materials about HIV is an important function of methadone programs. These materials should be to the point and appropriate for the target population. Possible risk reduction interventions for methadone patients are group work, cognitive-behavioural programs and motivational interviewing. Using proven techniques adapted for the specific problems associated with HIV risk-taking behaviour and HIV infection is appropriate at this point in time. Providing information about needle exchanges or providing injecting equipment is another role that methadone units may play in reducing their patients' risk of contracting or transmitting HIV.

Testing patients for HIV infection has become common in methadone clinics. A necessary part of HIV testing is pre- and post-test counselling. The purpose of pre- and post-test counselling is to help the patient understand and cope with what might be a very traumatic experience. It is also an opportunity for risk reduction counselling. The management of HIV positive patients and patients with AIDS requires an understanding of their situation and the problems associated with it. Managing these patients can be stressful for unit staff — stresses which are not unlike those experienced by others who work with the terminally ill.

12

METHADONE MAINTENANCE DURING PREGNANCY

INTRODUCTION

s heroin dependence became increasingly more widespread during the 1960s, it was inevitable that pregnant women in this predicament would present for care. At first, neither drug treatment clinics nor maternity wards knew how to deal with the serious complications that arose in these women and their infants (Suffet & Brotman, 1984). For example, in the early 1970s, the Food and Drug Administration in the USA recommended 21-day methadone detoxification programs as the treatment of choice for the pregnant addict. However, when reports started appearing in the literature of an association between withdrawal and stillbirth, as well as a range of other complications, this recommendation was dropped (Chavkin, 1990). Since then, the treatment of choice for the opioid-dependent pregnant woman has been methadone maintenance (MM) throughout pregnancy (Finnegan, 1983; 1991).

In this chapter we examine the rationale and evidence for the use of methadone maintenance as a treatment for opioid-dependent pregnant women and provide an overview of the clinical issues involved in caring for these women and their potential offspring.

Important clinical issues in methadone maintenance for this population include: an appropriate methadone dose; specialised antenatal care; the role of counselling in treatment; the human immunodeficiency virus (HIV); viral hepatitis infections; and the management of birth and the abstinence syndrome in the neonate. The focus of this review is restricted to the care of pregnant women in methadone maintenance programs and the immediate impact that methadone maintenance has on their newborn children. Previous reviews in this area have been relied upon (e.g. Finnegan, 1983; Householder et al., 1982) because of the extent and variety of material that is relevant to this topic. Finnegan (1980; 1991), a recognised authority in this field, has provided comprehensive accounts of the clinical issues. We would refer the interested reader to her work for detail concerning obstetrics and medical care that are beyond the scope of the topic as discussed here.

RATIONALE AND EVIDENCE FOR THE USE OF METHADONE MAINTENANCE DURING PREGNANCY

The Opioid-Dependent Pregnant Woman

A woman dependent on illicit opioids must be considered medically to be in a high-risk category when she is pregnant. Such a woman is at risk for the usual health-related problems found among injecting drug users (e.g. hepatitis, HIV infection, endocarditis etc.) as well as anaemia, cystitis and a variety of problems specifically related to pregnancy, including premature labour and abruption of the placenta which may result in the death of both woman and foetus (see Finnegan, 1983; 1991, for more details). During pregnancy, these women often do not have the benefit of the three important conditions for a healthy pregnancy: adequate rest, nutrition and antenatal care (Finnegan, 1988). As well as being at risk medically, opioid-dependent pregnant women also suffer from a range of other problems (Finnegan, Hagan & Kaltenbach, 1991; Waldby, 1988). These include various psychological (low self-esteem, depression, anxiety states) and social problems (poverty, homelessness, legal crises, domestic violence). Many of these women have lost children to child welfare agencies in the past and, as a consequence, feel reluctant to contact health care agencies and remain suspicious when they do. They are well aware that they belong to one of the most highly stigmatised groups of women in society (Jessup, 1990; Waldby, 1988).

It is not surprising that the foetus of a drug-dependent woman does not always fare well in its deprived environment. Besides the impediment of lack of adequate nutrition, rest and antenatal care, the foetus has to contend with problems created by the cycle of withdrawal and intoxication associated with the mother's dependent opioid use. Intoxication and withdrawal both place stress upon the foetus. Opioid withdrawal during pregnancy is dangerous and has been associated with foetal death; this is especially the case if the woman is experiencing withdrawal while she is in labour (Finnegan, 1983). According to Hoegerman et al. (1990), of even greater concern is the uncertainty about adulterants with which illicit drugs may have been cut in moving down the distribution network. Some of the contaminants found in black market heroin may be teratogenic. (A substance is said to be teratogenic when exposure may cause morphological changes in the developing foetus.) Opioids themselves have no known teratogenic effects on the human foetus (Finnegan, 1983).

Many women also present late in pregnancy, because they often misinterpret any signs or symptoms they may have. Menstrual problems, especially amenorrhoea, are common among heroin-dependent women (Finnegan, 1980). After entering methadone maintenance, menstruation usually returns to normal within six to 12 months. This observation leads to the conclusion that it is aspects associated with the illicit drug using lifestyle that are responsible for a high incidence of menstrual problems among these women. The concomitant nutritional deficiencies, infections (e.g. hepatitis, pelvic infections) and psychosocial stresses of illicit drug use are thought to contribute to this phenomenon. The high incidence of menstrual abnormalities among these women has given rise to one of the perennial mythologies of the heroin subculture — that a woman is unlikely to become pregnant while she is using heroin (Waldby, 1988). This mythology, in turn, is in part responsible for a neglect of contraception as a safeguard against unwanted pregnancy. When heroin-using women do become pregnant they are not expecting it and often mistake the early signs and symptoms (nausea, headaches, fatigue, etc.) for withdrawal symptoms or the effects of dirty drugs (i.e. harmful contaminants). This means that they often do not become aware that they are pregnant, and do not present for treatment, until relatively late.

Methadone Maintenance in Pregnancy: The Rationale

The rationale for the use of methadone maintenance for pregnant women who are opioid dependent has two main components (Mackie-Ramos & Rice, 1988): methadone replaces illicit opioids of uncertain composition and dose with a pure substitute at a stable dose; and enrolment in a methadone maintenance program allows the woman to receive the antenatal care and advice necessary for a successful pregnancy. Detoxification from all drugs is unrealistic for most of this population and often results in the mother experiencing an abstinence syndrome leading to foetal distress, which is more harmful than a medically supervised methadone dependence (Finnegan, 1991). Pregnant women who are maintained on methadone have no need to engage in drug-related crime or prostitution, usually improve their nutritional intake, reduce their risk for HIV infection, are more willing to attend for antenatal care, and can spend more time preparing for birth and becoming a parent because they are relieved of the burden of drug seeking.

Methadone Maintenance in Pregnancy: The Evidence

Research evidence has consistently shown that methadone maintenance is superior on a number of outcome measures to not being in treatment for this population. As well as a reduction in drug use and crime, methadone maintenance retains patients in treatment, providing them with sufficient antenatal care to achieve as successful a birth as possible given the circumstances. The gains to be expected are comparative: a better outcome is expected on these measures than if these women remained heroin dependent and received little or no antenatal care. When assessed in this way, methadone maintenance for pregnant women, when delivered properly, is a highly successful intervention.

Most of the problems experienced by infants born to opioid-dependent mothers are due to premature birth and being small for gestational age (Ellwood et al., 1987; Finnegan, 1983; 1991). The evidence to date clearly and consistently shows that infants born to methadone-maintained mothers are born later and are larger for gestational age than those born to opioid-dependent women not in treatment (Finnegan, 1980; Giles et al., 1989; Householder et al., 1982). Pregnant women in methadone maintenance programs attend for more antenatal care than do women out of treatment (Finnegan, 1983; Giles et al., 1989) and both this and the improved outcomes mentioned above are related to time spent in methadone maintenance (Doberczak et al., 1987; Ellwood et al., 1987; Suffet & Brotman, 1984). The amount of antenatal care received is an important predictor of outcome for both mother and foetus (Suffet & Brotman, 1984; Wilson, 1989).

Although some of the problems experienced by infants born to opioid-dependent mothers are drug-related (e.g. neonatal abstinence syndrome), most of the morbidity and mortality for these newborns is due to the harm associated with the heroin-using lifestyle. The specific effects of opioids such as heroin on the neonate are difficult to specify due to insurmountable methodological problems in carrying out research in this area. The effects of heroin are confounded by the harm associated with the lifestyle (intoxication–withdrawal cycle, drug contaminants, infections, poverty, etc.), the difficulty in specifying and quantifying drugs taken, and the influence of inadequate care (Deren, 1986; Hoegerman et al., 1990; Householder et al., 1982; Kaltenbach & Finnegan, 1989; Kreek, 1983b). For example, the almost universal incidence of cigarette smoking in this population must have some influence on birth weight (Doberczak et al., 1987; Ellwood et al., 1987; Giles et al., 1989). According to Wilson (1989), studies on the subsequent intellectual development of infants exposed to heroin *in utero* suggest that inadequate antenatal care is common for children who turn out to be severely impaired. There have been no demonstrated long-term disadvantages for infants born to methadone-maintained women when lifestyle factors are taken into account (e.g. Lifschitz et al., 1985).

In any discussion of the efficacy of methadone maintenance for pregnant women, it has to be kept in mind that it is not so long ago that infants born to heroin-dependent mothers had little chance of survival (Finnegan, 1988). The dramatic increase in survival and reduction in morbidity in this group is due to developments that have taken place in the capacity to successfully care for high-risk neonates. These developments and the use of methadone maintenance in combination with good antenatal care means that many of these women will give birth to infants at term. For example, Finnegan (1988) reports that of 196 recent admissions to her program 72% of women gave birth to infants at term, 12% were born prematurely, 8% suffered medical complications, and 8% died *in utero*.

CLINICAL ISSUES I: THE ANTENATAL PERIOD

Methadone Dose and Pregnancy

The ideal use of methadone for the heroin-dependent pregnant woman would be to stabilise her on a low dose of methadone (<40 mg) early in her pregnancy, to slowly reduce the methadone dose (5 mg per fortnight) between the 14th and 32nd weeks, and for mother and infant to be drug-free at birth (Finnegan, 1980, 1991; 1983; Gerada et al., 1990). Withdrawal is best carried out during this period because it may induce abortion before the 14th week and premature labour or withdrawal-induced foetal stress after the 32nd week. Patients who insist on detoxification or who have been maintained on very high doses of methadone (>80 mg) should be allowed to attempt full or partial detoxification. However, it has to be acknowledged that full detoxification is an unrealistic option for most heroin-dependent women and that pregnancy does not significantly alter this. Most women on a methadone withdrawal regimen like the one described above would quickly relapse to heroin use, which is far more dangerous than maintenance with methadone under medical supervision (Finnegan, 1980). Finnegan (1991), who has extensive experience with this population, reports a 100% failure to achieve abstinence in her program in Philadelphia, either because patients were unable to bear the diminishing doses of methadone, or could not proceed due to the likely onset of premature labour. Tranquillisers, like diazepam, are contraindicated for the relief of withdrawal symptoms for pregnant women undergoing detoxification because of possible negative effects on the foetus. If a patient is unable to continue with withdrawal, then her methadone dose should be readjusted upwards in slow increments until she reaches a level she feels comfortable with.

Methadone Dose and Neonatal Withdrawal

If withdrawal is not possible, then the next most desirable option, according to some authors, is maintenance on as low a dose of methadone as possible (Batey et al., 1990; Gerada et al., 1990; Suffet & Brotman, 1984). There are two reasons for this recommendation: the lowest dose of methadone will have the least negative effects upon the foetus; and the lower the dose of methadone, the less withdrawal distress will be experienced by the newborn infant. However, neither of these two reasons bear a simple relationship to the research evidence. For example, in the case of the effect of high doses of methadone on the foetus, Doberczak et al. (1987) found that higher doses of methadone were associated with greater increases in maternal weight during pregnancy. As Kreek (1983b) has pointed out, it is not clear from the evidence available what the effects of different methadone dosage regimens are on the developing foetus and the evidence will not be clear until studies are done on women who do not use alcohol, nicotine or other drugs during their pregnancy. Further, the risks associated with relapse to heroin use or substitution with other drugs such as benzodiazepines, which might complicate withdrawal in the neonate, have to be considered. When factors like these are taken into account, it would seem advisable to adopt the principle of providing sufficient methadone to meet the needs of the patient, based on the more general principle that what is good for the mother is generally good for the foetus. Finnegan (1991) points out that it is counter-productive to treat mother and foetus as if they were 'separate and competing entities'. In any case, as yet there is no evidence to suggest that either pregnancy or outcome for the neonate is related in any way to methadone dose with doses up to 100 mg daily (Finnegan, 1980, 1991; Thakur et al., 1990).

Although some studies have found an association between maternal methadone dose and severity of neonatal withdrawal (e.g. Collins, 1990; 1992; Suffet & Brotman, 1984), this relationship has not been consistently observed (Mack et al., 1991; Finnegan, 1991). When considering matters related to the neonatal abstinence syndrome, it has to be kept in mind that this syndrome in an infant born to a methadone-maintained woman is a relatively benign and treatable manifestation in comparison to the complications that may arise in a heroin-dependent or poly-drug abusing woman who has received insufficient antenatal care (Finnegan cited in Gastel & Collins, 1983). It would seem inadvisable to restrict methadone dose below a certain level in order to avoid a withdrawal syndrome in the neonate, although this may be used as an incentive to encourage women to keep their doses as low as possible.

Assessment and Initial Methadone Dose

Under no circumstances should a pregnant woman be administered naloxone to diagnose opioid dependence because of the hazards involved for both woman and foetus (Finnegan, 1991). Assessment should be based on the taking of a careful history and physical examination (as detailed in Chapter 5). Finnegan (1991) recommends the following procedure for commencing methadone maintenance in a hospital setting. As soon as the beginning of withdrawal is apparent, 10 mg of methadone is administered, followed by 5 mg every four to six hours until the symptoms are alleviated. The next day, the previous day's totalled dose is administered and again supplemented as needed. Most patients can be adequately stabilised on 20 to 35 mg, though increases may be necessary after discharge from hospital. An adequate maintenance dose will depend on length of dependence, how long the patient has been on methadone maintenance, and the concurrent prescription of other drugs known to enhance the metabolism of methadone (e.g. phenytoin — see Chapter 6 for a discussion of this phenomenon). Dose should be increased in small increments if there is relapse to heroin use, ongoing illicit drug use or indications of increased methadone metabolism in the third trimester.

It should be emphasised that no matter what course is chosen for methadone maintenance for a pregnant woman, dose adjustments should be made with care. As already noted, the effects of opioids on the woman will also affect the foetus and both withdrawal and intoxication may lead to serious complications. For these reasons, initial stabilisation on methadone has often taken place during a short period of hospitalisation so that the patient can be closely observed and have her medical condition assessed (e.g. Ellwood et al., 1987; Finnegan, 1991), especially if she has presented late in her pregnancy (Gerada et al., 1990). However, successful programs are possible on an outpatient basis (Giles et al., 1989; Batey et al., 1990). When a woman is inducted as an outpatient, Batey et al. (1990) recommend an initial methadone dose of 20 to 40 mg (depending upon assessment) because rapid stabilisation is necessary to promptly halt illicit opioid use. Patients on this intake regimen are then closely monitored on a daily basis to ensure a quick response to either intoxication or withdrawal.

Methadone Metabolism in the Pregnant Woman

Pregnancy is one of a number of factors known to influence the effects of methadone in human beings (Finnegan, 1983; Kreek, 1983a, 1983b; Pond et al., 1985) (see Chapter 6 for a discussion of other factors). Pond et al. (1985) in a study of nine pregnant women found that for all the subjects the concentration of methadone in plasma at its lowest point during the 24-hour dosing cycle (trough plasma level) was lower when adjusted for dose than what it was when measured post-partum. Three of these women began to experience withdrawal symptoms towards the end of their pregnancies and these symptoms were associated with significant differences in trough plasma levels pre- and post-partum. These differences in methadone plasma levels were greater than could be expected when changes in dose and increases in body weight and fluid were taken into account.

The authors hypothesised that towards the end of pregnancy the foetus begins to metabolise methadone and that this accounts for the unexpected drop in plasma levels, although this has yet to be demonstrated (see Finnegan, 1983). The observation of decreased plasma levels and unexpected withdrawal symptoms in some women during the third trimester is a consistent one (Finnegan, 1983 Kreek, 1983a, 1983b). This phenomenon is arguably responsible, in part, for the high level of relapse observed during the third trimester. Fifty per cent of the participants in Waldby's study (1988) relapsed at this time, although she suggests that anxiety about approaching birth and parenthood is also an important factor.

Two solutions have been proposed for the woman who begins to experience withdrawal in the third trimester: split-dosing and an increase in dose. Split-dosing has been recommended as a way in which to maintain plasma levels at a more steady level and has been found to be satisfactory in achieving this goal (Hoegerman et al., 1990; Pond et al., 1985; Sutton & Hinderliter, 1990; Wittman & Segal, 1991). Wittman & Segal (1991), in a study of seven women whose methadone dose was inadequate during the third trimester, found through the use of ultrasound that the foetus in such cases becomes agitated by the end of the usual 24-hour dosing cycle and shows restricted movement after the woman has been dosed. They found that split-dosing reduced these fluctuations in foetal movement. If split-dosing were to be considered seriously as an option, then allowing these women to take at least one of their doses home with them would also have to be taken into consideration. Increasing the methadone dose is another solution (Pond et al., 1985). As mentioned above, although the ideal would seem to be reducing the dose of methadone to as low as possible, the risk of relapse to illicit drug use and its associated risks for the woman and foetus have to be taken into account when considering this issue.

Groups for Methadone-Maintained Pregnant Women

Although attendance at general or specific purpose groups (educational, psychotherapeutic, etc.) is usually low or non-existent among the general methadone maintenance patient population, in the case of pregnant women they are desirable and, under the right circumstances, reasonably well attended (Batey et al., 1990; Finnegan, 1991; Finnegan et al., 1991; Holmes, 1989; Mackie-Ramos & Rice, 1988). Mackie-Ramos and Rice (1988) point out that these women have two things in common: they are drug dependent and they are pregnant. Attending a group allows them to discuss their problems and become informed about pregnancy, birth and parenting with women who share their own experience. Attendance at groups may remain quite low, however, if no incentive is given. At a specialist Drugs in Pregnancy Service at a Sydney hospital, the provision of incentives and clever scheduling has been successful in encouraging attendance. An effective formula has been to schedule the group between morning dosing time and an afternoon antenatal clinic held for patients, and to provide lunch and child care while the group is meeting (J. Holmes, pers. comm., 15 October 1991).

As well as offering antenatal education and parenting skills training, groups for drug-dependent women also need to address specific issues pertinent to their situation. Anxieties about the effect of past drug use, methadone and past and current infections (e.g.

hepatitis) upon their future child are very common. Batey et al. (1990) suggest that many of these women may have a range of unresolved psychological problems arising out family experiences and at the hands of the legal and welfare systems. Other current psychological problems (e.g. anxiety and depression) are also likely. In this sense, then, groups for these women may need to be more like group therapy sessions than the usual antenatal classes. This does not preclude or replace the need for individual counselling where necessary.

Finnegan et al. (1991) do not recommend mixed sex groups. Many drug-dependent women have been sexually or physically abused at some time in their lives and will not feel free to communicate in the presence of males. In a group restricted to women, group members are able to express themselves freely without fearing male censure. The issue of group composition is a specific component of the more general issue of whether male partners should be treated in the same methadone maintenance program. Finnegan (1991) and Batey et al. (1990) recommend that partners be enrolled in the same program. Finnegan prefers a family-oriented treatment approach, while Batey et al. suggest that having the partner in the same methadone maintenance reduces conflict. Conflict with regard to access to methadone maintenance does appear to be a serious problem for these couples. Waldby (1988) documents several case histories where the basis of a couple's relationship (drug-dependent lifestyle) was threatened by the woman's entry to methadone maintenance. It is common for pregnant women to have priority access to methadone maintenance in many places throughout the world. This quick access to treatment often leaves the couple in a situation in which the woman is trying to abstain from illicit drug use yet her partner cannot find a program that will accept him. A family-oriented treatment approach obviates this difficulty by treating both the woman and her partner.

The issue of involving partners in treatment in specialist programs for pregnant women, however, does not meet with consensus from workers in the field. The high incidence of domestic violence in this population has led some workers to see the need for the methadone maintenance unit to function as a safe place for women, a role that may at times be difficult to fulfil if the unit is also dispensing to the partner concerned (J. Holmes, pers. comm., 15 October, 1991).

Antenatal Care

Two of the reasons why drug-dependent women do not seek out

antenatal care is that they fear a negative reaction from clinic staff and that their child might be taken from them (Gerada et al., 1990). It is important, therefore, that such women receive non-judgemental antenatal care (Finnegan, 1980). It must be remembered in this regard that health care workers ignorant of the research concerning the positive role of methadone in the management of opioid dependence may regard methadone as no different from heroin. For these reasons, the ideal situation is where an methadone maintenance unit specialising in the care of pregnant women works with an antenatal care unit. It has been found in the past that women in methadone maintenance attend more often for antenatal visits than heroin-dependent women out of treatment, but that they still do not attend as regularly as women who are not drug dependent. Giles et al. (1989) have suggested scheduling more frequent visits for drug-dependent women, both in and out of methadone maintenance treatment, as a way of making up for low attendance rates. The importance of this aspect of care cannot be overemphasised given the consistent observation that amount of antenatal care is associated with fewer complications and a number of measures of positive outcome.

CLINICAL ISSUES II: HIV, VIRAL HEPATITIS AND PREGNANCY

HIV

PERINATAL TRANSMISSION

It is now clear that a woman infected with HIV can perinatally transmit the infection to her infant (e.g. Brown et al., 1989b; Thornton et al., 1990). It is thought that perinatal transmission may take place by one of three routes: by infection *in utero*; by exposure to blood and other cervical secretions at birth; and through breast milk (Peckham & Newell, 1990). If the mother is infected, current knowledge suggests that perinatal transmission will take place in between 20% to 40% of cases (World Health Organization, 1990). The type of delivery does not seem to affect the rate of transmission (Chadwick, 1988; Peckham & Newell, 1990). Determining whether transmission has taken place is difficult because of the presence of maternal HIV-antibodies in the infant's blood after birth. All such infants will, therefore, be positive in HIV serological tests until they are between nine and 18 months of age. Infected children may begin to show signs of HIV-related disease during that period (World Health Organization, 1990). Most infected infants begin to show signs of such disease before two years of age (Chadwick, 1988; Peckham & Newell, 1990).

THE CONSEQUENCES OF PERINATAL TRANSMISSION

The World Health Organization estimates that worldwide there have been 0.5 million cases of AIDS in children (National Centre in HIV Epidemiology and Clinical Research, 1991). However, with nine to 11 million people estimated to be infected with HIV around the world, this figure is expected to increase. The potential extent of this problem is exemplified in the experience in the USA (Hoegerman et al., 1990 summarises this literature). In the USA, perinatal transmission accounts for nearly all cases of HIV infection in children and most HIV-positive women are either injecting drug users or partners of injecting drug users.

THE EFFECT OF PREGNANCY ON WOMEN WITH HIV INFECTION

On the basis of the first few studies done on pregnant women who were HIV positive it was concluded that pregnancy hastened the progression from being asymptomatic to showing more or less severe signs and symptoms of HIV-related disease. This, however, is no longer believed to be the case (Chadwick, 1988), but there is little evidence available, and the situation with regard to women who have already developed symptoms of HIV-related disease is unknown (Peckham & Newell, 1990). An example of one of the studies that has been done among drug-dependent women to date is a prospective study of 24 HIV positive, methadone-maintained women in New York, in which Selwyn et al. (1989a) observed that only one woman in the group progressed in her HIV-disease status during her pregnancy. The only difference between this group of women and a matched group of controls was that the HIV positive women were found to suffer more from infectious diseases not included among AIDS-defining infections while they were pregnant (mainly bacterial pneumonia). HIV positive women do not appear to suffer an unexpected level of birth complications as a result of their serostatus. Complications that are observed in this population appear to be related to injecting drug use during pregnancy (Peckham & Newell, 1990; Selwyn et al., 1989a).

Green (1989) has pointed out that when advising women who are HIV positive or who have AIDS about the risks that pregnancy might pose for them, the advice that anyone can give will only be as good as the scientific evidence available at the time. At the moment, this evidence suggests that for asymptomatic HIV positive women there is little risk of pregnancy contributing to progression in their status. However, as Green goes on to point out, it may still be the case that there are some women for whom pregnancy and giving birth will hasten the progression of their HIV-disease status. As yet we neither know if this is this case, and if it is, what the defining characteristics of these women might be.

HIV INFECTION AND TERMINATION

Green (1989) and the World Health Organization (1990) have outlined the issues involved in termination of pregnancy for HIV positive women and women with AIDS. Termination is in fact the only intervention that can be offered to a woman who finds herself in this situation, but it should not be automatically assumed that termination will be her choice. The various risks involved for her and her potential infant should be clearly explained. However, the choice remains hers and she should be supported in that choice (World Health Organization, 1990). The effect of termination on HIV-disease status is, at the time of writing, unknown (Green, 1989). The possibility of termination being an option may depend on the legal situation in the local jurisdiction, and the religious and cultural beliefs of the woman concerned (World Health Organization, 1990).

If termination is chosen, then the woman should receive both HIV and termination counselling (Green, 1989). As Green remarks, this brings together into one session two of the most difficult issues for both counsellor and client. One important issue that will have to be explained and dealt with is the need for infection control procedures at the termination. These procedures will be thought necessary by the staff performing the procedure and are likely to be a source of distress for the woman having the termination.

HIV POSITIVE PREGNANT WOMEN IN METHADONE MAINTENANCE PROGRAMS

Given that many drug-dependent women do not discover that they are pregnant until well into the second trimester, it is possible that for some HIV positive women termination may not be an option. Further, just as many infected women may not know they are pregnant, many women who are pregnant may not know they are infected (Campbell, 1990). For these reasons, HIV testing should be encouraged, although the ultimate decision to be tested or not remains the patient's. All women who are tested should receive both pre- and post-test counselling (see Chapter 11). Women who are HIV positive or who have AIDS should be treated no differently from other women in an methadone maintenance program, but it should be recognised that they may have special needs and concerns.

A pregnant woman who is HIV-infected has special counselling needs in addition to those of the drug-dependent pregnant woman and the HIV positive person (Green, 1989; World Health Organization, 1990). She will need to consider the prospect that her child might also be infected and that she might have to care for a child who is often ill. Education about HIV and its possible effects on the woman and her prospective infant is important (Peckham &

Newell, 1990). Anxiety about whether her child will be infected will probably continue for at least a year after birth, given the difficulty in determining HIV infection during this period. Whether her child is infected or not, she will also have to consider the future and who might be available to care for her child should she die herself. At the birth, the staff involved in the delivery will take a range of infection control precautions that should be explained to the woman and her concerns about this should be addressed. The discovery that perinatal transmission has taken place (due to the presence of HIV-related infection) is likely to have a devastating effect on the mother concerned, who will need a lot of support (Thornton et al., 1990). Finally, HIV discrimination (i.e. abuse of the rights of HIV-positive individuals and people with AIDS) has increasingly become a matter for concern and unfortunately health care workers have been involved in some of the more serious cases. Methadone unit staff can play an active role as advocates for HIV positive women and in educating other health care workers about the true risks involved in caring for this population so that they will be treated with the compassion they deserve.

HIV INFECTION AND BREASTFEEDING

Although the World Health Organization (1990) recommends breastfeeding by HIV positive women in countries where sanitary conditions create great risks for the bottle-fed child, in countries like Australia where such risks are low, breastfeeding by HIV positive women is not recommended (Finnegan, 1991; Gerada et al., 1990).

EQUIVOCAL HIV TEST RESULTS AMONG PREGNANT WOMEN

Pregnant women may return indeterminate results on some HIV-antibody tests. An indeterminate test result means that it is unclear whether the person has HIV antibodies in their blood or not. A small proportion of women (9/970) who test negative for HIV antibodies before pregnancy have been found to return indeterminate results during pregnancy which then revert to negative after the birth of the child (Collins & Capus, 1991). Such results may cause the woman concerned considerable anxiety and, where possible, further testing should be sought. Indeterminate results are not restricted to pregnant women and specific testing strategies have been developed to deal with such cases (see Celum et al., 1991; National HIV Reference Laboratory, 1991).

Viral Hepatitis

HEPATITIS B

The extent of infection with hepatitis B virus (HBV) among injecting drug users is extremely high both in Australia (e.g. Bell et al., 1990) and overseas, and this is also true of drug-injecting pregnant women (Mutchnick et al., 1991; Thornton et al., 1990). In the majority of individuals, infection with HBV results in a mild, acute illness of short duration. However, 5% to 10% of those infected will become chronically infected and these individuals are at high risk for liver disease (Millard, 1988; Mutchnick et al., 1991). For mothers who are suffering either chronic or acute infection at birth, in 15% to 70% of cases their infants will be infected. Most (85%) perinatally HBV-infected infants go on to become chronically infected and are at high risk for liver disease. It is thought that transmission takes place at birth rather than *in utero*, because very few neonates show signs of infection and will not yield positive test results indicating current active infection until two to four months of age. This window period allows for immunoprophylaxis (hepatitis B immunoglobulin and vaccine) which is extremely effective. Millard (1988) does not recommend breastfeeding by chronically HBV-infected women as it might interfere with immunoprophylaxis. Millard (1988) points out that this advice is sometimes not indicated for countries where sanitary conditions pose great risks for bottle-fed infants, as in the case, mentioned earlier, of HIV infection and breastfeeding.

HEPATITIS C

After tests recently became available for antibodies to the Hepatitis C virus (HCV) (previously known as non-A, non-B), it was discovered that this infection was as common as HBV among injecting drug users. Three different samples of methadone maintenance patients in Sydney have tested positive for HCV antibodies in 86% to 89% of cases (Bell et al., 1990c; Collins & Capus, 1991; Latt et al., 1992). Perinatal transmission has been observed (Mutchnick et al., 1991), but the rates of this mode of transmission and the risks involved in breastfeeding are unknown at present, as is the long-term outcome of infants infected with HCV (Millard, 1988).

The possible consequences of this high rate of infection with HCV among injecting drug users is a matter of concern given that current estimates suggest that 50% of individuals infected with hepatitis C via blood transfusion turn out to be chronically infected and that half of these will suffer cirrhosis (Farrell, 1991 cited in Latt et al., 1992).

CLINICAL ISSUES III: BIRTH AND THE POSTNATAL PERIOD

Analgesia and Anaesthesia During Labour and Birth

ethadone-maintained women should be given standard analgesia when required during labour (Batey et al., 1990; Gerada et al., 1990). Methadone as taken during methadone maintenance does not provide pain relief. This remains true even if the woman needs to receive her daily dose of methadone during labour. According to Collins (1991), opioids for pain relief should be avoided where possible during labour because it may increase the opioid load on the infant at birth. Other interventions, such as the use of nitrous oxide and non-opioid epidural anaesthesia, are preferable. Increasing the opioid load on the infant during labour may lead to a sedated neonate which in turn may lead to the administration of naloxone, the usual procedure for dealing with this condition. The use of naloxone with infants born to opioid-dependent women (methadone or heroin) may precipitate an acute neonatal abstinence syndrome and should only be administered under the supervision of senior medical staff who have experience with this population.

While in labour, the patient should be given her daily methadone dose at about the time she normally takes it, although it is best to avoid dosing during the second stage of labour (Collins, 1991). Once the woman has given birth, the use of opioids for pain relief is again indicated and, in such cases, the normal adult dosing regimen should be employed in addition to methadone (Collins, 1991).

The Opioid Withdrawal Syndrome in the Neonate

NEONATAL ABSTINENCE SYNDROME: DESCRIPTION

As already mentioned, Finnegan (cited in Gastel & Collins, 1983) has pointed out that the withdrawal syndrome observed in infants born to methadone-maintained women has to be kept in perspective. Compared to the problems observed in the neonates of heroin-dependent women out of treatment, the condition is relatively benign and responds readily to appropriate treatment. The neonatal abstinence syndrome, then, is:

> ...a generalised disorder characterized by signs and symptoms of central nervous system hyperirritability, gastrointestinal dysfunction, and respiratory distress, and by vague autonomic symptoms that include yawning, sneezing, mottling, and fever. Initially, the infants appear only to be restless. Tremors begin when the infants are

disturbed and progress to the point where they occur when the infants are not disturbed. High-pitched cry, increased muscle tone, and further irritability develop. When examined, the infants have deep tendon reflexes and an exaggerated Moro reflex. The rooting reflex is increased, and the infants are frequently seen sucking their fists or thumbs, yet when fed the infants have extreme difficulty and regurgitate frequently because of uncoordinated and ineffectual sucking and swallowing reflexes. Because of loose stools, decreased intake, and regurgitation, the infants are susceptible to dehydration and electrolyte imbalance (Finnegan, 1983 p. 410).

This syndrome usually begins within 72 hours but may appear for up to two weeks after birth. The timing of onset is influenced by many factors including the drug(s) used by the mother, the dose taken, when the drug(s) was last taken in relation to birth, the nature of labour, anaesthesia and analgesia used during labour, the gestational age of the infant, nutritional factors, and the presence of disease in the infant. Many patterns of development of symptoms are also observed, from the mild through to the severe, and from the transient through to the more longer lasting (Finnegan, 1983). As we have seen, some reports suggest that the neonatal abstinence syndrome is associated with maternal methadone dose (e.g. Collins, 1992; Suffet & Brotman, 1984). Approximately 30% of infants recently born to methadone-maintained women at one Sydney specialist program required treatment for the syndrome after birth (Collins & Capus, 1991).

A recent case report by Sutton and Hinderliter (1990) describes a protracted withdrawal syndrome in two infants born to methadone-maintained women who were taking large doses of illicit diazepam regularly. The two infants experienced a withdrawal syndrome typical for methadone abstinence, which was successfully dealt with by paregoric (camphorated tincture of opium), but at one week the symptoms reappeared despite this medication. The authors attributed this phenomenon to diazepam withdrawal. Diazepam passes through the placenta and accumulates in the foetus. Its half-life is longer in the infant than the adult and this reappearance of withdrawal, they argue, is consistent with a second abstinence syndrome due to another drug. The observations made in these two cases are consistent with the discussion of these issues by Finnegan (1980) and highlight the necessity of knowing the drug history of the woman concerned so that the appropriate pharmacological intervention can be used.

Neonatal Abstinence Syndrome: Treatment

It is important that all neonates at risk for withdrawal are assessed systematically with a scoring chart designed for that purpose (Batey et al., 1990; Finnegan, 1983; see Finnegan, 1980 for such a chart). According to the instructions for the assessment instrument in use, once treatment is warranted (as indicated by a consistently high score above a certain level on a specified number of occasions) it should begin immediately. The treatment of choice is pharmacotherapy and the most commonly used drugs are paregoric (opium tincture) and phenobarbitone (Finnegan 1983). Although once used, diazepam is no longer recommended (Finnegan, 1980; 1988). In Sydney, the two specialist programs treating pregnant women recommend phenobarbitone for all cases (Batey et al., 1990); an orally administered solution of morphine for opioid withdrawal; and the use of phenobarbitone for benzodiazepine, barbiturate and alcohol withdrawal (Collins, 1992). Hoegerman et al. (1990) recommends methadone 1 mg to 2 mg twice daily. All of these interventions require initial dosing to achieve relief and then tapering off the dose slowly to avoid further withdrawal.

Finnegan (1980; Finnegan et al., 1991) recommends involving mothers in the treatment of their babies' withdrawal to promote mother-infant attachment and to help the mother alleviate her guilt feelings and develop her self-efficacy. In cases of less severe withdrawal (abstinence syndrome scores less than critical level for pharmacological intervention), simple measures may be shown to the mother such as reducing stimuli, swaddling and the provision of a pacifier. In other cases where a course of pharmacotherapy is indicated, treatment on an outpatient basis is possible, with the mother administering the medication to her child (Collins, 1992). More generally, Finnegan et al. (1991) point out that teaching these women to care for their babies involves:

> ...educating the mother about her infant's needs and by teaching comforting techniques and how to interact with her infant in a positive, responsive manner. This intervention is essential because infants exposed to drugs in utero tend to be difficult to feed, have poor sucking reflex and are often irritable and difficult to console... Without intervention, mothers with limited care-giving skills and resources attempt to parent infants difficult to care for and who provide little positive reinforcement (p. 236).

It is not uncommon for hospital staff who lack experience with drug-dependent women to become angry at them when an infant experiences discomfort after birth as a result of the mothers drug use, or treatment in the case of methadone maintenance. Methadone unit staff are a source of support and advocacy in these situations.

Methadone Maintenance and Breastfeeding

Breastfeeding is suggested for methadone-maintained women (Batey et al., 1990; Finnegan, 1980). According to Finnegan (1980), breastfeeding contributes to the development of mother–infant attachment, provides the infant with maternal antibodies, is nutritionally tailored to the infant and is thought by some to assist in reducing the severity of the neonatal abstinence syndrome (e.g. Hoegerman et al., 1990; Mack et al., 1991). Pond et al. (1985) found only very low levels of methadone in breast milk, even at high maintenance doses. They found that the highest dose an infant would receive via breast milk would be about 0.01 mg to 0.03 mg of methadone in a day. Doses this low would not be expected to have any clinical effects (see also Finnegan, 1980). However, Finnegan (1980) suggests that this may change by three to six months of age due to the volume of milk consumed and therefore recommends that the infant should be weaned at this stage.

CONCLUSION

While at first sight methadone maintenance for pregnant women might seem a controversial intervention, the evidence clearly suggests that for many opioid-dependent women it is the least harmful option. Methadone programs for pregnant women have much in common with the usual methadone maintenance program and in this regard, where not otherwise indicated, the issues outlined in the rest of this book also apply to these specialist programs.

Finnegan (1980; 1991) has consistently argued that methadone by itself is not a sufficient intervention for the dependent pregnant woman. The evidence and clinical opinion cited in this chapter clearly supports this proposition. It is the combination of methadone maintenance, specialised antenatal care, education and counselling that keeps these women in treatment and makes possible a maximum number of trouble-free births. Although apparently an expensive option, as Ellwood et al. (1987) have pointed out, when the substantial cost of neonatal intensive care for infants born to drug-dependent women not in treatment is taken into account, comprehensive methadone maintenance programs for this population begin to look not only effective as an intervention but cost-effective as well.

SUMMARY

Opioid-dependent pregnant women are a high-risk group. These women do not usually have adequate nutrition, rest or antenatal care. The daily use of illicit opioids (such as heroin) expose the woman and her foetus to dangerous fluctuations in blood heroin levels, a range of unknown drugs and contaminants, and a range of infections associated with injecting drug use, including hepatitis and HIV.

Opioid-dependent women not in treatment usually give birth prematurely and their babies are small for their gestational age. These children suffer from a variety of complications due to their prematurity and until relatively recently many of them died soon after birth. Developments over the past few decades in the ability to care for neonates at risk has decreased the mortality rate among infants of heroin-dependent mothers.

Methadone maintenance replaces an illicit drug of dependence of unknown quality and uncertain supply with a pure opioid that is administered under medical supervision. Providing a pregnant woman with a daily dose of methadone means that she and her foetus are no longer subject to the peaks and troughs of heroin blood levels nor an unknown range of contaminants, some of which are known to be teratogenic. Enrolment in an methadone maintenance program also allows the delivery of adequate antenatal care.

The research evidence to date unconditionally supports comprehensive methadone maintenance programs for opioid-dependent pregnant women. When compared to similar groups out of treatment, women in methadone maintenance programs have longer pregnancies, have fewer complications at birth and have infants who are larger for their gestational age.

Even though the ideal treatment course for an opioid-dependent pregnant woman would be to initiate low dose methadone maintenance and then to withdraw her during the safest period for detoxification (14 to 32 weeks) so that she would be drug-free at birth, few women can achieve total abstinence without relapse or obstetrical complications intervening. Therefore, the treatment of choice for most women is methadone maintenance throughout their pregnancy.

Although it has been argued that methadone dose should be kept as low as possible for methadone maintenance during pregnancy in the interests of not harming the foetus or causing unnecessary withdrawal in the neonate, it has to be acknowledged that what is in the best interest of the mother is best for the foetus. Dose of methadone has to be offset against risks posed by relapse and obstetrical complications associated with withdrawal.

Pregnancy may affect the metabolism of methadone in human beings, especially during the third trimester when lower than expected levels of methadone in blood plasma may be observed. Some women report the onset of unexpected withdrawal symptoms during this period that may need to be dealt with by splitting or increasing methadone dose.

Initial dose of methadone should be low (10 mg) for pregnant women and increased with care.

Groups for pregnant women in methadone maintenance are feasible and desirable. Such groups function as antenatal and parenting classes as well as group therapy sessions. These groups are most successful when they are restricted to women only.

Debate remains about the desirability of treating the partners of pregnant women at specialist methadone maintenance units for pregnant women. While treating only the women places stress on their relationships with their partners, the presence of men in the clinic may at times be detrimental to optimal treatment delivery.

Antenatal care for women in methadone maintenance should be non-judgmental. Where possible special clinic times specifically for methadone maintenance patients should be scheduled and operated by staff experienced in working with this population.

HIV is transmitted perinatally in 20% to 40% of cases. As yet there have been few cases of perinatal transmission in Australia, but the overseas evidence suggests that as infection rates increase there will be significant numbers of children infected by this route. In the USA, where perinatal infection is not uncommon, injecting drug use is the main risk factor in most cases.

Current knowledge suggests that pregnancy does not hasten the onset of HIV-related illnesses in asymptomatic HIV positive women. The effect of pregnancy on women with AIDS-related complex or AIDS is not known. The effects of termination are not known in this regard, but it is thought that the potential effect would be less than that of pregnancy.

A woman who is infected with HIV and decides to proceed with her pregnancy will need intensive support and counselling. As well as having to deal with issues concerning her own death and possible infection in her child, a woman in this situation may suffer discrimination because of her serostatus.

The incidence of both hepatitis B and C is very high among

injecting drug users (around 80% to 90%). Infants born to women who are acutely or chronically infected with hepatitis B at the time of birth should be provided with hepatitis B immunoglobulin and vaccine shortly after birth. The consequences and possibility of perinatal hepatitis C infection are currently unknown.

Women on methadone maintenance should not be denied analgesia or anaesthesia during labour or birth. Opioids should be avoided during labour but are indicated after the woman has given birth. In such cases, the adult analgesic dose should be administered in addition to the usual daily methadone.

Many infants born to methadone-maintained women will exhibit an abstinence syndrome, usually within 72 hours of being born. The severity of the neonatal abstinence syndrome should be assessed using an instrument designed for this purpose. The syndrome responds well to paregoric, morphine, methadone or phenobarbitone.

Breastfeeding is not contraindicated for women on methadone maintenance. The amount of methadone present in breast milk is minute and unlikely to harm an infant in the first three to six months of life. Breast milk provides the infant with maternal antibodies and the feeding itself encourages mother–infant attachment between a difficult to care for infant and a mother who might not readily know what her child's needs are.

13

CONCURRENT PSYCHIATRIC DISORDERS

INTRODUCTION

Intervention for specific concurrent (or comorbid) psychiatric disorders among the opioid dependent has been shown to improve overall outcome in a number of domains of functioning, including drug use (see Chapter 8). A failure to diagnose these disorders may render the effect of methadone maintenance treatment less than optimal, and result in prolonged illicit drug use. Therefore, as part of establishing the extent of the health care needs of methadone maintenance patients, this chapter examines the evidence on the prevalence of psychiatric diagnoses (other than opioid dependence) within this population. To foreshadow the conclusions, it has been a consistent finding from studies of the prevalence of psychiatric disorders among the opioid dependent that the rates of a number of disorders are increased above population rates. The disorders that are more frequent are the depressive disorders, antisocial personality disorder, and alcohol abuse and alcohol dependence. The following sections address the rates of psychiatric disorders overall, and then address the specific diagnoses that are found to be more prevalent.

RESULTS OF PREVALENCE STUDIES

he Epidemiologic Catchment Area (ECA) study (Regier et al., 1990) was a large-scale survey of the prevalence of psychiatric disorders conducted recently in the USA. The study and its results are important because they provide estimates of the prevalence of specific psychiatric disorders for the USA population which could then be used as base rates with which to compare prevalence data for samples of opioid-dependent individuals (Regier et al., 1990). Without estimates for the general population, it is difficult to assess how elevated the apparently high rates found in the studies discussed are. The fact that nearly all the studies to be discussed have been carried out in the USA makes the ECA findings especially useful for this purpose.

The ECA findings are also of interest themselves. As can be seen from Table 5, in the general population the lifetime rate for any psychiatric disorder (excluding drug and alcohol disorders) was 22.5%, whereas 13.5% had an alcohol disorder and 6% some other drug use disorder. Only 0.7% of the population reported an opioid use disorder (Regier et al., 1990). When those with an opioid use disorder were compared with the general population, estimates of comparative risk for specific disorders can be made through the use of odds ratio. In the Regier et al. (1990) study, opioid users were found to be seven times more likely to have experienced a psychiatric disorder than the general population (odds ratio = 6.7), and these data are presented in Table 5.

Prevalence rate estimates of specific psychiatric disorders among the opioid dependent are also summarised in Table 5. These estimates are derived from a number of studies which have been conducted in North America. When compared to the rates obtained for the general population in the USA in the ECA study, opioid-dependent individuals had higher overall rates of lifetime and current psychiatric disorders and higher rates for depression, ASP and alcohol disorders (Regier et al., 1990). For specific disorders, opioid users were at nine times the risk for schizophrenia (OR = 8.8),* at five times the risk for an affective disorder (OR = 5), at three times the risk for anxiety disorders (OR = 2.8), at 24 times the risk for antisocial personality disorder (OR = 24.3), and at 13 times

---

* Due to the small numbers involved, the increased risk for schizophrenia was not statistically significant and should therefore be regarded with caution. Other prevalence studies among opioid users have not consistently found an increased risk

Table 5. Estimates of Prevalence of Psychiatric Comorbidity in the Opioid Dependent and in the General Population

Author	Sample type (No. in sample)	Prevalence rate (current [a] or lifetime [b])	Any psychiatric diagnosis %	Depressive disorder %	Anxiety disorder %	Alcohol use disorder %	Antisocial personality disorder %
Rounsaville et al. (1982)	Opioid dependent [c] (533)	Current	70	26	3	14	27
Khantzian & Treece (1985)	Opioid dependent [c] (133)	Current	93	56	11	14	35
Woody et al. (1983; 1985)	Methadone patients (110)	Lifetime	–	43	7	26	15
Strain et al. (1991)	Methadone patients (66)	Lifetime	47	23	2	49	30
Regier et al. (1990)	Opioid users (142)	Lifetime	65	31	32	66	37
Reigier et al. (1990)	General population sample (20,291)	Current	13.0	5.2	7.3	2.8	(.5
		Lifetime	22.5	8.3	14.6	13.5	2.6
		'Relative risk' [d] of lifetime diagnosis	6.7	5.0	2.8	12.8	24.3

Notes. [a] 'Current' indicates that the individual currently has the disorder; [b] 'Lifetime' indicates that the individual had disorder at some time in life. [c] Refers to a mixed sample of opioid-dependent individuals some of whom were in, and some of whom were not in, treatment. [d] The figures on 'relative risk' are odds ratios reported by Regier et al. (1990) and they indicate the increased likelihood that a person meeting diagnostic criteria for opiate abuse or dependence will also meet criteria for the diagnoses indicated.

the risk for an alcohol disorder (OR = 12.8). These estimates, which are based on comparisons between those with an opioid use disorder and the general population, are generally confirmed by studies that have looked at self-selected samples of opioid addicts.

The ECA study also found that individuals diagnosed with a drug (other than alcohol) use disorder who were in treatment had significantly higher rates of psychopathology than those who were not in treatment (Regier et al., 1990). Similar results were reported by Rounsaville and Kleber (1985a) who compared prevalence rates for samples of opioid addicts in and out of treatment and also found a significant difference in number of psychiatric disorders. This difference was mainly accounted for by diagnoses of depressive disorders. In addition to depression, legal difficulties and poorer

for schizophrenia (for example, Khantzian & Treece, 1985; Rounsaville et al., 1982). However, Regier et al. (1990) did find that individuals with a diagnosis of schizophrenia were at increased risk for substance disorder diagnoses when compared to the general population, though this again did not reach significance.

social functioning predicted being in the treatment sample, whereas estimates of drug consumption did not. As Rounsaville and Kleber (1985a) point out, findings such as these suggest that it is not heavy drug use that motivates drug users to seek out treatment but difficulties like social, legal and psychological problems.

One notable feature of the data presented from the studies reviewed in Table 5 is the variance in rates. Some of the disparity observed between the rates presented may be attributed to a number of factors including: the population assessed; sample size assessed; the diagnostic criteria used; the interview schedule and format employed; and the timing of the diagnostic interview. The effect of these and other factors on the results of studies addressing the co-occurrence of comorbid psychiatric disorders among substance abusers has been considered in some detail by Weiss et al. (1992).

Overall, the results presented in Table 5 suggest that for samples of opioid users in the USA psychiatric comorbidity is prevalent and because of this prevalence it constitutes a serious problem for the management of patients in that country. The extent to which this is true for other countries has yet to be established. In Australia, the finding of two recent studies carried out by the National Drug and Alcohol Research Centre suggest that rates of psychiatric comorbidity are also probably high among opioid users seeking or already in treatment (Darke et al., in press; Swift et al., 1990). Both of these studies found high levels of psychopathology as measured by the General Health Questionnaire (GHQ), an instrument which provides an overall estimate of psychopathology. In each of the two samples, 60% of subjects reported significant levels of psychopathology. Research is now required to establish the prevalence of the various psychiatric disorders among populations of opioid-dependent individuals in countries other than the USA. Until such data become available it must be assumed that the prevalence of these disorders is likely to be heightened in opioid abusing and dependent samples relative to the population at large.

DEPRESSION

B y far the most common and consistent finding of prevalence studies of psychiatric comorbidity among opioid users is of high rates of depressive disorders (Khantzian & Treece, 1985; Regier et al., 1990; Rounsaville et al., 1982; Weissman et al., 1976). As noted above, the ECA study found that people diagnosed with an opioid use disorder are five times more likely to have had a depressive disorder than are the general population (Regier et al., 1990), and that women are found to be more commonly diagnosed with depression than are men (see previous section). Rounsaville and Kleber (1985a) also found that opioid users in treatment are more likely to be diagnosed with depression than their counterparts who have not sought treatment. A diagnosis of depression has been found to predict poorer psychosocial functioning (Rounsaville et al., 1986b) and to increase the risk of relapse to heroin use in the event of life crises among methadone maintenance patients.

The relationship between having a depressive disorder and being in methadone maintenance treatment has to be considered along with three studies which have found a decline in the incidence of depression over time in samples of methadone maintenance patients assessed at entry to treatment and periodically thereafter (Dorus & Senay, 1980; Steer & Kotzker, 1980; Strain et al., 1991). It is well known that some form of crisis often precipitates a decision to seek out treatment, and it may be the case that prevalence studies that assess patients on entry to treatment may overestimate the relationship between being in treatment and being depressed. The stabilisation that being in methadone maintenance brings to a person's life may be enough in many cases to eliminate depressive disorders that are reactions to stressful situations associated with a heroin-using lifestyle (e.g. housing, legal, relationship problems). Patients who remain depressed after stabilisation on methadone may be in need of specialist treatment. (The relationship between opioid dependence and depression is discussed in more detail later in this chapter. See pp. 266–67)

ANTISOCIAL PERSONALITY DISORDER

According to Robins et al. (1991a):

Antisocial personality is a disorder that begins in childhood with a variety of behavior problems at home and in school and continues into adult life with failure to conform to social norms in many areas including work, family, and other interpersonal relationships. Persons with the disorder tend to be aggressive and impulsive and are thought to lack normal capacities for love, guilt, and cooperation with authority figures. Many of them come into conflict with the legal system (p. 258).

The ECA population estimate for the lifetime and current rates of antisocial personality disorder are 2.6% and 0.6% respectively (Regier et al., 1990). As already mentioned, men (4.5%) are far more likely than women (0.8%) to have had this disorder at some time in their lives; however, along with becoming more prevalent in recent times, the differences between the rates for men and women have also been lessening (Robins et al. 1991a). As also noted above, individuals diagnosed with an opioid use disorder were found to be 24 times more likely to be diagnosed with antisocial personality disorder than the general population (Regier et al., 1990). These differences between men and women and the high rates for opioid users have been consistently found in studies of drug users.

As can be seen from Table 5, consistently high rates of antisocial personality disorder have been found in opioid-dependent samples. Other studies have found rates as high as 55% (Kosten et al., 1982), suggesting that there may be some variability in the application of diagnostic criteria. Rounsaville et al. (1982) demonstrated this point when they diagnosed antisocial personality disorder using two different sets of criteria and found a marked difference in rate. When DSM-III criteria were used, 53.9% of the sample was diagnosed with antisocial personality disorder, but when the Research Diagnostic Criteria were used, only 26.5% were so diagnosed. There were two main reasons for the differences in rate found. The first was that the DSM-III criteria (and the DSM-III-R) included many items that describe the typical heroin addict's lifestyle (drug dealing, theft, unemployment, defaulting on debts, recklessness) which may, in many cases, be a function of opioid dependence rather than any underlying personality disorder.

As Weiss et al. (1992) point out, the Research Diagnostic Criteria do not diagnose anti-social personality disorder if some of the symptoms of that disorder are clearly attributable to the substance abuse itself. According to Gerstley and her colleagues (1990), this could be resolved by ensuring that the criteria for antisocial behaviour are independent of drug dependence. The second criticism of the DSM-III criteria is that they focus on overt behaviour and do not include enough items that have been traditionally labelled psychopathic traits, such as the inability to experience love and guilt (for example, Gerstley et al., 1990; Task Force on DSM-IV, 1991). It should also be noted that there is a much larger debate about the usefulness of the diagnosis, and whether it is justifiable to infer that there is an underlying psychiatric disorder from criminal, deviant and antisocial behaviour. This debate has gone on since the first use of diagnostic categories such as 'psychopath' and 'sociopath' early this century and continues today with 'antisocial personality disorder', which is the heir to these older terms (Blackburn, 1988; Courtwright, 1982; Robins et al., 1991).

Though there may be debates about which criteria to use and whether the application of a diagnosis of antisocial personality disorder is medicalising deviance, the more important point for methadone maintenance treatment providers is that the diagnosis may have implications for treatment. As noted in Chapter 8, methadone maintenance patients with a diagnosis of antisocial personality disorder do not respond to psychotherapy unless they also have a concurrent diagnosis of depression. (Patients with diagnoses of antisocial personality disorder do respond to methadone maintenance treatment, however, in that they reduce their drug use and criminal activity (Woody et al., 1985b).) A concurrent depressive disorder may not be that uncommon in some patients with a diagnosis of antisocial personality disorder. For example, Rounsaville et al. (1982) found that most subjects who were diagnosed with antisocial personality disorder were also diagnosed as having a depressive disorder. The inability to establish a therapeutic alliance with a therapist may be the main reason for this lack of response to psychotherapy. As yet, there is no known method of engaging individuals diagnosed with antisocial personality disorder in psychotherapeutic treatment because of the features associated with this disorder (Quality Assurance Project, 1991).

The ECA study has found that the symptoms of antisocial personality disorder tend to remit as sufferers enter their third and fourth decade of life which, as Robins et al. (1991) suggest, may mean that if the factors associated with remission can be determined, they may provide indications for possible treatment. On the basis of the evidence available at the time of writing, it would appear that for those patients in methadone maintenance with a diagnosis of antisocial personality disorder and no diagnosis of depression, psychotherapy should not be offered as it is not likely to bring about any changes. Methadone maintenance, however, is indicated for these individuals because of the consistent finding that injecting drug users with a diagnosis of antisocial personality disorder tend to engage in higher levels of risk behaviour associated with the transmission of HIV (see Chapter 4).

SEX DIFFERENCES IN RATES OF PSYCHIATRIC DISORDERS

n the ECA study of the USA general population sample, it was found, contrary to previous findings, that men (36%) had suffered more psychiatric disorders in their lives than had women (30%). The two sexes had equal prevalence rates for having had a disorder in the past year (20%) (Robins et al., 1991b). However, when the types of disorders represented among each sex were examined, important differences emerged. More women than men were diagnosed with anxiety disorders, depression and somatisation disorder. More men than women were diagnosed with antisocial personality disorder, alcohol use disorders and other drug use disorders. The main reason for the excess of lifetime psychiatric disorder among men was that men made up such a large proportion of alcohol disorder diagnoses.

The differences between men and women in the general population are mirrored in the findings of studies carried out with opioid-dependent populations. Women have been found to suffer from more anxiety disorders (Rounsaville et al., 1982) and more depressive disorders than men (Croughan et al., 1982; Khantzian & Treece, 1985; Rounsaville et al., 1982; Strain et al., 1991), whereas men tend to be more likely to be diagnosed with antisocial personality disorder (Croughan et al., 1982; Khantzian & Treece, 1985; Rounsaville et al., 1982). These data are consistent with the findings of the two Australian studies (Darke et al., in press; Swift et al., 1990) which found that women had significantly higher levels of psychopathology as measured by the GHQ than did men. These findings suggest that women and men suffer from different kinds of psychological problems and therefore may have different needs. As will be seen below, generally speaking, it would seem that women may be more amenable to psychotherapeutic interventions than men, although to date the major psychotherapy studies have only looked at their effectiveness with men.

PSYCHIATRIC SEVERITY AND RESPONSE TO TREATMENT

s described in Chapter 8, a global estimate of psychiatric severity has been found to predict the response of patients to psychotherapy as an adjunct to methadone maintenance treatment

(Woody et al., 1984). Patients assessed as having high severity psychiatric problems were found to do better in methadone maintenance treatment if they received psychotherapy than if they did not. This finding is significant when it is placed in the context of other findings that indicate that patients with more severe psychiatric problems do not respond well to treatment for their drug problems.

The relationship between severity of psychiatric problems and poor response to treatment has been observed for methadone maintenance treatment (McLellan et al., 1984; Ramer et al., 1971; Rounsaville et al., 1986b; Woody et al., 1984), and more generally for a range of treatments for drug and alcohol disorders (McLellan et al., 1984). However, research by McLellan et al. (1984) suggests that opioid users with severe psychiatric problems may also be better off in methadone maintenance treatment than in the other major treatment modality for this population — the therapeutic community. They found that low-severity patients did quite well with brief treatment courses in either modality, and that the medium-severity patients did well in either with longer treatment courses. Among high-severity patients, the treatment response was poor to both methadone maintenance and therapeutic communities, but there were small positive gains after exposure to methadone maintenance, whereas the group exposed to therapeutic communities tended to get worse. McLellan et al. (1984) suggest that methadone maintenance is indicated for high-severity patients and that this might be due to both anti-psychotic properties of methadone itself, and to the fact that methadone maintenance programs often provide ancillary psychotropic medication for such patients. Therapeutic communities tend to frown on the use of any medication, although the view that prescribed psychotropic medications are inappropriate in therapeutic communities has begun to change recently.

The relationship between psychiatric severity and response to treatment may not be as simple as the above research suggests. Ball and Ross (1991) failed to find any relationship between the two in their recent study of six methadone maintenance units in the USA. This finding is surprising when it is acknowledged that the sample size in their study was sufficiently large to detect such a relationship, if there was one, and that they used exactly the same measure (ASI) as that used in the other studies that found such a relationship.

Whether there is a consistent, predictable relationship between psychiatric severity and response to treatment or not, the implications of the majority of the findings to date are clear.

Applicants for methadone maintenance with severe psychiatric problems are suitable for admission, and those with florid psychotic disorders should be placed on maintenance neuroleptics (e.g. phenothiazines) in addition to methadone so that their psychosis can be controlled. The response to treatment of all patients with serious psychiatric disorder will, however, be attenuated unless their special needs are catered for by specialist treatment such as psychotherapy and psychotropic medication. These findings suggest that all applicants for methadone maintenance should be screened for psychiatric problems, and referred for proper assessment if the results of the screening indicate a significant level of psychopathology (McLellan et al., 1984; Rounsaville et al., 1986b).

RELATIONSHIP BETWEEN DEPENDENCE AND PSYCHOPATHOLOGY

Given the high prevalence of psychiatric disorder among the opioid dependent, what is the relationship that underlies the association between drug dependence and certain kinds of psychopathology? Meyer (1986) suggests that there are a number of ways in which the two might be related. Specifically, certain conditions (e.g. antisocial personality disorder or depression): (a) may lead to drug dependence; (b) may facilitate its onset and course; (c) may arise as a result of drug dependence; (d) may simply be associated with drug dependence (both being caused by some other factor); or (e) the two disorders may not be related at all. The evidence reviewed above suggest that the two do often occur together and the example of depression is instructive in this regard. Depression may: (a) lead to opioid use as an attempt at self-medication; (b) lead to a more severe dependence than is seen in non-depressed individuals; (c) it may arise as a result of being dependent and the lifestyle associated with it; (d) it may be a result of factors common to the genesis of both opioid dependence and depression (e.g. poverty, lack of social support, and chronic unemployment); (e) or be the result of a neurochemical imbalance that has nothing to do with opioid dependence.

The most important distinction, in terms of treatment options, is whether depression is an antecedent or consequence of opioid dependence. It is sometimes argued that if depression is a consequence of the stressors associated with an opioid-dependent lifestyle, then presumably the successful treatment of the dependence should, in time, lead to the resolution of the symptoms of depression. The evidence concerning the relationship between time in methadone maintenance and a decline in depression (reviewed in Chapter 8) supports this argument for some patients. However, it does not necessarily follow that depression which develops as a consequence of an opioid-dependent lifestyle will remit through treatment for dependence. Depressive disorders that arise as a result of stressful life events may develop a dynamic of their own and become chronic without treatment. According to the opposite viewpoint — that drug dependence is a consequence of pre-existing depression (often known as the self-medication hypothesis) — the successful treatment of opioid dependence would necessitate treating the underlying psychopathology (Khantzian, 1985b).

The data from the ECA study provides some information on the nature of the relationship between opioid dependence and the development of comorbid psychiatric states. Christie et al. (1988) found that for a sub-group of young adults, a pre-existing anxiety or depressive disorder doubled the risk of later development of drug abuse disorders (excluding alcohol). Unfortunately, data specifically for opioid use disorders were not presented in the study, but the data do suggest psychiatric disorders may precede drug abuse.

Another study carried out in Canada on a sample of people presenting for a range of alcohol and drug problems found some variation in the relationship between age of onset for drug problems and other psychiatric disorders (Ross et al., 1988). In nearly every case of antisocial personality disorder, the onset of the disorder preceded the onset of drug problems, which was not surprising given that one of the criteria for antisocial personality disorder was that it must have started in childhood. For anxiety and depressive disorders, it was less likely that the psychiatric disorder preceded drug abuse problems, although a substantial proportion (23%–40%) reported the reverse relationship. These two studies, taken together, suggest that different sequences in the onset of drug use and other psychiatric disorders are possible, and that there is a need for further research to clarify this relationship and its prognostic implications.

SUMMARY

pioid dependent individuals suffer depressive disorders, antisocial personality disorder and alcohol abuse and dependence at much higher rates than occur in the general community. Sex differences in rates of psychiatric disorders have been recorded among methadone maintenance patients, with depression being more common among women and antisocial personality disorder among men.

Depressive disorders are common among methadone maintenance patients. However, there is some evidence that a proportion of these disorders remit in response to methadone maintenance, suggesting that they might be the result of the life crises associated with an opioid-dependent lifestyle. Patients who remain depressed after stabilisation on methadone are likely to need specialist assessment and treatment. Many methadone maintenance patients when assessed are diagnosed with antisocial personality disorder, with the majority by far being men. There is controversy over the usefulness of this diagnosis in general and, specifically, in its application to opioid-dependent individuals.

There is some evidence that individuals with drug and alcohol problems who also have severe psychiatric problems do not respond well to treatment, although the evidence is contradictory with regard to methadone maintenance treatment. The finding that the addition of psychotherapy can alter the response of these patients to methadone maintenance treatment suggests that concurrent psychiatric treatment should be offered in such cases.

The relationship between opioid dependence and concurrent psychopathology is not clear and needs to be researched more thoroughly. There is evidence that some disorders such as depression precede drug use and may predispose its sufferers to self-medicating drug use. Other evidence suggests that other cases of disorders such as depression may be due to the stresses and chaotic lifestyle associated with being dependent on illicit drugs.

The evidence concerning psychiatric comorbidity among methadone maintenance patients suggests that patients accepted for treatment should be assessed with a screening instrument for psychiatric disorders once they have been stabilised on methadone and referred for specialist assessment where indicated.

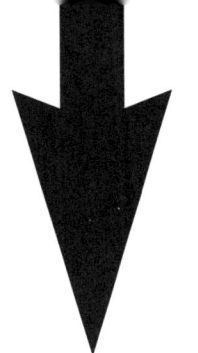

SECTION IV
CONCLUSIONS

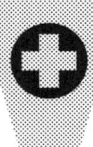

14

METHADONE MAINTENANCE IN AUSTRALIA

Most of the major research studies on methadone maintenance that have been reviewed in this book have been from the USA. From the point of view of Australian and other national policymakers, the questions must be raised: 'How applicable are the findings of American studies to the performance of methadone programs outside the USA?' and 'What qualifications may need to be made in using this research to inform policymakers on methadone maintenance treatment?' This chapter addresses these questions from an Australian perspective and provides a short history of methadone maintenance treatment in Australia and a brief review of the small amount of research that has been undertaken to describe the characteristics of methadone patients, program policies and procedures, and the outcome of treatment in terms of retention and drug use and criminal activity.

METHADONE TREATMENT IN AUSTRALIA

ethadone maintenance was introduced into Australia in 1970 by Dr Stella Dalton, whose advocacy of the treatment led to an increase in the provision of places in methadone programs during the 1970s. In the late 1970s and early 1980s the provision of places in methadone programs in Australia contracted because the treatment failed to live up to the high expectations that some had of it as a cure for heroin addiction (Burgess et al., 1990). The reasons for the disenchantment with methadone continue to be contentious: its critics attribute it to a failure of methadone to deliver on the promises of its proponents; its defenders attribute it to a failure to implement methadone *maintenance* in the form advocated by Dole and Nyswander.

Methadone treatment regained popularity in Australia during the mid-1980s, initially in the face of increasing demand for places in methadone programs by injecting drug users, and later in response to fears about an epidemic of HIV among injecting drug

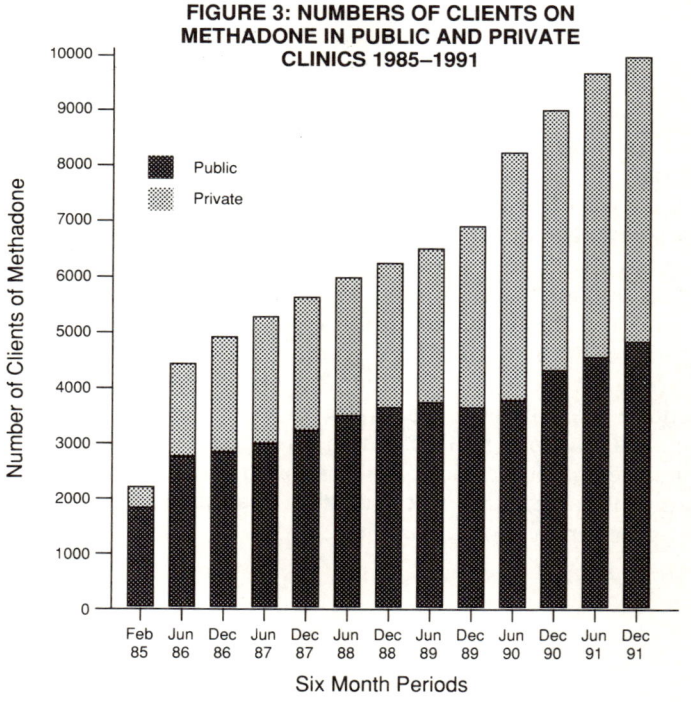

FIGURE 3: NUMBERS OF CLIENTS ON METHADONE IN PUBLIC AND PRIVATE CLINICS 1985–1991

users. As can be seen in Figure 3, the expansion of program places begun in 1984 accelerated after the National Drug Summit endorsed methadone as part of the strategy for treating heroin dependence in 1985. The methadone program continued to expand throughout the late 1980s, with an increase in the number of persons on methadone from 2 203 in February 1985 to 10 054 in September 1991 (pers. comm., Commonwealth Department of Community Services and Health, December 1991). Figure 3 also illustrates the extent to which this expansion has taken place mainly in private rather than public methadone clinics.

The rapid expansion of methadone programs in the late 1980s was accompanied by a proliferation of competing models, rationales and goals of methadone treatment. There are probably few workers today who would embrace either the metabolic disease model of Dole and Nyswander or the goal of long-term maintenance that it implies. A recent national survey of methadone programs (Baillie et al., 1991) suggests that many programs operate within a therapeutic model, according to which the goal of methadone treatment is abstinence from all opioid drugs, including methadone, which is to be achieved within a period of several years.

One consequence of the adoption of this therapeutic approach has been time-limited treatment with abstinence as a goal, and a reduction in methadone dose from the high levels originally used by Dole and Nyswander. These trends have been observed in both the USA (Gerstein & Harwood, 1990; D'Aunno & Vaughn, 1992) and Australia (Baillie et al., 1991). The reasons for the change are uncertain but they probably include a potent confluence of economics and ideology: the scarcity of places in methadone treatment has encouraged staff to create vacancies for new patients by discharging old ones, and a time limit on maintenance appeals to abstinence-oriented practitioners in the drug and alcohol field who are responsible for administering methadone programs.

The advent of HIV/AIDS, and its threatened spread to the general community via injecting drug users, has further complicated the therapeutic task of methadone programs. The expansion of methadone programs as part of the strategy to prevent the transmission of HIV has been accompanied by an increased emphasis on the goal of 'harm-reduction'. This has been variously interpreted but has often been taken to mean that priority should be given to preventing the transmission of HIV by unsafe injecting practices, such as needle sharing, rather than to achieving abstinence from opioid drugs.

The pluralism in Australian methadone program rationales and goals makes it difficult, and somewhat misleading, to provide an overall evaluation of the effectiveness of methadone treatment in Australia. Nonetheless, the necessity to make decisions about the allocation of treatment resources requires answers to the questions: 'Does the average heroin-dependent person who enters an Australian methadone program have a reasonable chance of benefiting from the experience?' 'If so, which opioid-dependent people are the most likely to benefit from the treatment?' and 'What are the best ways to provide methadone treatment to those who are most in need of it?'

RESEARCH ON METHADONE MAINTENANCE IN AUSTRALIA

There have been no controlled clinical trials and no large-scale prospective studies of methadone maintenance in Australia comparable to Treatment Outcome Prospective Study or the Drug Abuse Reporting Program. Australian research on methadone maintenance consists of a small number of observational studies that describe patient populations and report outcomes, usually without any comparison group. Assessments of the effectiveness of methadone maintenance in Australia have largely depended upon the assumption that the results of American research are applicable to Australian heroin users. In this section we examine the justification for such an assumption by examining available data on the characteristics of patients who attend methadone clinics in Australia, the types of programs that are available, and the limited amount of research that has been conducted on treatment outcome in Australian methadone programs.

PATIENT CHARACTERISTICS

One obvious and potentially important way in which Australian methadone patients differ from American patients is in ethnicity. Although the proportions differ according to city, American methadone patient populations include substantial proportions of Afro-Americans and Hispanics. By contrast, the ethnic diversity of the Australian population appears not to have been reflected in the patients found in methadone clinics, if one can judge from the absence of information on the ethnicity of Australian methadone patients. According to the one study that has reported on the ethnicity of patients (Reilly et al., 1987), only 12% of patients at a Sydney methadone clinic were from non-English speaking backgrounds.

Besides ethnicity, the majority of methadone patient populations reported in overseas studies are primarily unemployed males aged around 25 to 35 years, who have a long history of opioid dependence, and extensive criminal backgrounds. Surveys of Australian methadone patients reveal a similar population: two-thirds are males with an average age of 28 years; the mean period of addiction at entry to methadone treatment is seven years; three-quarters have had prior treatment contact; and four out of five have had a criminal conviction (Caplehorn, 1992). As in the USA, these characteristics have changed in the 20 years since the introduction of methadone treatment (Bell et al., 1990; Reilly et al.,1987; Reynolds et al., 1976). Methadone patients have become older, more women have applied for treatment, the patients' history of dependence is longer, and more patients are appearing with histories of criminal activity. On the whole, with the exception of ethnicity, Australian methadone patients are remarkably similar to patients in American studies.

PROGRAM CHARACTERISTICS

There is much less information on the characteristics of Australian methadone programs than there is on the characteristics of their patients. What is available suggests that many Australian programs have departed substantially from the original maintenance model of Dole and Nyswander. This has led some to urge caution in extrapolating the results of American studies of methadone maintenance to Australia (for example, Reilly et al., 1987). While acknowledging the need for caution, we believe that the variations in policies and procedures between American methadone clinics revealed in the Drug Abuse Reporting Program, the Treatment Outcome Prospective Study, Ball and Ross and General Accounting Office studies is substantially similar to the variations between programs in Australia.

A comparison of the results of a recent Australian national survey of agencies providing treatment for opioid users (Baillie et al., 1991) with the descriptions of American programs provided by Gerstein and Harwood (1990) and D'Aunno and Vaughn (1992) is instructive. It suggests that there has been a move in both countries towards time-limited programs that use lower doses of methadone and have abstinence as a treatment goal. In the Australian survey, information on the duration of methadone was incomplete but among the programs that supplied information the average duration was 15 months. The average doses of methadone varied between the different States, with South Australia and Victoria having half or more of their patients on doses below 40 mg per day, and 84% of the total sample receiving daily doses of less than 80 mg. Although direct comparisons are difficult, the dose ranges are similar to the 40 mg to 50 mg averages reported recently in the USA by Ball and Ross (1990), D'Aunno and Vaughn (1992) and the General Accounting Office study (1989).

TREATMENT OUTCOME IN AUSTRALIAN METHADONE PROGRAMS

The few Australian studies that have attempted to assess the outcome of methadone treatment have been uncontrolled retrospective or cross-sectional studies, usually without a comparison population, and often lacking data on drug use and crime among patients before they enter treatment. The following review examines the few prospective studies that have been done on treatment retention, and heroin use and crime.

Reynolds and Magro (1976) followed up a sample of 116 Sydney methadone patients two years after treatment. Eighty-three per cent of the original sample were located, and 68% per cent of those followed up (54% of the original cohort) were still in methadone treatment. No data were reported on the drug use of those still in treatment. Of those who were no longer in treatment, 27% were abstinent at the time of interview, 30% were irregular opiate users, 23% were dependent, and 17% were in prison. Those who stayed in the program continuously for two years had fewer criminal charges than those who left and re-entered treatment, or those who left and did not return to treatment. A later four-year follow-up from patient records rather than interviews found that approximately the same percentage of patients remained in treatment (Reynolds et al., 1975).

Dalton and her colleagues conducted two follow-up studies of 50 patients at one to two years (Dalton et al., 1976), and at six to eight years (Dalton & Duncan, 1979) after entry to a high-dose methadone program. The treatment goal was patient compliance with treatment. At the one to two year follow-up 36 of the original

50 patients were traced and interviewed, and one patient was known to have died. If the treatment drop-outs are counted the compliance rate was 66%. At the six to eight year follow-up, 43 of the original group were contacted, of whom five had died, and two could not be found. When the treatment drop-outs were included, the compliance rate was 62%.

At one to two years 75% of the patients who remained in treatment were not using illicit drugs, and 14% of the follow-up sample were not using any drugs, including methadone. At the six to eight year follow-up, 23 of the original sample were drug-free, 12 were using heroin occasionally, and eight were regularly using heroin. Thirty-one per cent of the original group (excluding the five who had died) had completed treatment and were doing well. Criminal activity was only reported at the one to two-year follow-up, with only four patients having been convicted of a crime as against 29 before treatment. There is, however, a problem with a comparison of the number of offences (rather than the rate) because of the difference in the length of time covered by the pre-treatment period and the one to two years of follow-up. Dalton et al. argued that if liberal criteria were used in judging outcome, 31 of the 43 patients who could be contacted six to eight years after entering treatment were 'leading a reasonably happy and productive life'. This claim is difficult to assess, however, because the data were not well presented, and treatment drop-outs were excluded from the data.

Powell et al., (1984) described 35 patients who entered a methadone program in the A.C.T. between 1979 and 1983. No data were presented on the outcome of 11 people who had been expelled or had left the program. Five had completed the program and were opiate-free, and two had transferred to programs interstate. No outcomes were reported on the 17 patients who were currently on methadone. The authors reported that nearly all of the patients had reduced their criminal activity, but no data were presented.

Foy et al., (1989) reported a prospective one year study of 47 patients who stayed in treatment for at least two weeks in a methadone program in Newcastle. Overall, 70% of the admissions either ended in expulsion for continued illicit drug use, or the patient leaving the program. The authors report that only 14% of the patients in the program were abstinent from opioid and other illicit drugs for at least three months. This outcome may be unnecessarily pessimistic about the benefits of methadone. The average dose of methadone was 51 mg per day, and the authors acknowledge that their program policies were the probable reason for the high drop-out rate from the program. There was also a substantial rate of injecting amphetamine use among this population which was one of the major reasons for being excluded from methadone treatment.

A recent study of 16 800 urine samples collected from five Sydney methadone units during 1986 to 1987 provided evidence of continuing heroin use among a substantial number of people in methadone treatment (Lewis & Chesher, 1990). The authors classified patients from these units into three categories of heroin use: light, moderate, and heavy. The 'heavy users' were those who, at most, used heroin once or twice a week, a much lower level than the daily use which is usually implied by the term 'heavy' heroin use. The results showed that 51% of all patients were 'heavy' users whose urine samples accounted for 90% of the drug use, and hence that about half of the patients monitored during this period had no or very little heroin use. This study indicated a substantial rate of continued relatively infrequent heroin use among about half of the methadone patients in the sample. It is impossible from the data, however, to relate the heroin use to program characteristics such as methadone dose or policy towards continued drug use. As a consequence we do not know whether these results were typical of patients in all five programs or whether they were confined to patients in a small number of the programs.

Caplehorn and Bell (1991) reported a study of retention in two Sydney methadone programs that had different dosage policies. Their results showed that the lower dose program had the lower retention rate, and that the difference between programs in retention persisted after adjustment for differences in patient characteristics. Their analysis showed that the maximum dose of methadone a patient received during the first 120 days of treatment was the best predictor of retention in treatment. The relative risk of leaving treatment decreased with dose: those with a dose between 60 mg and 80 mg had half the risk of leaving treatment of those given a dose less than 60 mg, and this risk halved again for those given a dose greater than 80 mg.

Bell et al., (1992) reported a two-year follow up study of the impact of methadone maintenance on the rate of conviction for drug and property offences recorded by police. Their cohort consisted of 313 patients from the cohort reported on by Caplehorn and Bell as well as a group of 80 people who applied for methadone maintenance at the same time but who either were refused entry or failed to complete the assessment process. The results showed a lower rate of convictions in the two-year follow up among those who did not enter methadone treatment. However, the interpretation of this result was complicated because half of those who initially failed to enter treatment subsequently did so, while half of those who entered treatment spent less than 12 months in the program. When results were examined for the whole cohort, the length of time in treatment predicted the rate of both drug and property convictions in the follow up period. The rate of both drug and property convictions approximately halved for each year in treatment. Moreover, statistical analyses indicated that this result was *not* due to a higher rate of drop out among people with a high rate of convictions prior to treatment. In fact, there was a trend for people with high rates of pre-assessment conviction to be retained longer in treatment. Taken together, the results of the Caplehorn and Bell (1991) and Bell et al. (1992) studies are consistent with the results of American prospective studies in showing that the higher the methadone dose, the longer the patient's stay in treatment, and the longer the patient's stay in treatment, the greater the reduction in the rate of criminal convictions.

Australian studies provide similar results to American and other overseas studies on the effectiveness of methadone, and the characteristics of treatment that predict outcome. Although they do not provide compelling evidence for effectiveness, when taken together with the American research, they suggest that, on average, Australian methadone treatment reduces illicit opiate use and criminal activity. There is also evidence of considerable variability in program policies, the most obvious of which is average dose, with a general departure from the model of methadone maintenance originally espoused by Dole and Nyswander. The variation in policies is mirrored in variation in outcome, with some studies reporting very low rates of patient retention, and others a substantial amount of continuing heroin use. There is clearly a need for good prospective studies on the effectiveness of methadone maintenance in Australia, and on the characteristics of methadone programs and their patients that predict differences in program effectiveness.

SUMMARY

n interpreting the methadone treatment outcome literature it is reasonable to assume that the results of overseas studies are relevant to the Australian context. The major difference between American and Australian treatment populations is in ethnic composition, the importance of which is diminished by the consistent findings from randomised controlled clinical trials in three different cultural contexts. Although there are variations in policies and outcomes between Australian methadone programs, this is probably similar to the variations observed between programs in the major American multi-centre studies. In addition, the relationships observed between program characteristics and treatment outcome has been similar in both the USA and Australia.

The few outcome studies of methadone treatment carried out in Australia are difficult to interpret because of the lack of data that either compares patients outcomes with their pretreatment performance, or with that of opioid addicts who did not receive treatment. There is, nonetheless, suggestive evidence that the time spent in Australian methadone programs is associated with a reduction in opiate use (Reynolds & Magro, 1976), and that methadone dosage is an important predictor of retention in treatment (Caplehorn & Bell, 1991; Reynolds et al., 1976; Waters et al., 1975). In addition, methadone programs which use low doses of methadone (Caplehorn & Bell, 1991; Foy et al, 1989) have higher treatment drop-out rates. Until such time as better designed Australian studies have been conducted, it is reasonable to assume that the American results can be extrapolated to Australia.

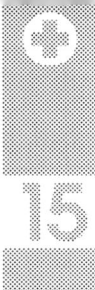

CONCLUSIONS

In this chapter the evidence reviewed in each of the previous chapters is summarised and its implications briefly discussed. First, an overall statement is made about the effectiveness of methadone maintenance as a treatment for opioid dependence. Second, general statements are made about some of the features of methadone maintenance programs which explain the variation in their effectiveness in retaining patients, and reducing drug use and criminality. Third, priorities for research on methadone maintenance treatment in Australia are outlined. The chapter concludes with a statement about the role of methadone maintenance in the treatment of opioid dependence in Australia.

AN OVERALL APPRAISAL OF EFFECTIVENESS

An overall evaluation of the effectiveness of methadone maintenance has been reached by examining the degree to which the observational and experimental evidence satisfies a modified set of criteria which were originally suggested by Hill (1965, 1977) as a way of making inferences about disease aetiology from observational data. These criteria were used by the USA Surgeon General in drawing the conclusion that cigarette smoking was a cause of lung cancer. They can be readily adapted to the task of making analogous causal inferences about treatment effectiveness. Although no single one of these criteria is necessary, the more of them that are met, the greater our confidence that a causal relationship exists between treatment and outcome.

Strength of association

Relationships that are strong indicate that the outcome of treatment is highly predictable. They are generally more deserving of trust than those based on a weak relationship because stronger relationships are less open to alternative explanations, such as assessment or selection bias, than are weaker ones.

The relationship between methadone maintenance and a reduction in both illicit opioid use and criminal behaviour is, on average, a reasonably strong one. The rate of each approximately halves with each year that a patient remains in treatment. The relationship between methadone and outcome is strongest in the small number of randomised controlled trials that compare its effectiveness with little or no treatment.

Consistency

A relationship is consistent if it is observed in studies conducted by different investigators, using different study methods, in different populations. Relationships that are consistent are less likely to be due to sampling error and methods of study.

A relationship between methadone treatment and reduced drug use and criminal behaviour has been consistently observed in controlled trials, quasi-experimental studies, comparative studies, and pre-post-studies in the USA, Sweden, and Hong Kong. The same relationship has been observed in a limited number of studies in Australia. This relationship is most consistent in studies of programs that use doses above 60 mg and which have maintenance as their treatment goal.

Specificity

Specificity exists when the relationship between treatment and outcome is such that if treatment is given, the outcome occurs, and if the outcome is observed, then one can confidently infer that treatment has been given. This criterion is desirable in that, if it exists, it suggests that there is a strong relationship between treatment and outcome. But it is not necessary in that its absence does not exclude the possibility that treatment makes a contribution to a good outcome.

A degree of specificity is evident in the relationship between methadone treatment and outcome. Its effects are most evident on those outcomes it has been designed to change: opioid use and criminal behaviour motivated by the need to finance illicit opioid use. Its effects are less marked on other outcomes such as non-opioid illicit drug use (e.g. cocaine and amphetamine) and vocational adjustment, unless this is specifically addressed in the program, as was the case in the Swedish methadone program.

A dose-response relationship

A dose-response relationship between exposure to treatment and outcome (for example, the longer the time in treatment, the more intensive the treatment) is desirable. Such a relationship increases confidence that there are some specific treatment components that are responsible for the benefits of treatment.

A dose-response relationship between methadone maintenance and reduced opioid use and criminality is shown in three ways. First, there is a relationship between the dose of methadone received and treatment retention and outcome. Both within individual programs and between programs, the higher the dose of methadone, the longer the retention in treatment and the better the outcome in terms of reduced drug use and criminal behaviour. Secondly, there is a relationship between treatment duration and benefit: the longer patients remain in treatment, the better the outcome. This relationship does not appear to be explained by a higher retention rate among patients who have a good prognosis. Thirdly, there is suggestive evidence that the strength of the relationship between methadone treatment and outcome also varies with the fidelity with which the Dole and Nyswander model of treatment has been implemented. That is, demonstrated effectiveness decreases to the degree that methadone moves away from the high dose *maintenance* treatment with extensive ancillary services initiated by Dole and Nyswander towards low dose programs which often aim to achieve abstinence within a period of several years.

Plausibility

A relationship is plausible if it is consistent with other relevant knowledge, such as, for example, the mechanisms of addiction. The consonance of a relationship with such mechanisms enhances our confidence in it.

The rationale for the effectiveness of methadone maintenance is plausible. Opioid dependence is characterised by an overweening preoccupation with the procurement of illicit opioid drugs to the detriment of the user's health and well-being. The provision of a legal opioid drug (methadone), in doses which avert withdrawal and reduce the positive effects of illicit opioid use, reduces the salience of opioid use and the necessity for users to spend most of their daily existence in the pursuit of opioid drugs.

Coherence

A relationship is coherent if it makes sense of other information about the natural history of the condition. The evidence on the effects of methadone maintenance is coherent with what is known about the natural history of opioid drug use: by the time patients present for treatment they have a long history of opioid use so it takes time for methadone maintenance to achieve its benefits; opioid dependence is a chronic condition with a high rate of relapse, so the effects of methadone maintenance treatment appear to last only while people remain in treatment.

Experiment

Although there is limited experimental evidence of the effectiveness of methadone maintenance, it is consistently positive. There are only three controlled trials of comprehensive methadone maintenance over periods of a year or more (Dole et al., 1969; Newman & Whitehill, 1979; Gunne & Grönbladh, 1981), all involving small numbers of patients and conducted in three very different cultural settings. All provide evidence of substantial differences in outcome on opioid drug use and crime that favours methadone maintenance treatment.

SOME CAVEATS

Taken as a whole, the evidence provides good reasons for believing that methadone maintenance is an effective form of treatment for opioid dependence *on average*. The phrase 'on average' implies a number of caveats that need to be spelt out.

First, methadone is not a panacea for heroin dependence. On average, about half of those who enter treatment either leave or are discharged for continued illicit drug use within 12 months, and a substantial but variable proportion of those who stay in treatment continue to use heroin and other illicit drugs, albeit at much reduced rates.

These outcomes will be regarded as 'poor' if judged by the unrealistic expectation that all patients should achieve enduring abstinence from all opioid drugs, a standard implicitly demanded of methadone maintenance by some of its critics. In evaluating the treatment of heroin dependence, we need to compare the outcome of methadone treatment with what would have happened without it (Gerstein & Harwood, 1990). If this is done, it becomes apparent that methadone maintenance is the best of the available alternatives. Other forms of treatment attract and retain fewer patients, and do not produce superior outcomes among those who complete treatment; and a failure to provide any sort of treatment carries a high risk of premature mortality and serious morbidity for users, and high social and economic costs to the community (Collins & Lapsley, 1991; Gerstein & Harwood, 1990).

Second, different methadone programs vary in their policies and in their effectiveness in reducing drug use and criminal acts. The factors responsible for this variability are not well understood, although the available evidence strongly suggests that they include the dose of methadone given, the duration of treatment, and the characteristics of the patients in the programs. Other relevant factors probably include the quality of the therapeutic relationships between patients and staff, and the intensiveness of ancillary services.

Third, the most effective methadone programs are those that resemble the model introduced by Dole and Nyswander, namely, higher doses of methadone in the context of a comprehensive treatment program with maintenance rather than abstinence as a treatment goal. The effectiveness is much less certain for programs that reduce methadone dose and impose abstinence from methadone as a treatment goal. Indeed, there is no good evidence that such programs are effective in achieving the goal of abstinence among a substantial proportion of patients within one to two years. Uncertainty also exists about the effectiveness of the newer low-threshold and low-intervention programs (which lower the admission criteria, reduce ancillary services, and reduce the expectation that patients will decrease their heroin use) which are proposed as a way of preventing the transmission of HIV by needle sharing and unsafe sexual behaviour.

Fourth, the benefits of methadone maintenance continue only as long as patients remain in treatment. Patients who discontinue treatment relapse to opioid use at a high rate. There have been very few studies of people who have successfully 'graduated' from methadone programs to indicate whether planned attempts at withdrawal and rehabilitation are more likely to succeed.

RESEARCH PRIORITIES

The available information on program policies, procedures and outcomes suggests that a substantial proportion of methadone maintenance programs in Australia and the USA provide sub-optimal treatment. Such programs appear to use inadequate doses of methadone for an arbitrarily limited period with the aim of achieving enduring abstinence from all opioid drugs, including methadone. From the point of view of improving existing methadone programs, a research priority is to provide better descriptions of existing programs, and better evaluations of their effectiveness, as measured by their ability to retain patients in treatment, to reduce drug use and criminal behaviour, and to improve the health and well-being of patients while they are in treatment. The effect of the recent increases in the availability of methadone maintenance and changes in policies in response to HIV also need to be critically examined.

A number of research priorities follow from the conclusion that the most effective form of methadone treatment is potentially indefinite *maintenance* using an adequate dose of methadone (see Chapter 6). If this model were to be widely implemented then some individuals now entering treatment would be maintained on methadone for lengthy periods. This would accelerate the rate of the number of patients on methadone maintenance, which has been steadily increasing over the past seven years (see Figure 3 in Chapter 14).

The increasing number of patients enrolled in methadone maintenance programs has important policy implications. It is unlikely that the community will continue to fund the indefinite expansion of methadone maintenance treatment based on the Dole and Nyswander (1967) model, especially during times of economic recession. Hard decisions will have to be made, and sensible methods found to efficiently and equitably rations limited treatment resources. The gravity and difficulty of this task may be heightened by the possibility that the prevalence of HIV among injecting drug users will slowly but steadily increase.

Ideally, the rationing of methadone maintenance places should be informed by credible estimates of the costs and benefits of methadone maintenance and other forms of treatment for people who are opioid-dependent. Crude estimates of the costs of methadone maintenance suggests that it costs about $3000 per patient per year, a figure that may at first sight seem expensive. The community may be more likely to support such expenditure if it were better informed about the economic costs of *not* treating opioid dependence (illness, criminal behaviour, foregone earnings capacity, etc.), and the economic benefits of providing methadone maintenance and other forms of treatment, as against increasing expenditure on law enforcement, and the legal and correctional systems.

A good start has been made by Collins and Lapsley (1991) at estimating the tangible and intangible economic costs of illicit drug dependence in Australia. This study indicated that the tangible and intangible costs of all illicit drug use were of the order of $1.44 billion, compared with $6.03 billion for alcohol and $6.84 billion for tobacco. The estimated net cost to the Federal budget of illicit drugs was $281.9 million compared with $623 million for alcohol and $104.6 million for tobacco. The authors stressed that all these cost estimates were conservative because of the absence of essential information on the impact of alcohol and other drug use on productivity. In addition, the lack of and the poor quality of data on illicit drug use did not enable the economic costs of opioid and other forms of illicit drug dependence to be distinguished. In the light of these cost estimates, good economic appraisals of the costs and benefits of methadone maintenance and other forms of treatment for opioid dependence are a high research priority.

From the perspective of practitioners, methadone maintenance research must focus on more efficient ways of providing treatment to as many opioid dependent people as possible. Researchers need to investigate better ways of matching patients to treatment and more imaginative methods of reducing the cost of methadone maintenance treatment without impairing its effectiveness. One popular suggestion has been to 'stream' patients within existing programs by matching the entry criteria and the level of intervention to the patients' goals. For example, 'harm-reduction' programs may provide maintenance doses of methadone and little or no ancillary services to patients who do not want a comprehensive program. This would reduce needle sharing and other behaviour that puts the drug user at risk of contracting or transmitting HIV. On the other hand, for patients who want to discontinue opioid use, this proposal recommends more traditional comprehensive methadone maintenance programs; and for patients who have achieved stable long-term maintenance, the intensity of intervention and surveillance of drug use could be reduced by transferring their management to suitably trained medical practitioners.

Clinical research is also needed to improve the post-methadone outcome of patients who wish to stop taking methadone, whether it is after many years of stable maintenance or earlier on in the course of their treatment. This may be accomplished, for example, by the development of structured after-care programs within existing methadone maintenance programs, or by improved co-operation between methadone maintenance and drug-free treatment programs. Exploring ways of identifying and treating psychiatric comorbidity among methadone patients is also a research priority because of the impact that psychiatric disorders have on the outcome of methadone maintenance.

All of these suggestions for modifications to methadone maintenance aim to increase its effectiveness by increasing the number of people to whom it is provided. The challenge is to do this in such a way that the effectiveness of methadone maintenance treatment is not impaired by the proliferation of less effective forms of maintenance treatment as has happened over the first 25 years of its history. The best way of doing so is to ensure that all new programs of methadone maintenance are independently evaluated from the time of their introduction.

A FINAL NOTE

This book originated with a request from the New South Wales State Government to review the research literature on methadone maintenance in order to formulate a policy which was based (as much as possible) on evidence. In the process of undertaking this task we became aware that methadone maintenance is unique in the way in which it is regarded by politicians, health administrators, health care providers, and the general community. As Newman (1991) has recently noted, methadone maintenance treatment continues to be regarded as an 'illegitimate' or questionable type of intervention, despite the fact that it achieves its objectives and meets the needs of both its patients and the community in managing opioid dependence and minimising old (hepatitis and overdose deaths) and new risks to health (HIV).

In the light of the evidence for its effectiveness, it is unacceptable that methadone maintenance treatment continues to have to justify its existence when less well evaluated and supported forms of alcohol and drug treatment are publicly funded. It is similarly unacceptable that its fate continues to be affected by the views of those in the community who continue to insist upon the unattainable treatment goal of abstinence in the absence of effective methods of achieving it. We believe that the available evidence suggests that the public provision of methadone maintenance treatment has economic benefits for the community. Even if it did not, the community has a moral responsibility to provide access to effective treatment for those who become dependent on opioid drugs and request assistance in overcoming their dependence.

BIBLIOGRAPHY

Abdul-Quader, A.S., Friedman, S.R., Des Jarlais, D., Marmor, M.M., Maslansky, R., & Bartelme, S. (1987) Methadone maintenance and behavior by intravenous drug users that can transmit HIV. *Contemporary Drug Problems, 14*, 425–434.

Abrahms, J.L. (1979) A cognitive-behavioural versus nondirective group treatment program for opioid-addicted persons: An adjunct to methadone maintenance. *International Journal of the Addictions, 14*, 503–511.

Aiken, L.S., LoSciuto, L.A., Ausetts, M.A. & Brown, B.S. (1984a) Paraprofessional versus professional drug counsellors: Diverse routes to the same role. *International Journal of the Addictions, 19*, 153–173.

Aiken, L.S., LoSciuto, L.A., Ausetts, M.A. & Brown, B.S. (1984b) Paraprofessional versus professional drug counsellors: The progress of clients in treatment. *International Journal of the Addictions, 19*, 383–401.

American Psychiatric Association. (1987) *Diagnostic and Statistical Manual of Mental Disorders (DSM-III-R).* (3rd Edition, Revised) Washington: American Psychiatric Association.

Andrews, G., Armstrong, M.S., Brodaty, H., Hall, W., Harvey, P.R., & Tennant, C.C. (1982) Preparing outlines of current treatments in psychiatry. *Australian Clinical Review*, June, 20–22.

Andrews, H.L. & Himmelsbach, C.K. (1944) Relation of the intensity of the morphine abstinence syndrome to dosage. *Journal of Pharmacology and Experimental Therapeutics, 81*, 288–293.

Anglin, M.D. (1988) The efficacy of civil commitment in treating narcotic addiction.

In C.G. Leukefeld & F.M. Tims (Eds), *Compulsory Treatment of Drug Abuse: Research and Clinical Practice*. NIDA Research Monograph 86. Maryland: National Institute on Drug Abuse.

Anglin, M.D., & McGlothlin, W.H. (1984) Outcome of narcotic addict treatment in California. In F.M. Tims & J.P. Ludford (Eds), *Drug Abuse Treatment Evaluation: Strategies, Progress, and Prospects*. NIDA Research Monograph, 51. Maryland: National Institute on Drug Abuse.

Anglin, M.D., Speckart, G.R., Booth, M.W., & Ryan, T.M. (1989) Consequences and costs of shutting off methadone. *Addictive Behaviors, 14*, 302–326.

Attewell, P. & Gerstein, D.R. (1979) Government policy and local practice. *American Sociological Review, 44*, 311–327.

Australian Social Issues Research. (1991) *A Descriptive Study of New South Wales Public Methadone Clinics*. Report prepared for the Drug & Alcohol Directorate, New South Wales Department of Health, Australia.

Aylett, P. (1982) Methadone dose assessment in heroin addiction. *International Journal of the Addictions, 17*, 1329–1336.

Baekeland, F. & Lundwall, L. (1975) Dropping out of treatment: A critical review. *Psychological Bulletin, 82*, 738–783.

Baillie, A.J., Webster, P. & Mattick, R.P. (1991) *National Survey of Treatment Procedures for Opiate Users*. NDARC Working Paper No. 5. Sydney: National Drug & Alcohol Research Centre.

Baker, A. & Dixon, J. (1991) Motivational interviewing for HIV risk reduction. In W.R. Miller & S. Rollnick (Eds), *Motivational Interviewing: Preparing People to Change Addictive Behavior*. U.S.A.: Guilford.

Baker, A., Heather, N., & Wodak, A. (1991) The application of self-control strategies to reducing HIV risk-taking behaviour in intravenous drug users. In N. Heather, W.R. Miller, & J. Greeley (Eds), *Self-control in the Addictive Behaviours*. Melbourne: Maxwell Macmillan.

Baldwin, R. (1987) The cost of methadone maintenance programs: A comparison between public hospital clinics and private practitioner programs in New South Wales. *Australian Drug and Alcohol Review, 6*, 185–193.

Bale, R.N., Van Stone, W.W., Kuldau, J.M., Engelsing, T.M.J., Elashoff, R.M., & Zarcone, V.P. (1980) Therapeutic communities vs methadone maintenance. A prospective controlled study of narcotic addiction treatment: Design and one-year follow-up. *Archives of General Psychiatry, 37*, 179–193.

Ball, J.C. & Ross, A. (1991) *The Effectiveness of Methadone Maintenance Treatment: Patients, Programs, Services, and Outcome*. New York: Springer-Verlag.

Ball, J.C., Lange, W.R., Myers, C.P., & Friedman, S.R. (1988) Reducing the risk of AIDS through methadone maintenance treatment. *Journal of Health and Social Behavior, 29*, 214–226.

Batey, R.G., Patterson, T. & Sanders, F. (1990) Practical issues in the methadone management of pregnant heroin users. *Drug and Alcohol Review, 9*, 303–310.

Batki, S.L., Sorensen, J.L., Faltz, B., & Madover, S. (1988) Psychiatric aspects of treatment of IV drug users with AIDS. *Hospital and Community Psychiatry, 39*, 439–443.

Becker, M.H., & Joseph, J.G. (1988) AIDS and behavioral change to reduce risk: A review. *American Journal of Public Health, 78*, 394–410.

Bell, J. (1990) The influence of assessment process on retention in a methadone program. Paper presented to National Methadone Conference, Sydney, Australia.

Bell, J, Batey, R.G., Farrell, G.C., Crewe, E.B., Cunningham, A.L. & Byth, K., (1990c) Hepatitis C virus in intravenous drug users. *Medical Journal of Australia, 153*, 274–276.

Bell, J., Bowron, P., Lewis, J., & Batey, R. (1990b) Serum levels of methadone in maintenance clients who persist in illicit drug use. *British Journal of Addiction, 85*, 1599–1602.

Bell, J., Digiusto, E. & Byth, K. (in press) Who should receive methadone maintenance? *British Journal of Addiction.*

Bell, J., Fernandes, D. & Batey, R. (1990a) Heroin users seeing methadone treatment. *Medical Journal of Australia, 152,* 361–364.

Bell, J. Hall, W. & Byth, K. (1992) Changes in criminal activity after entering methadone maintenance. *British Journal of Addiction, 87,* 251–258.

Bell, J., Seres, V., Bowron, P., Lewis, J., & Batey, R. (1988) The use of serum methadone levels in patients receiving methadone maintenance. *Clinical Pharmacology and Therapeutics, 43,* 623–629.

Bellis, D.J. (1990) Fear of AIDS and risk reduction among heroin-addicted female prostitutes: Personal interviews with 72 southern California subjects: *Journal of Alcohol and Drug Education, 35* (3), 26–37.

Benet, L.Z. & Sheiner, L.B. (1985) Pharmacokinetics: The dynamics of drug absorption, distribution, and elimination. In A.G. Gilman, L.S. Goodman, & F. Murad (Eds), *The Pharmacological Basis of Therapeutics.* (7th Edition) USA: Macmillan.

Berken, G.H., Stone, M.M. & Stone, S.K. (1978) Methadone in schizophrenic rage: A case study. *American Journal of Psychiatry, 135,* 248–249.

Berridge, V. (1990) Comments on Stimson's 'AIDS and HIV'. AIDS and HIV: The historical perspective. *British Journal of Addiction, 85,* 343–344.

Berry, G.J. (1972) Dose-related responses to methadone, including placebo therapy. In Proceedings of the Fourth National Conference on Methadone Treatment. New York: National Association for the Prevention of Addiction to Narcotics.

Berry, G.J. & Kuhn, K.L. (1973) Dose-related response to methadone: Reduction of maintenance dose. In Proceedings of the Fifth National Conference on Methadone Treatment. New York: National Association for the Prevention of Addiction to Narcotics.

Bickel, W.K., Higgins, S.T., & Stitzer, M.L. (1986) Choice of blind methadone dose increases by methadone maintenance patients. *Drug and Alcohol Dependence, 18,* 165–171.

Blachly, P.H. (1973) Naloxone for diagnosis in methadone programs. *Journal of the American Medical Association, 224,* 334–335.

Blackburn, R. (1988) On moral judgements and personality disorders: The myth of psychopathic personality revisited. *British Journal of Psychiatry, 153,* 505–512.

Blanke, R.V. (1986) Accuracy in urinalysis. In R.L. Hawks & C.N. Chiang, (Eds), *Urine Testing for Drugs of Abuse.* NIDA Research Monograph 73. Maryland: National Institute on Drug Abuse.

Blix, O. & Grönbladh, L. (1988) AIDS and IV heroin addicts: The preventive effect of methadone maintenance in Sweden. Paper presented to 4th International Conference on AIDS, Stockholm, 1988.

Blum, K. (1984) *Handbook of Abusable Drugs.* USA: Gardner Press.

Borkovec, T.D. (1990) Control groups and comparison groups in psychotherapy outcome research. In L.S. Onken & J.D. Blaine (Eds), *Psychotherapy and Counseling in the Treatment of Drug Abuse.* NIDA Research Monograph 104. Maryland: National Institute on Drug Abuse.

Bracy, S.A., & Simpson, D.D. (1982–83) Status of opioid addicts 5 years after admission to drug abuse treatment. *American Journal of Drug and Alcohol Abuse, 9,* 115–127.

Brockmeyer, N.H., Mertins, L. & Goos, M. (1991) Pharmacokinetic interaction of antimicrobial agents with levomethadon in drug-addicted AIDS patients. *Klinische Wochenschrift, 69,* 16–18.

Brooner, R.K., Bigelow, G.E., Strain, E., & Schmidt, C.W. (1990) Intravenous drug abusers with antisocial personality disorder: Increased HIV risk behavior. *Drug and Alcohol Dependence, 26,* 39–44.

Bross, I. (1967) Pertinency of an extraneous variable. *Journal of Chronic Diseases, 20,* 487–495.

Brown, B., & Beschner, G. (1989) AIDS and HIV infection — implications for drug abuse treatment. *Journal of Drug Issues, 19,* 141–162.

Brown, B.S., Jansen, D.R. & Benn, G.J. (1975) Changes in attitude toward methadone. *Archives of General Psychiatry, 32,* 214–218.

Brown, B.S., Watters, J.K. & Iglehart, A.S. (1982–83) Methadone maintenance dosage levels and program retention. *American Journal of Drug and Alcohol Abuse, 9,* 129–139.

Brown, L.S., Chu, A., Nemoto, T., Ajuluchukwu, D. & Primm, B.J. (1989a) Human immunodeficiency virus infection in a cohort of intravenous drug users in New York City: Demographic, behavioral, and clinical features. *New York State Journal of Medicine, 89,* 506–510.

Brown L.S., Mitchell, J.L., DeVore, S.L. & Primm, B.J. (1989b) Female intravenous drug users and perinatal HIV transmission. *New England Journal of Medicine, 320,* 1493–1494.

Buning, E.C., Van Brussel, G.H.A. & Van Stanten, G.V. (1990) The 'methadone by bus' project in Amsterdam. *British Journal of Addiction, 85,* 1247–1250.

Burgess, P.M, Gill, A.J., Pead, J. & Holman, C.P. (1990) Methadone: Old problems for new programmes. *Drug and Alcohol Review, 9,* 61–66.

Burgess, P.M., Stripp, A.M., Pead, J. & Holman, C.P. (1989) Severity of opiate dependence in an Australian sample: Further validation of the SODQ. *British Journal of Addiction, 84,* 1451–1459.

Calsyn, D.A. & Saxon, A.J. (1987) A system for uniform application of contingencies for illicit drug use. *Journal of Substance Abuse Treatment, 4,* 41–47.

Calsyn, D. A., Saxon, A. J., Blaes, P., & Lee-Meyer, S. (1990) Staffing patterns of American methadone maintenance programs. *Journal of Substance Abuse Treatment, 7,* 255–259.

Calsyn, D.A., Saxon, A.J. & Barndt, C. (1991b) Urine screening practices in methadone maintenance clinics: A survey of how the results are used. *Journal of Nervous and Mental Disease, 179,* 222–227.

Calsyn, D.A., Saxon, A.J., Freeman, G. & Whittaker, S. (1991a) Needle-use practices among intravenous drug users in an area where needle purchase is legal. *AIDS, 5,* 187–193.

Campbell, C.A. (1990) Women with AIDS. *Social Sciences and Medicine, 30,* 407–415.

Caplehorn, J.R.M., Bell, J., Kleinbaum, D.G. & Gebski, V.J. (forthcoming) Methadone dose and heroin use during maintenance treatment.

Caplehorn, J.R.M., McNeil, D.R. & Kleinbaum, D.G. (in press) Clinic policy and retention in methadone maintenance. *International Journal of the Addictions.*

Caplehorn, J.R.M. (1992) A comparison of private and public methadone maintenance patients. *Drug and Alcohol Review, 11,* 43–49.

Caplehorn, J.R.M. & Bell, J. (1991) Methadone dosage and retention of patients in maintenance treatment. *Medical Journal of Australia, 154,* 195–199.

Celum, C.L., Coombs, R.W., Lafferty, W., Inui, T.S., Louie, P.H., Gates, C.A., McCreedy, B.J., Egan, R., Grove, T., Alexander, S., Koepsell, T., Weiss, N., Fisher, L., Corey, L. & Holmes, K.K. (1991) Indeterminate human immunodeficiency virus type 1 Western blots: Seroconversion risk, specificity of supplemental tests, and an algorithm for evaluation. *Journal of Infectious Diseases, 164,* 656–664.

Chadwick, E.G. (1988) AIDS in pregnancy and the newborn. In I.J. Chasnoff (Ed), *Drugs, Alcohol, Pregnancy and Parenting.* London: Kluwer.

Chaisson, R.E., Bacchetti, P., Osmond, D., Brodie, B., Sande, M.A., & Moss, A.R. (1989) Cocaine use and HIV infection in intravenous drug users in San Francisco. *Journal of the American Medical Association, 261,* 561–565.

Charney, D.S., Heninger, G.R. & Kleber, H.D. (1986) The combined use of clonidine and naltrexone as a rapid, safe, and effective treatment of abrupt withdrawal from methadone. *American Journal of Psychiatry, 143,* 831–837.

Chavkin, W. (1990) Drug addiction and pregnancy: Policy crossroads. *American Journal of Public Health, 80,* 483–487.

Christie, K.A., Burke Jr., J.D., Regier, D.A., Rae, D.S., Boyd, J.H. & Locke, B.Z. (1988) Epidemiologic evidence for early onset of mental disorders and higher risk of drug abuse in young adults. *American Journal of Psychiatry, 145*, 971–975.

Chu, A., Brown, L.S., Banks, S., Nemoto, T., & Primm, B.J. (1989) Intravenous heroin use: Its association with HIV infection in patients in methadone treatment. In L.S. Harris (Ed), *Problems of Drug Dependence 1989*. NIDA Research Monograph, 95, 447–448.

Cole, S.G. & James, L.R. (1975) A revised treatment typology based on the DARP. *American Journal of Drug & Alcohol Abuse, 2*, 37–49.

Coleman, S.B. & Davis, D.I. (1978) Family therapy and drug abuse: A national survey. *Family Process, 17*, 21–29.

Collins, D.J. & Lapsley, H.M. (1991) *Estimating the Economic Costs of Drug Abuse in Australia*, National Campaign Against Drug Abuse Monograph Series No. 15. Canberra: Australian Government Publishing Service.

Collins, E. (1990) Outcomes for the children of mothers who used heroin/methadone during pregnancy. Paper presented to National Methadone Conference, Sydney, 1990.

Collins, E. (1991) Drugs in Pregnancy Service (DIPS) Women. Sydney: Drugs in Pregnancy Service, King George V Hospital.

Collins, E. (1992) Pregnancy. Paper presented to 1992 National Methadone Conference, Sydney.

Collins, E. & Capus, C. (1991) Human immunodeficiency virus (HIV) & hepatitis status of pregnant drug dependent women. Paper presented at 9th Australian Perinatal Society Annual Congress, Melbourne, 1991.

Commonwealth Department of Community Services and Health. (1988) *National Methadone Guidelines*. Canberra: Australian Government Publishing Service.

Commonwealth Department of Community Services and Health. (1991) *National Methadone Guidelines*. Canberra: Australian Government Publishing Service.

Cook, T. D. and Campbell, D.T. (1979) *Quasi-Experimentation: Design and Analysis Issues for Field Settings*. Chicago: Rand McNally.

Cooper, J.R. (1989) Methadone treatment and acquired immunodeficiency syndrome. *Journal of the American Medical Association, 262*, 1664–1668.

Cooper, J.R., Altman, F., Brown, B.S. & Czechowicz, D. (Eds), (1983c) *Research on the Treatment of Narcotic Addiction: State of the Art*. Maryland: NIDA, U.S. Department of Health and Human Sciences.

Cooper, J.R., Altman, F. & Keeley, K. (1983a) Discussion summary [of Judson & Goldstein, Uses of Naloxone in the diagnosis and treatment of heroin addiction]. In J.R. Cooper, F. Altman, B.S. Brown, & D. Czechowicz (Eds), *Research on the Treatment of Narcotic Addiction: State of the Art*. Maryland: NIDA, U.S. Department of Health and Human Sciences.

Cooper, J.R., Altman, F., & Keeley, K. (1983b) Discussion summary [of W.A. Hargreaves, Methadone dosage and duration for maintenance treatment]. In J.R. Cooper, F. Altman, B.S. Brown, & D. Czechowicz (Eds), *Research on the Treatment of Narcotic Addiction: State of the Art*. Maryland: NIDA, U.S. Department of Health and Human Sciences.

Corty, E., Ball, J.C. & Myers, C.P. (1988) Psychological symptoms in methadone maintenance patients: Prevalence and change over treatment. *Journal of Consulting and Clinical Psychology, 56*, 776–777.

Craig, R.J. (1980) Effectiveness of low-dose methadone maintenance for the treatment of inner city heroin addicts. *International Journal of the Addictions, 15*, 701–710.

Crits-Christoph, P., Beebe, K.L. & Connolly, M.B. (1990) Therapist effects in the treatment of drug dependence: Implications for conducting comparative treatment studies. In L.S. Onken & J.D. Blaine (Eds), *Psychotherapy and Counseling in the Treatment of Drug Abuse*. NIDA Research Monograph 104. Maryland: National Institute on Drug Abuse.

Croughan, J.L., Miller, J.P., Wagelin, D. & Whitman, B.Y. (1982) Psychiatric illnesses in male and female narcotic addicts. *Journal of Clinical Psychiatry, 43*, 225–228.

Curet, E., Langrod, J., Page, J., & Lowinson, J.H. (1985) Issues of transference in methadone maintenance treatment. *International Journal of the Addictions, 20*, 435–448.

Cushman, P. (1978a) Abstinence following detoxification and methadone maintenance treatment. *American Journal of Medicine, 65*, 46–52.

Cushman, P. (1978b) Methadone maintenance: Long-term follow-up of detoxified patients. *Annals of the New York Academy of Sciences, 311*, 165–172.

Cushman, P. (1981) Detoxification after methadone treatment. In J.H. Lowinson & P. Ruiz (Eds), *Substance Abuse: Clinical Problems and Perspectives*. U.S.A.: Williams & Wilkins.

Cushman, P. & Dole, V.P. (1973) Detoxification of rehabilitated methadone-maintained patients. *Journal of the American Medical Association 226*, 747–752.

D'Amanda, C. (1983) Program policies and procedures associated with treatment outcome. In J.R. Cooper, F. Altman, B.S. Brown, & D. Czechowicz (Eds), *Research on the Treatment of Narcotic Addiction: State of the Art*. Maryland: NIDA, U.S. Department of Health and Human Sciences.

D'Aunno, T. & Vaughn, T.E. (1992) Variations in methadone treatment practices: Results from a national study. *Journal of the American Medical Association, 267*, 253–258.

Dalton, M.S., & Duncan, D. (1979) Fifty opiate addicts treated with methadone blockade. Eight year follow up. *Medical Journal of Australia, 1*, 153–154.

Dalton, M.S., Duncan, D., & Taylor, N. (1976) Methadone blockade in the treatment of opiate addiction: A follow-up study. *Medical Journal of Australia, 5*, 755.

Darke, S. (in press) Injecting drug users and the Human Immunodeficiency Virus: What do we know? *Drug and Alcohol Review*.

Darke S., Baker, A., Dixon, J., Wodak, A. & Heather, N. (1992) Drug use and HIV risk-taking behaviour among clients in methadone maintenance treatment. *Drug and Alcohol Dependence, 29*, 263–268.

Darke, S., Hall, W., & Carless, J. (1990) Drug use, injecting practices and sexual behaviour of opioid users in Sydney, Australia. *British Journal of Addiction, 85*, 1603–1609.

Darke, S., Hall, W., Heather, N. & Ward, J. (1992a) Development and validation of a multi-dimensional instrument for assessing outcome of treatment among opiate users: The Opiate Treatment Index. *British Journal of Addiction*.

Darke, S., Hall, W., Heather, N., Ward, J., & Wodak, A. (1991) The reliability and validity of a scale to measure HIV risk-taking behaviour among intravenous drug users. *AIDS, 5*, 181–185.

Darke, S., Hall, W., Ross, M. & Wodak, A. (forthcoming) Benzodiazepine use and HIV risk-taking behaviour among injecting drug users.

Darke, S., Wodak, A., Hall, W., Heather, N. & Ward, J. (in press) Prevalence and predictors of psychopathology among opioid users. *British Journal of Addiction*.

Dawes, R.M., Faust, D. & Meehl, P.E. (1989) Clinical versus actuarial judgment. *Science, 243*, 1668–1674.

De Angelis, G.G. (1972) Testing for drugs — advantages and disadvantages. *International Journal of the Addictions, 7*, 365–385.

Deren, S. (1986) Children of substance abusers: A review of the literature. *Journal of Substance Abuse Treatment, 3*, 77–94.

Des Jarlais, D.C. (1992a) The first and second decades of AIDS among injecting drug users. *British Journal of Addiction, 87*, 347–353.

Des Jarlais, D.C. (1992b) Methadone and prevention the spread of HIV infection. A global perspective. Paper presented at the 1992 National Methadone Conference, Sydney, Australia, March 1992.

Des Jarlais, D.C., Abdul-Quader, A. & Tross, S. (1991) The next problem: Maintenance of AIDS risk reduction among intravenous drug users. *International*

Journal of the Addictions, 26, 1279–1292.

Des Jarlais, D.C., Friedman, S.R., & Casriel, C. (1990) Target groups for preventing AIDS among intravenous drug users: 2. The "hard" data studies. *Journal of Consulting and Clinical Psychology, 58,* 50–56.

Des Jarlais, D.C., Friedman, S.R., Novick, D.M., Sotheran, J.L., Thomas, P., Yancovitz, S.R., Mildvan, D., Weber, J., Kreek, M.J., Maslansky, R., Bartelme, S., Spira, T., & Marmor, M. (1989) HIV-1 infection among intravenous drug users in Manhattan, New York City, from 1977 through 1987. *Journal of the American Medical Association, 261,* 1008–1012.

Des Jarlais, D.C., Joseph, H. & Dole, V.P. (1981) Long-term outcomes after termination from methadone maintenance treatment. *Annals of the New York Academy of Sciences, 362,* 231–238.

Desmond, D.P. & Maddux, J.F. (1983) Optional versus mandatory psychotherapy in methadone maintenance. *International Journal of the Addictions, 18,* 281–290.

Doberczak, T.M., Thornton, J.C., Bernstein, J. & Kandall, S.R. (1987) Impact of maternal drug dependency on birth weight and head circumference of offspring. *American Journal of Diseases of Children, 141,* 1163–1167.

Dobinson, I. & Ward, P. (1985) *Drugs and Crime: A Survey of N.S.W. Prison Property Offenders 1984.* Sydney: Bureau of Crime Statistics & Research, Department of the Attorney General and of Justice.

Dobinson, I. & Ward, P. (1987) *Drugs and Crime — Phase II: A Study of Individuals Seeking Drug Treatment.* Sydney: N.S.W. Bureau of Crime Statistics and Research, Attorney General's Department.

Dolan, M.P., Black, J.L., Deford, H.A., Skinner, J.R., & Robinowitz, R. (1987) Characteristics of drug abusers that discriminate needle-sharers. *Public Health Reports, 102,* 395–398.

Dole, V.P. (1988) Implications of methadone maintenance for theories of narcotic addiction. *Journal of the American Medical Association, 260,* 3025–3029.

Dole, V.P. (1989) Methadone treatment and the acquired immunodeficiency syndrome epidemic. *Journal of the American Medical Association, 262,* 1681–1682.

Dole, V.P. (1991) Interim methadone clinics: An undervalued approach. *American Journal of Public Health, 81,* 1111–1112.

Dole, V.P. & Joseph, H.J. (1977) Methadone maintenance: Outcome after termination. *New York State Journal of Medicine, 77,* 1409–1412.

Dole, V.P. & Joseph, H.J. (1978) Long-term outcome of patients treated with methadone maintenance. *Annals of the New York Academy of Sciences, 311,* 181–189.

Dole, V.P. & Nyswander, M. (1965) A medical treatment for diacetylmorphine (heroin) addiction. *Journal of the American Medical Association, 193,* 80–84.

Dole, V.P. & Nyswander, M. (1967) Heroin addiction — a metabolic disease. *Archives of Internal Medicine, 120,* 19–24.

Dole, V.P. & Nyswander, M. (1976) Methadone maintenance treatment: A ten-year perspective. *Journal of the American Medical Association, 235,* 2117–2119.

Dole, V.P., Nyswander, M.E. & Kreek, M.J. (1966) Narcotic blockade. *Archives of Internal Medicine, 118,* 304–309.

Dole, V.P., Nyswander, M., & Warner, A. (1968) Successful treatment of 750 criminal addicts. *Journal of the American Medical Association, 206,* 2708–2711.

Dole, V.P., Robinson, J.W., Orraca, J., Towns, E., Searcy, P., & Caine, E. (1969) Methadone treatment of randomly selected criminal addicts. *New England Journal of Medicine, 280,* 1372–1375.

Donoghoe, M.C. (1992) Sex, HIV and the injecting drug user. *British Journal of Addiction, 87,* 405–416.

Donoghoe, M.C., Stimson, G.V. & Dolan, K.A. (1989) Sexual behaviour of injecting drug users and associated risks of HIV infection for non-injecting sexual partners. *AIDS Care, 1* (1), 51–58.

Dorus, W. & Senay, E.C. (1980) Depression, demographic dimensions, and drug abuse. *American Journal of Psychiatry, 137*, 699–704.

Drummer, O.H., Syrjanen, M., Opeskin, K. & Cordner, S. (1990) Deaths of heroin addicts starting on a methadone maintenance programme. *The Lancet, 335*, 108.

Durante, A. (1991) HIV infection in injecting drug users. *AIDS Care, 3*, 439–441.

Durran:, M. (1989) The role of family therapy for substance abusers and their families. *International Congress: Alcohol, Other Drugs and the Family*. Sydney: Alcohol and Drug Foundation, NSW.

Edwards, G., Arif, A. & Hodgson, R. (1981) Nomenclature and classification of drug- and alcohol-related problems: A WHO memorandum. *Bulletin of the World Health Organization, 59* (2), 225–242.

Ellwood, D.A., Sutherland, P., Kent, C. & O'Connor, M. (1987) Maternal narcotic addiction: Pregnancy outcome in patients managed by a specialized drug-dependency antenatal clinic. *Australian & New Zealand Journal of Obstetrics & Gynaecology, 27*, 92–98.

Feucht, T.E., Stephens, R.C., & Roman, S.W. (1990) The sexual behavior of intravenous drug users: Assessing the risk of sexual transmission of HIV. *The Journal of Drug Issues, 20*, 195–213.

Finnegan, L.P. (Ed), (1980) *Drug Dependence in Pregnancy: Clinical Management of Mother and Child*. London: Castle House.

Finnegan, L.P. (1983) Clinical perinatal and development effects of methadone. In J.R. Cooper, F. Altman, B.S. Brown & D. Czechowicz (Eds), *Research on the Treatment of Narcotic Addiction: State of the Art*. Maryland: National Institute on Drug Abuse.

Finnegan, L.P. (1988) Drug addiction and pregnancy: The newborn. In I.J. Chasnoff (Ed), *Drugs, Alcohol, Pregnancy and Parenting*. London: Kluwer.

Finnegan, L.P. (1991) Treatment issues for opioid-dependent women during the perinatal period. *Journal of Psychoactive Drugs, 23*, 191–201.

Finnegan, L.P., Hagan, T. & Kaltenbach, K.A. (1991) Scientific foundation of clinical practice: Opiate use in pregnant women. *Bulletin of the New York Academy of Medicine, 67*, 223–239.

Fisher, D.G. & Anglin, M.D. (1987) Survival analysis in drug program evaluation. Part I. Overall program effectiveness. *International Journal of the Addictions, 22*, 115–134.

Foy, A., Drinkwater, V. & White, A. (1989) A prospective clinical audit of methadone maintenance therapy at The Royal Newcastle Hospital. *Medical Journal of Australia, 151*, 332–337.

Freedman, R.R. & Czertko, G. (1981) A comparison of thrice weekly LAAM and daily methadone in employed heroin addicts. *Drug and Alcohol Dependence, 8*, 215–222.

Freedman, S.R. & Des Jarlais, D.C. (1991) HIV among drug injectors: the epidemic and the response. *AIDS Care, 3*, 239–250.

Friedland, G. (1989) Parenteral drug users. In R.A. Kaslow & D.P. Francis (Eds), *The Epidemiology of AIDS: Expression, Occurrence, and Control of Human Immunodeficiency Virus Type 1 Infection*. New York: Oxford University Press.

Friedman, S.R., Des Jarlais, D.C., Sotheran, J.L., Garber, J., Cohen, H., & Smith, D. (1987) AIDS and self-organization among intravenous drug users. *International Journal of the Addictions, 22*, 201–219.

Garbutt, G.D. & Goldstein, A. (1972) Blind comparison of three methadone dosages in 180 patients. In Proceedings of the Fourth National Conference on Methadone Treatment. New York: National Association for the Prevention of Addiction to Narcotics.

Gardner, R. (1970) Methadone misuse and death by overdosage. *British Journal of Addiction, 65*, 113–118.

Gastel, B. & Collins, T.E. (1983) Discussion summary [of L.P. Finnegan, Clinical perinatal and development effects of methadone.]. In J.R. Cooper, F. Altman,

B.S. Brown & D. Czechowicz (Eds), *Research on the Treatment of Narcotic Addiction: State of the Art*. Maryland: National Institute on Drug Abuse.

Gearing, F.R. & Schweitzer, M.D. (1974) An epidemiologic evaluation of long-term methadone maintenance treatment for heroin addiction. *American Journal of Epidemiology*, 100, 101–112.

General Accounting Office. (1990) Report to the Chairman, Select Committee on Narcotics Abuse and Control, House of Representatives. *Methadone Maintenance: Some Treatment Programs Are Not Effective; Greater Federal Oversight Needed*. General Accounting Office, Washington, DC.

Gerada, C., Dawe, S. & Farrell, M. (1990) Management of the pregnant opiate user. *British Journal of Hospital Medicine*, 43, 138–141.

Gerstein, D.R. & Harwood, H.J. (Eds), (1990) *Treating Drug Problems, Vol. I. A Study of the Evolution, Effectiveness, and Financing of Public and Private Drug Treatment Systems*. Washington: National Academy Press.

Gerstley, L.J., Alterman, A.I., McLellan, A.T., & Woody, G.E. (1990) Antisocial personality disorder in patients with substance abuse disorders: A problematic diagnosis. *American Journal of Psychiatry, 147*, 173–178.

Giles, W., Patterson, T., Sanders, F., Batey, R., Thomas, D. & Collins, J. (1989) Outpatient methadone programme for pregnant heroin using women. *Australian & New Zealand Journal of Obstetrics and Gynaecology, 29*, 225–229.

Ginzburg, H.M. (1983) Use of clonidine or lofexidine to detoxify from methadone maintenance or other opioid dependencies. In J.R. Cooper, F. Altman, B.S. Brown, & D. Czechowicz (Eds), *Research on the Treatment of Narcotic Addiction: State of the Art*. Maryland: NIDA, U.S. Department of Health and Human Sciences.

Glasner, P.D., & Kaslow, R.A. (1990) The epidemiology of human immunodeficiency virus infection. *Journal of Consulting and Clinical Psychology, 58*, 13–21.

Gold, M.L., Sorensen, J.L., McCanlies, N., Trier, M. & Dlugosch, G. (1988) Tapering from methadone maintenance: Attitudes of clients and staff. *Journal of Substance Abuse Treatment, 5*, 37–44.

Goldberg, R.J., Greenwood, J.C. & Taintor, Z. (1976) Alpha conditioning as an adjunct treatment for drug dependence. *International Journal of the Addictions, 11*, 1085–1089.

Goldstein, A. (1971) Blind dosage comparisons and other studies in a large methadone program. *Journal of Psychedelic Drugs, 4*, 177–181.

Goldstein, A. (1972a) Blind comparison of once-daily and twice daily dosage schedules in a methadone program. *Clinical Pharmacology and Therapeutics, 13*, 59–63.

Goldstein, A. (1972b) Heroin addiction and the role of methadone in its treatment. *Archives of General Psychiatry, 26*, 291–297.

Goldstein, A. (1991) Heroin addiction: Neurobiology, pharmacology, and policy. *Journal of Psychoactive Drugs, 23*, 123–133.

Goldstein, A. & Brown, B.W. (1970) Urine testing schedules in methadone maintenance treatment of heroin addiction. *Journal of the American Medical Association, 214*, 311–315.

Goldstein, A. & Judson, B.A. (1973) Efficacy and side effects of three widely different methadone doses. In Proceedings of the Fifth National Conference on Methadone Treatment. New York: National Association for the Prevention of Addiction to Narcotics.

Goldstein, A. & Judson, B.A. (1974) Three critical issues in the management of methadone programs. In P.G. Bourne (Ed), *Addiction*. New York: Academic Press.

Goldstein, A. & Judson, B.A. (1983) Critique [of W.A. Hargreaves, Methadone dosage and duration for maintenance treatment]. In J.R. Cooper, F. Altman, B.S. Brown, & D. Czechowicz (Eds), *Research on the Treatment of Narcotic Addiction: State of the Art*. Maryland: NIDA, U.S. Department of Health and Human Sciences.

Goldstein, A., Hansteen, R.W., & Horns, W.H. (1975) Control of methadone dosage by patients. *Journal of the American Medical Association, 234*, 734–737.

Goldstein, A., Horns, W.H. & Hansteen, R.W. (1977) Is on-site urine testing of therapeutic value in a methadone treatment program? *International Journal of the Addictions, 12,* 717–728.

Gossop, M. (1988) Clonidine and the treatment of the opiate withdrawal syndrome. *Drug and Alcohol Dependence, 21,* 253–259.

Gossop, M. & Grant, M. (1991) A six country survey of the content and structure of heroin treatment programmes using methadone. *British Journal of Addiction, 86,* 1151–1160.

Gossop, M. & Strang, J. (1991) A comparison of the withdrawal responses of heroin and methadone addicts during detoxification. *British Journal of Psychiatry, 158,* 697–699.

Gossop M., Battersby, M. & Strang, J. (1991) Self-detoxification by opiate addicts: A preliminary investigation. *British Journal of Psychiatry, 159,* 208–212.

Gotthel, E., Caddy, G.R. & Austin, D.L. (1976) Fallibility of urine drug screens in mon toring methadone programs. *Journal of the American Medical Association, 236,* 1035–1038.

Graff, H. & Ball, J.C. (1976) The methadone clinic: Function and philosophy. *International Journal of Social Psychiatry, 22,* 140–146.

Green, J. (1989) Counselling and pregnancy. In J. Green & A. McCreaner, A. (1989) *Counselling in HIV Infection and AIDS.* Oxford: Blackwell.

Green. L. & Gossop, M. (1988) Effects of information on the opiate withdrawal syncrome. *British Journal of Addiction, 83,* 305–309.

Grevert, P. & Weinberg, A. (1973) A controlled study of the clinical effectiveness of urire test results in a methadone maintenance program. In *Proceedings of the 5th National Conference on Methadone Treatment.* New York.

Grmex, M.D. (1990) *History of AIDS: Emergence and Origin of a Modern Pandemic.* U.S.A.: Princeton University Press.

Grönbladh, L. & Gunne, L-M. (1989) Methadone-assisted rehabilitation of Swedish heroin addicts. *Drug and Alcohol Dependence, 24,* 31–37.

Gunne, L-M. & Grönbladh, L. (1981) The Swedish methadone maintenance program: A controlled study. *Drug and Alcohol Dependence, 7,* 249–256.

Hall, S.M. (1979) The abstinence phobia. In N.A. Krasnegor (Ed), *Behavioral Analysis of Substance Abuse.* NIDA Research Monograph 25. U.S.: National Institute on Drug Abuse.

Hall, S.M. (1983) Methadone treatment: A review of the research findings. In J.R. Cooper, F. Altman, B.S. Brown & D. Czechowicz (Eds), *Research on the Treatment of Narcotic Addiction: State of the Art.* Maryland: NIDA, U.S. Department of Health and Human Sciences.

Hall. S.M., Loeb, P.C. & Kushner, M. (1984) Methadone dose decreases and anxiety reduction. *Addictive Behaviors, 9,* 11–19.

Hall W. & Einfeld, S. (1990) On doing the "impossible": Inferring that a putative causal relationship does not exist. *Australian and New Zealand Journal of Psychiatry, 24,* 217–226.

Hall, W., Darke, S., Ross, M. & Wodak, A. (in press) Patterns of drug use and risk-taking among injecting amphetamine and opioid drug users in Sydney, Australia. *British Journal of Addiction.*

Hardal, P.J. & Lander, J.J. (1976) Methadone treatment: Program evaluation and dose response relationships. *International Journal of the Addictions, 11,* 363–375.

Hansen, H.J., Caudill, S.P. & Boone, J. (1985) Crisis in drug testing: Results of CDC blind study. *Journal of the American Medical Association, 253,* 2382–2387.

Harford, R.J. & Kleber, H.D. (1978) Comparative validity of random-interval and fixed-interval urinalysis schedules. *Archives of General Psychiatry, 35,* 356–359.

Hargreaves, W. A. (1983) Methadone dosage and duration for maintenance treatment. In J.R. Cooper, F. Altman, B.S. Brown, & D. Czechowicz (Eds), *Research on the Treatment of Narcotic Addiction: State of the Art.* Maryland: NIDA, U.S. Department of Health and Human Sciences.

Harris, R.E., Langrod, J., Hebert, J.R., Lowinson, J., Zang, E., & Wynder, E.L. (1990) Changes in AIDS risk behavior among intravenous drug abusers in New York City. *New York State Journal of Medicine, 90*, 123-126.

Hartgers, C., Buning, E.C., van Santen, G.W., Verster, A.D., & Coutinho, R.A. (1989) The impact of the needle and syringe-exchange programme in Amsterdam on injecting behaviour. *AIDS, 3*, 571–576.

Hartmann, F., Poirier, M-P, Bourdel, M-C., Loo, H., Lecomte, J-M. & Schwartz, J-C. (1991) Comparison of acetorphan with clonidine for opiate withdrawal symptoms. *American Journal of Psychiatry, 148*, 627–629.

Hasin, D.S., Grant, B.F., Endicott, J. & Harford, T.C. (1988a) Cocaine and heroin dependence compared in poly-drug abusers. *American Journal of Public Health, 78*, 567–569.

Hasin, D.S., Grant, B.F., Harford, T.C. & Endicott, J. (1988b) The drug dependence syndrome and related disabilities. *British Journal of Addiction, 83*, 45–55.

Havassy, B. & Hall, S. (1981) Efficacy of urine monitoring in methadone maintenance. *American Journal of Psychiatry, 138*, 1497–1500.

Havassy, B. & Hargreaves, W.A. (1979) Self-regulation of dose in methadone maintenance with contingent privileges. *Addictive Behaviors, 4*, 31–38.

Havassy, B. & Hargreaves, W.A. (1981) Allowing methadone clients control over dosage: A 48-week controlled trial. *Addictive Behaviors, 6*, 283–288.

Havassy, B.E. & Tschann, J.M. (1983) Client initiative, inertia, and demographics: More powerful than treatment interventions in methadone maintenance? *International Journal of the Addictions, 18*, 617–631.

Hazelrigg, M.D., Cooper, H.M. & Borduin, C.M. (1987) Evaluating the effectiveness of family therapies: An integrative review and analysis. *Psychological Bulletin, 101*, 428–442.

Higgins, S.T., Stitzer, M.L., McCaul, M.E., Bigelow, G.E. & Liebson, I.A. (1985) Pupillary response to methadone challenge in heroin users. *Clinical Pharmacology and Therapeutics, 37*, 460–463.

Hill, A.B. (1965) The environment and disease: Association or causation. *Proceedings of the Royal Society of Medicine, 58*, 295–300.

Hill, A. B. (1977) *A Short Textbook of Statistics*. London: Hodder and Stoughton.

Hoegerman, G., Wilson, C.A., Thurmond, E. & Schnoll, S.H. (1990) Drug-exposed neonates. *Western Journal of Medicine, 152*, 559–564.

Holman, C.P. & Brown, J.P. (Eds), (1989) *The Pleasant View Manual on Addiction*. Melbourne: Pleasant View Publications.

Holmes, J. (1989) Women, narcotics, pregnancy. Paper presented at The Women, Alcohol and Other Drugs Conference, Adelaide.

Holmstrand, J., Änggård, E., & Gunne, L-M. (1978) Methadone maintenance: Plasma levels and therapeutic outcome. *Clinical Pharmacology and Therapeutics, 23*, 175–180.

Horns, W.H. & Goldstein, A. (1975) Plasma levels and symptom complaints in patients maintained on daily dosage of methadone hydrochloride. *Clinical Pharmacology and Therapeutics, 17*, 636–649.

Householder, J., Hatcher, R., Burns, W. & Chasnoff, I. (1982) Infants born to narcotic-addicted mothers. *Psychological Bulletin, 92*, 453–468.

Houston, C.C. & Milby, J. (1983) Drug-seeking behaviour and its mediation: Effects of aversion therapy with narcotic addicts on methadone. *International Journal of the Addictions, 18*, 1171–1177.

Howell, E.F. & Niven, R.G. (1989) The argument for HIV-antibody testing in chemical dependence treatment programs. *Journal of Psychoactive Drugs, 21*, 415–417.

Hubbard, R.L., Marsden, M.E., Rachal, J.V., Harwood, H.J., Cavanagh, E.R., & Ginzburg, H.M. (1989) *Drug Abuse Treatment: A National Study of Effectiveness*. U.S.A.: University of North Carolina Press.

Hubbard, R.L., Rachal, J.V., Craddock, S.G., & Cavanaugh, E.R. (1984) Treatment

Outcome Prospective Study (TOPS): Client characteristics and behaviors before, during, and after treatment. In F.M. Timms, & J.P. Ludford (Eds), *Drug abuse Treatment Evaluation: Strategies, Progress, and Prospects*. NIDA Research Monograph, 51.

Hume, D. (1739) *A Treatise on Human Nature*. (originally published 1739) Ed L.A. Selby-Bigge. Oxford: Oxford University Press, 1888.

Hunt, D.E., Lipton, D.S., Goldsmith, D.S., Strug, D.L. & Spunt, B. (1985–86) "It takes your heart": The image of methadone maintenance in the addict world and its effect on recruitment into treatment. *International Journal of the Addictions, 20*, 1751–1771.

Iguchi, M.Y., Stitzer, M.L., Bigelow, G.E. & Liebson, I.A. (1988) Contingency management in methadone maintenance: Effects of reinforcing and aversive consequences on illicit poly drug use. *Drug and Alcohol Dependence, 22*, 1–7.

Jacobsen, L.K. & Kosten, T.R. (1989) Naloxone challenge as a biological predictor of treatment outcome in opiate addicts. *American Journal of Drug and Alcohol Abuse, 15*, 355–366.

Jaffe, J H. (1970) Further experience with methadone in the treatment of narcotics users. *International Journal of the Addictions, 5*, 375–389.

Jaffe, J H. (1985) Drug addiction and drug abuse. In A.G. Gilman, L.S. Goodman & F. Murad (Eds), *The Pharmacological Basis of Therapeutics*. (7th Edition) USA: Macmillan.

Jaffe, J.H. & Martin, W.R. (1985) Opioid analgesics and antagonists. In A.G. Gilman, L.S. Goodman, & F. Murad (Eds), *The Pharmacological Basis of Therapeutics*. (7th Edition) USA: Macmillan.

Jessup, M. (1990) The treatment of perinatal addiction: Identification, intervention, and advocacy. *Western Journal of Medicine, 152*, 553–558.

Joe, G.W., Simpson, D.D. & Hubbard, R.L. (1991) Treatment predictors of tenure in methadone maintenance. *Journal of Substance Abuse, 3*, 73–84.

Johns, A.R. & Gossop, M. (1985) Prescribing methadone for the opiate addict: A problem of dosage conversion. *Drug and Alcohol Dependence, 16*, 61–66.

Jones, B.E. & Prada, J.A. (1975) Drug-seeking behavior during methadone maintenance. *Psychopharmacologia, 41*, 7–10.

Judson, B.A. & Goldstein, A. (1982) Prediction of long-term outcome for heroin addicts admitted to a methadone maintenance program. *Drug and Alcohol Dependence, 10*, 383–393.

Judson, B.A. & Goldstein, A. (1983) Uses of naloxone in the diagnosis and treatment of heroin addiction. In J.R. Cooper, F. Altman, B.S. Brown, & D. Czechowicz (Eds), *Research on the Treatment of Narcotic Addiction: State of the Art*. Maryland: NIDA, U.S. Department of Health and Human Sciences.

Judson, B.A., Himmelberger, D.U., & Goldstein, A. (1979) Measurement of urine temperature as an alternative to observed urination in a narcotic treatment program. *American Journal of Drug and Alcohol Abuse, 6*, 197–205.

Judson, B.A., Himmelberger, D.U. & Goldstein, A. (1980) The naloxone test for opiate dependence. *Clinical Pharmacology and Therapeutics, 27*, 492–501.

Judson, B.A., Ortiz, S., Crouse, L., Carney, T.M. & Goldstein, A. (1980) A follow-up study of heroin addicts five years after first admission to a methadone treatment program. *Drug and Alcohol Dependence, 6*, 295–313.

Käll, K.I., & Olin, R.G. (1990) HIV status and changes in risk behaviour among intravenous drug users in Stockholm 1987–1988. *AIDS, 4*, 153–157.

Kaltenbach, K. & Finnegan, L.P. (1989) Children exposed to methadone in utero: Assessment of developmental and cognitive ability. *Annals of the New York Academy of Sciences, 562*, 360–362.

Kanof, P.D., Aronson, M.J., Ness, R., Cochrane, K.J., Horvath, T.B. & Handelsman, L. (1991) Levels of opioid physical dependence in heroin addicts. *Drug and Alcohol Dependence, 27*, 253–262.

Kaslow, R.A. & Francis, D.P. (1989) Epidemiology: General considerations. In R.A.

Kaslow & D.P. Francis (Eds), *The Epidemiology of AIDS: Expression, Occurrence, and Control of Human Immunodeficiency Virus Type 1 Infection*. U.S.A. Oxford University Press.

Kaufman, E. & Blaine, G.B. (1974) Full services in methadone treatment. *American Journal of Drug and Alcohol Abuse, 1*, 213–231.

Kelly, J.A. & Murphy, D.A. (1991) Some lessons learned about risk reduction after ten years of the HIV/AIDS epidemic. *AIDS Care, 3*, 251–257.

Kelly, J.A., & St. Lawrence, J.S. (1988) *The AIDS Health Crisis: Psychological and Social Interventions*. New York: Plenum.

Kelly, J.A., St. Lawrence, J.S., Hood, H.V., & Brasfield, T.L. (1989) Behavioral intervention to reduce AIDS risk activities. *Journal of Consulting and Clinical Psychology, 57*, 60–67.

Khantzian, E.J. (1985a) Psychotherapeutic interventions with substance abusers — the clinical context. *Journal of Substance Abuse Treatment, 2*, 83–88.

Khantzian, E.J. (1985b) The self-medication hypothesis of addictive disorders: Focus on heroin and cocaine dependence. *American Journal of Psychiatry, 142*, 1259–1264.

Khantzian, E.J. & Treece, C. (1985) DSM-III psychiatric diagnosis of narcotic addicts: Recent findings. *Archives of General Psychiatry, 42*, 1067–1071.

Kleber, H.D. (1977) Detoxification from methadone maintenance: The state of the art. *International Journal of the Addictions, 12*, 807–820.

Kleber, H.D. (1981) Detoxification from narcotics. In J.H. Lowinson & P. Ruiz (Eds), *Substance Abuse: Clinical Problems and Perspectives*. U.S.A.: Williams & Wilkins.

Kleber, H.D. (1984) Is there a need for "professional psychotherapy" in methadone programs? *Journal of Substance Abuse Treatment, 1*, 73–76.

Kleber, H.D. & Gould, L.C. (1971) Urine testing schedules in methadone maintenance. *Journal of the American Medical Association, 215*, 2115–2116.

Klee, H., Faugier, J., Hayes, C., & Morris, J. (1991a) The sharing of injecting equipment among drug users attending prescribing clinics and those using needle-exchanges. *British Journal of Addiction, 86*, 217–233.

Klee, H., Faugier, J., Hayes, C. & Morris, J. (1991b) Risk reduction among injecting drug users: Changes in the sharing of injecting equipment and in condom use. *AIDS Care, 3*, 63–73.

Klee, H., Faugier, J., Hayes, C., Boulton, T., & Morris, J. (1990a) Factors associated with risk behaviour among injecting drug users. *AIDS Care, 2*, 133–145.

Klee, H., Faugier, J., Hayes, C., Boulton, T., & Morris, J. (1990b) AIDS-related risk behaviour, polydrug use and temazepam. *British Journal of Addiction, 85*, 1125–1132.

Klee, H., Faugier, J., Hayes, C., Boulton, T., & Morris, J. (1990c) Sexual partners of injecting drug users: The risk for HIV infection. *British Journal of Addiction, 85*, 413–418.

Kosten, T.A., Jacobsen, L.K. & Kosten, T.R. (1989) Severity of precipitated opiate withdrawal predicts drug dependence by DSM-III-R criteria. *American Journal of Drug and Alcohol Abuse, 15*, 237–250.

Kosten, T.R., Rounsaville, B.J. & Kleber, H.D. (1982) DSM-III personality disorders in opiate addicts. *Comprehensive Psychiatry, 23*, 572–581.

Kosten, T.R., Rounsaville, B.J. & Kleber, H.D. (1986) A 2.5-year follow-up of depression, life crises, and treatment effects on abstinence among opioid addicts. *Archives of General Psychiatry, 43*, 733–737.

Kosten, T.R., Rounsaville, B.J., Babor, T.F., Spitzer, R.L. & Williams, J.B.W. (1987) Substance-use disorders in DSM-III-R. *British Journal of Psychiatry, 151*, 834–843.

Kreek, M.J. (1979) Methadone in treatment: Physiological and pharmacological issues. In R.I. Dupont, A. Goldstein, J. O'Donnell, & B. Brown, (Eds), *Handbook on Drug Abuse*. USA: National Institute on Drug Abuse.

Kreek, M.J. (1983a) Factors modifying the pharmacological effectiveness of methadone. In J.R. Cooper, F. Altman, B.S. Brown & D. Czechowicz (Eds), *Research on the Treatment of Narcotic Addiction: State of the Art.* Maryland: National Institute on Drug Abuse.

Kreek, M.J. (1983b) Critique [of L.P. Finnegan, Clinical perinatal and development effects of methadone.]. In J.R. Cooper, F. Altman, B.S. Brown & D. Czechowicz (Eds), *Research on the Treatment of Narcotic Addiction: State of the Art.* Maryland: National Institute on Drug Abuse.

Krivanek, J. (1988) *Heroin: Myths and Reality.* Sydney: Allen & Unwin.

Kuna, D.J., Salkin, W. & Weinberger, K. (1976) Biofeedback, relaxation training, and methadone clients: An inquiry. *Contemporary Drug Problems, 5,* 565–572.

Kuncel, E.E. (1981) Effects of intensive counseling on client outcome in a methadone maintenance program. *International Journal of the Addictions, 16,* 415–424.

Latt, N., Lin, R., Farrell, G., Batey, R. & Crewe, E. (1992) Vertical transmission of hepatitis C virus in HIV-negative intravenous drug users (IVDU's): Does it occur? Paper presented at the International Association for the Study of the Liver Biennial Scientific Meeting, Brighton, United Kingdom, 1992.

Levine, D.P. & Sobel, J.D. (Eds), (1991) *Infections in Intravenous Drug Abusers.* New York: Oxford University Press.

Lewis, D.K., Watters, J.K., & Case, P. (1990) The prevalence of high-risk sexual behavior in male intravenous drug users with steady female partners. *American Journal of Public Health, 80,* 465–466.

Lewis, J.H. & Chesher, G.B. (1990) Patterns of heroin use in the methadone programme in Sydney, 1986–1987. *Drug and Alcohol Review, 9,* 219–224.

Lewis, V.S., Petersen, D.M., Geis, G. & Pollack, S. (1972) Ethical and social-psychological aspects of urinalysis to detect heroin use. *British Journal of Addiction, 67,* 303–307.

Lifschitz, M.H., Wilson, G.S., Smith, E.O. & Desmond, M.M. (1985) Factors affecting head growth and intellectual function in children of drug addicts. *Pediatrics, 75,* 269–274.

Ling, W., Charuvastra, C., Kaim, S.C., & Klett, C.J. (1976) Methadyl acetate and methadone as maintenance treatments for heroin addicts. *Archives of General Psychiatry, 33,* 709–720.

Loimer, N., Schmid, R., Grünberger, J., Jagsch, R., Linzmayer, L. & Presslich, O. (1991) Psychophysiological reactions in methadone maintenance patients do not correlate with methadone plasma levels. *Psychopharmacology, 103,* 538–540.

Longwell, B., Miller, J. & Nichols, A.W. (1978) Counselor effectiveness in a methadone maintenance program. *International Journal of the Addictions, 13,* 307–315.

LoSciuto, L., Aiken, L.S., Ausetts, M.A. & Brown, B.S. (1984) Paraprofessional versus professional drug abuse counselors: Attitudes and expectations of the counselors and their clients. *International Journal of the Addictions, 19,* 233–252.

Lowinson, J., Berle, B. & Langrod, J. (1976) Detoxification of long-term methadone patients: Problems and prospects. *International Journal of the Addictions, 11,* 1009–1018.

Lowinson, J.H. & Millman, R.B. (1979) Clinical aspects of methadone treatment. In R.I. Dupont, A. Goldstein, J. O'Donnell, & B. Brown, (Eds), *Handbook on Drug Abuse.* USA: National Institute on Drug Abuse.

Loxley W., Marsh, A. & Lo, S.K. (1991) Age and injecting drug use in Perth, Western Australia: The Australian national AIDS and injecting drug use study. *AIDS Care, 3,* 363–372.

Luborsky, L., Crits-Christoph, P., McLellan, A.T., Woody, G.E., Piper, W., Liberman, B., Imber, S. & Pilkonis, P. (1986) Do therapists vary much in their success? Findings from four outcome studies. *American Journal of Orthopsychiatry, 56,* 501–512.

Luborsky, L., McLellan, A.T., Woody, G.E., O'Brien, C.P. & Auerbach, A. (1985)

Therapist success and its determinants. *Archives of General Psychiatry, 42*, 602–611.

Mack, G., Thomas, D., Giles, W. & Buchanan, N. (1991) Methadone levels and neonatal withdrawal. *Journal of Paediatrics & Child Health, 27*, 96–100.

Mackie-Ramos, R-L. & Rice, J-M. (1988) Group psychotherapy with methadone-maintained pregnant women. *Journal of Substance Abuse Treatment, 5*, 151–161.

Macks, J. (1988) Women and AIDS: Countertransference issues. *Social Casework, 69*, 340–347.

Maddux, J.F., Esquivel, M., Vogtsberger, K.N. & Desmond, D.P. (1991) Methadone dose and urine morphine. *Journal of Substance Abuse Treatment, 8*, 195–201.

Magura, S. & Lipton, D.S. (1988) The accuracy of drug use monitoring in methadone treatment. *Journal of Drug Issues, 18*, 317–326.

Magura, S., Casriel, C., Goldsmith, D.S., Strug, D.L. & Lipton, D.S. (1988) Contingency contracting with polydrug-abusing methadone patients. *Addictive Behaviors, 13*, 113–118.

Magura, S., Freeman, R.C., Siddiqi, Q., & Lipton, D.S. (1992) The validity of hair analysis for detecting cocaine and heroin use among addicts. *International Journal of the Addictions, 27*, 51–69.

Magura, S., Goldsmith, D., Casriel, C., Goldstein, P.J. & Lipton, D.S. (1987) The validity of methadone clients' self-reported drug use. *International Journal of the Addictions, 22*, 727–749.

Magura, S., Grossman, J.I., Lipton, D.S., Siddiqi, Q., Shapiro, J., Marion, I., & Amann, K.R. (1989a) Determinants of needle sharing among intravenous drug users. *American Journal of Public Health, 79*, 459–462.

Magura, S., Shapiro, J.L., Grossman, J.I., & Lipton, D.S. (1989b) Education/support groups for AIDS prevention with at-risk clients. *Social Casework, 70*, 10–20.

Magura, S., Shapiro, J.L., Grossman, J.I., Siddiqi, Q., Lipton, D.S., Amann, K.R., Koger, J., & Gehan, K. (1990b) Reactions of methadone patients to HIV antibody testing. *Advances in Alcohol & Substance Abuse, 8* (3/4), 97–111.

Magura, S., Shapiro, J.L., Siddiqi, A., & Lipton, D.S. (1990a) Variables influencing condom use among intravenous drug users. *American Journal of Public Health, 80*, 82–84.

Magura, S., Siddiqi, Q., Shapiro, J., Grossman, J.I., Lipton, D.S., Marion, I.J., Weisenfeld, L., Amann, K.R. & Koger, J. (1991) Outcomes for an AIDS prevention program for methadone patients. *International Journal of the Addictions, 26*, 629–655.

Manno, J.E. (1986a) Interpretation of urinalysis results. In Hawks, R.L. & Chiang, C.N. (Eds), *Urine Testing for Drugs of Abuse*. NIDA Research Monograph 73. Maryland: National Institute on Drug Abuse.

Manno, J.E. (1986b) Specimen collection and handling. In Hawks, R.L. & Chiang, C.N. (Eds), *Urine Testing for Drugs of Abuse*. NIDA Research Monograph 73. Maryland: National Institute on Drug Abuse.

Markus, E., Lange, A. & Pettigrew, T.F. (1990) Effectiveness of family therapy: A meta-analysis. *Journal of Family Therapy, 12*, 205–221.

Marmor, M., Des Jarlais, D.C., Cohen, H., Friedman, S.R., Beatrice, S.T., Dubin, N., El-Sadr, W., Mildvan, D., Yancovitz, S.R., Mathur, U., & Holzman, R. (1987) Risk factors for infection human immunodeficiency virus among intravenous drug abusers in New York City. *AIDS, 1*, 39–44.

Martin, G.S., Serpelloni, G., Galvan, U., Rizzetto, A., Gomma, M., Morgante, S. & Rezza, G. (1990) Behavioural change in injecting drug users: Evaluation of an HIV/AIDS education programme. *AIDS Care, 2*, 275–279.

Martin, W.R., Jasinski, D.R., Haertzen, C.A., Kay, D.C., Jones, B.E., Mansky, P.A. & Carpenter, R.W. (1973) Methadone — a reevaluation. *Archives of General Psychiatry, 28*, 286–295.

Mattick, R. & Hall, W. (Eds), (in press) *A Treatment Outline for Opioid Dependence*. Canberra: National Campaign Against Drug Abuse Monograph.

Mattick R.P. & Grenyer, B.F. (1990) Quality assurance in drug and alcohol treatment: The development of standards for treatment content. *Drug and Alcohol Review, 9*, 75–79.

McAuliffe, W.E. (1990) A randomized controlled trial of recovery training and self-help for opioid addicts in New England and Hong Kong. *Journal of Psychoactive Drugs, 22*, 197–209.

McAuliffe, W.E. & Ch'ien, J.M.N. (1986) Recovery training and self help: A relapse-prevention program for treated opiate addicts. *Journal of Substance Abuse Treatment, 3*, 9–20.

McCarthy, J.J. & Borders, O.T. (1985) Limit setting on drug abuse in methadone maintenance patients. *American Journal of Psychiatry, 142*, 1419–1423.

McCutchan, J.A. (1990) Virology, immunology, and clinical course of HIV infection. *Journal of Consulting and Clinical Psychology, 58*, 5–12.

McGloth in, W.H. & Anglin, M.D. (1981a) Long-term follow-up of clients of high- and low-dose methadone programs. *Archives of General Psychiatry, 38*, 1055–1063.

McGlothlin, W.H. & Anglin, M.D. (1981b) Shutting off methadone: Costs and benefits. *Archives of General Psychiatry, 38*, 885–892.

McKegarey, N., Barnard, M., & Watson, H. (1989) HIV-related risk behaviour among a non-clinic sample of injecting drug users. *British Journal of Addiction, 84*, 1481–1490.

McLellan, A.T. (1983) Patient characteristics associated with outcome. In J.R. Cooper, F. Altman, B.S. Brown, & D. Czechowicz (Eds), *Research on the Treatment of Narcotic Addiction: State of the Art*. Maryland: NIDA, U.S. Department of Health and Human Sciences.

McLellan, A.T., Childress, A.R., Ehrman, R., O'Brien, C.P. & Pashko, S. (1986) Extinguishing conditioned responses during opiate dependence treatment: Turning laboratory findings into clinical procedures. *Journal of Substance Abuse Treatment, 3*, 33–40.

McLellan, A.T., Childress, A.R., Griffith, J. & Woody, G.E. (1984) The psychiatrically severe drug abuse patient: Methadone maintenance or therapeutic community? *American Journal of Drug and Alcohol Abuse, 10*, 77–95.

McLellar, A.T., Luborsky, L., Woody, G.E. & O'Brien, C.P. (1980) An improved evaluation instrument for substance abuse patients. *Journal of Nervous and Mental Diseases, 168*, 26–33.

McLellar, A.T., Luborsky, L., Woody, G.E., O'Brien, C.P. & Druley, K.A. (1983) Predicting response to alcohol and drug abuse treatments: Role of psychiatric severity. *Archives of General Psychiatry, 40*, 620–625.

McLellan A.T., Woody, G.E., Luborsky, L., & Goehl, L. (1988) Is the counselor an "active ingredient" in substance abuse rehabilitation? An examination of treatment success among four counselors. *Journal of Nervous and Mental Disease, 176*, 423–430.

McMaster Department of Clinical Epidemiology. (1981) How to read clinical journals IV: To determine etiology and causation. *Canadian Medical Association Journal, 124*, 985–990.

Meltzer, I.D. & Katz, S.E. (1980) Methadone patients: Dosage, psychopathology, and research participation. *International Journal of the Addictions, 15*, 1097–1102.

Mersky, S.A. (1989) Testing for human immunodeficiency virus in chemical dependence treatment programs. *Journal of Psychoactive Drugs, 21*, 407–413.

Metzger, D., Woody, G., De Philippis, D., McLellan, A.T., O'Brien, C.P. & Platt, J.J. (1991) Risk factors for needle sharing among methadone-treated patients. *American Journal of Psychiatry, 148*, 636–640.

Metzger, D.S. & Platt, J.J. (1987) Methadone dose levels and client characteristics in heroin addicts. *International Journal of the Addictions, 22*, 187–94.

Meyer, R.E. (1986) How to understand the relationship between psychopathology and addictive disorders: Another example of the chicken and the egg. In R.E. Meyer (Ed), *Psychopathology and Addictive Disorders*. U.S.A.: Guilford.

Milby, J.B. (1988) Methadone maintenance to abstinence: How many make it? *Journal of Nervous and Mental Disease, 176,* 409–422.

Milby, J.B., Gurwitch, R.H., Hohmann, A.A., Wiebe, D.J., Ling, W., McLellan, A.T. & Woody, G.E. (1987) Assessing pathological detoxification fear among methadone maintenance patients: The DFSS. *Journal of Clinical Psychology, 43,* 528–538.

Milby, J.B., Gurwitch, R.H., Wiebe, D.J., Ling, W., McLellan, A.T. & Woody, G.E. (1986) Prevalence and diagnostic reliability of methadone maintenance detoxification fear. *American Journal of Psychiatry, 143,* 739–743.

Millard, D.D. (1988) Viral hepatitis in pregnancy. In I.J. Chasnoff (Ed), *Drugs, Alcohol, Pregnancy and Parenting.* London: Kluwer.

Miller, W.R. & Brown, J.M. (1991) Self-regulation as a conceptual basis for the prevention and treatment of addictive behaviours. In N. Heather, W.R. Miller & J. Greeley (Eds), *Self-control in the Addictive Behaviours.* Australia: Maxwell Macmillan.

Miller, W.R. & Rollnick, S. (1991) *Motivational Interviewing: Preparing People to Change Addictive Behavior.* New York: Guilford.

Miller, W.R. & Sovereign, R.G. (1989) The check-up: A model for early intervention in addictive behaviors. In T. Løberg, W.R. Miller, P.E. Nathan & G.A. Marlatt (Eds), *Addictive Behaviors: Prevention and Early Intervention.* Amsterdam: Swets & Zeitlinger.

Mintz, J., O'Brien, C.P., O'Hare, K. & Goldschmidt, J. (1975) Double-blind detoxification of methadone maintenance patients. *International Journal of the Addictions, 10,* 815–824.

Montalvo, Jr., J.G., Scrignar, C.B., Alderette, E., Harper, B. & Eyer, D. (1972) Flushing, pale-colored urines, and false negatives: Urinalysis of narcotic addicts. *International Journal of the Addictions, 7,* 355–364.

Morlet, A., Darke, S., Guinan, J.J., Wolk, J., & Gold, J. (1990) Intravenous drug users who present to the Albion Street (AIDS) Centre for diagnosis and management of human immunodeficiency virus infection. *Medical Journal of Australia, 152,* 78–80.

Muraskin, W. (1988) The silent epidemic: The social, ethical, and medical problems surrounding the fight against hepatitis B. *Journal of Social History, 22,* 277–298.

Murphy, S., & Rosenbaum, M. (1989) Money for methadone: II. Unintended consequences of limited-duration methadone maintenance. *Journal of Psychoactive Drugs, 20,* 397-402.

Mutchnick, M.G., Lee, H.H. & Peleman, R.R. (1991) Liver disease associated with intravenous drug abuse. In D.P. Levine & J.D. Sobel (Eds), *Infections in Intravenous Drug Abusers.* New York: Oxford University Press.

Nathan, J.A., & Karan, L.D. (1989) Substance abuse treatment modalities in the age of HIV spectrum disease. *Journal of Psychoactive Drugs, 21,* 423–429.

National Centre on HIV Epidemiology and Clinical Research. (1991) *Cumulative Analysis of AIDS Cases in Australia,* August 1991. Sydney: NCHIVECR.

National HIV Reference Laboratory. (1991) *Bulletin 1991.* Melbourne: National HIV Reference Laboratory.

Nelkin, D. (1973) *Methadone Maintenance: A Technological Fix.* New York: George Braziller.

Newman, R.G. (1974) The role of ancillary services in methadone maintenance treatment. *American Journal of Drug and Alcohol Abuse, 1,* 207–212.

Newman, R.G. (1977) *Methadone Treatment in Narcotic Addiction.* New York: Academic Press.

Newman, R.G. (1983a) Critique [of R. Resnick, Methadone detoxification from illicit opiates and methadone maintenance]. In J.R. Cooper, F. Altman, B.S. Brown, & D. Czechowicz (Eds), *Research on the Treatment of Narcotic Addiction: State of the Art.* Maryland: NIDA, U.S. Department of Health and Human Sciences.

Newman, R.G. (1983b) The need to redefine "addiction". *New England Journal of Medicine, 308,* 1096–1098.

Newman, R.G. (1991) What's so special about methadone maintenance? *Drug and Alcohol Review, 10*, 225–232.

Newman, R.G. & Peyser, N. (1991) Methadone treatment: Experiment and experience. *Journal of Psychoactive Drugs, 23*, 115–121.

Newman, R.G., & Whitehill, W.B. (1979) Double-blind comparison of methadone and placebo maintenance treatments of narcotic addicts in Hong Kong. *Lancet*, September 8, 485–488.

Newman, R.G. & Des Jarlais, D.C. (1991) Criteria for judging methadone maintenance programs. *Journal of the American Medical Association, 265*, 2190–2191.

Newmeyer, J.A. (1988) Why bleach? Development of a strategy to combat HIV contagion among San Francisco intravenous drug users. In R.J. Battjes & R.W. Pickens (Eds), *Needle sharing among intravenous drug abusers: National and international perspectives*. NIDA Research Monograph, 80, 151–159.

Nicolosi, A., Molinari, S., Musicco, M., Saracco, A., Ziliani, N., & Lazzarin, A. (1991) Positive modification of injecting behavior among intravenous heroin users from Milan and Northern Italy 1987–1989. *British Journal of Addiction, 86*, 91–102.

Nolimal, D., & Crowley, T.J. (1989) HIV risk behavior: Antisocial personality disorder, drug use patterns, and sexual behavior among methadone maintenance admissions. In L.S. Harris (Ed), *Problems of Drug Dependence 1989*. NIDA Research Monograph, 95, 401–402.

Nolimal, D. & Crowley, T.J. (1990) Difficulties in a clinical application of methadone-dose contingency contracting. *Journal of Substance Abuse Treatment, 7*, 219–224.

Novick, D.M., Joseph, H., Croxson, T.S., Salsitz, E.A., Wang, G., Richman, B.L., Poretsky, L., Keefe, J.B., & Whimbey, E. (1990) Absence of antibody to human immunodeficiency virus in long-term, socially rehabilitated methadone maintenance patients. *Archives of Internal Medicine, 150*, 97–99.

Novick, D.M., Kreek, M.J., Fanizza, A.M., Yancovitz, S.R., Gelb, A.M., & Stenger, R.J. (1981) Methadone disposition in patients with chronic liver disease. *Clinical Pharmacology and Therapeutics, 30*, 353–362.

Novick, D.M., Ochshorn, M., Ghali, V., Croxson, T.S., Mercer, W.D., Chiorazzi, N., & Kreek, M.J. (1989) Natural killer cell activity and lymphocyte subsets in parenteral heroin abusers and long-term methadone maintenance patients. *The Journal of Pharmacology and Experimental Therapeutics, 250*, 606–610.

O'Brien, C.P., Greenstein, R., Ternes, J. & Woody, G.E. (1978) Clinical pharmacology of narcotic antagonists. *Annals of the New York Academy of Sciences, 311*, 232–239.

Olsen, G.D., Wilson, J.E., & Robertson, G.E. (1981) Respiratory and ventilatory effects of methadone in healthy women. *Clinical Pharmacology and Therapeutics, 29*, 373–380.

Panerinto, W., Arnon, D., Silver, F., Orbe, M. & Kissin, B. (1977) Detoxification from methadone maintenance in a family-oriented program. *British Journal of Addiction, 72*, 255–259.

Peachey, J.E. & Lei, H. (1988) Assessment of opioid dependence with naloxone. *British Journal of Addiction, 83*, 193–201.

Peckham, C.S. & Newell, M-L. (1990) HIV-1 infection in mothers and babies. *AIDS Care, 2*, 205–211.

Perkins, M.E. & Bloch, H.I. (1971) A study of some failures in methadone treatment. *American Journal of Psychiatry, 128*, 47–51.

Perry, S., Fishman, B., Jacobsberg, L., Young, J. & Frances, A. (1991) Effectiveness of psychoeducational interventions in reducing emotional distress after human immunodeficiency virus antibody testing. *Archives of General Psychiatry, 48*, 143–147.

Phillips, G.T., Gossop, M. & Bradley, B. (1986) The influence of psychological factors on the opiate withdrawal syndrome. *British Journal of Psychiatry, 149*, 235–238.

Phillips, G.T., Gossop, M.R., Edwards, G., Sutherland, G., Taylor, C. & Strang, J.

(1987) The application of the SODQ to the measurement of the severity of opiate dependence in a British sample. *British Journal of Addiction, 82,* 691–699.

Pond, S.M., Kreek, M.J., Tong, T.G., Raghunath, J. & Benowitz, N.L. (1985) Altered methadone pharmacokinetics in methadone-maintained pregnant women. *Journal of Pharmacology and Experimental Therapeutics, 233,* 1–6.

Powell, K., Mench, F.H., Smith, J.R., & O'Malley, J.O. (1984) Methadone maintenance in the A.C.T. from January 1979 – 31st July 1983. *Australian Alcohol/Drug Review, 3,* 35–38.

Power, R., Hartnoll, R., & Daviaud, E. (1988) Drug injecting, AIDS, and risk behaviour: Potential for change and intervention strategies. *British Journal of Addiction, 83,* 649–654.

Prochaska, J.O. & DiClimente, C.C. (1986) Toward a comprehensive model of change. In W.R. Miller & N. Heather (Eds), *Treating Addictive Behaviors: Processes of Change.* New York: Plenum Press.

Quality Assurance Project. (1991) Treatment outlines for antisocial personality disorder. *Australian and New Zealand Journal of Psychiatry, 25,* 541–547.

Rachels, J. (1986) *The Elements of Moral Philosophy.* Philadelphia: Temple University Press.

Raczynski, J.M., Wiebe, D.J., Milby, J.B. & Gurwitch, R.H. (1988) Behavioral assessment of narcotic detoxification fear. *Addictive Behaviors, 13,* 165–169.

Ramer, B.S., Zaslove, M.O. & Langan, J. (1971) Is methadone enough? The use of ancillary treatment during methadone maintenance. *American Journal of Psychiatry, 127,* 80–84.

Rawson, R.A., Washton, A.M., Resnick, R.B. & Tennant, F.S. (1984) Clonidine hydrochloride detoxification from methadone treatment: The value of naltrexone aftercare. *Advances in Alcohol and Substance Abuse, 3,* 41–49.

Regier, D.A., Farmer, M.E., Rae, D.S., Locke, B.Z., Keith, S.J., Judd, L.L. & Goodwin, F.K. (1990) Comorbidity of mental disorders with alcohol and other drug abuse: Results from the Epidemiologic Catchment Area (ECA) study. *Journal of the American Medical Association, 264,* 2511–2518.

Reilly, D., O'Connor, D., Wodak, A., & Clarke, C. (1987) *Methadone Treatment: A Profile of Clients in a New South Wales Program.* Sydney: New South Wales Drug and Alcohol Authority In-house Series.

Renner, J.A. (1984) Methadone maintenance: Past, present, and future. *Addictive Behaviours, 3,* 75–90.

Resnick, R. (1983) Methadone detoxification from illicit opiates and methadone maintenance. In J.R. Cooper, F. Altman, B.S. Brown, & D. Czechowicz (Eds), *Research on the Treatment of Narcotic Addiction: State of the Art.* Maryland: NIDA, U.S. Department of Health and Human Sciences.

Reynolds, I. & Magro, D. (1975) *The Use of Methadone as a Treatment Tool for Opiate Addicts: A Two-year Follow-up Study.* Sydney: Division of Health Services Research, Health Commission of New South Wales.

Reynolds, I., & Magro, D. (1976) The use of methadone as a treatment tool for opiate addicts: A two-year follow-up study. *Medical Journal of Australia, 2,* 560–562.

Reynolds, I., Di Giusto, J., & McCulloch, R. (1976) *A Review of New South Wales Health Commission Treatment for Narcotic Dependent Persons.* Sydney: Division of Health Services Research, Health Commission of New South Wales.

Robins, L.N., Locke, B.Z. & Regier, D.A. (1991b) An overview of psychiatric disorders in America. In L.N. Robins & D.A. Regier (Eds), *Psychiatric Disorders in America: The Epidemiologic Catchment Area Study.* New York: The Free Press.

Robins, L.N., Tipp, J. & Przybeck, T. (1991a) Antisocial personality. In L.N. Robins & D.A. Regier (Eds), *Psychiatric Disorders in America: The Epidemiologic Catchment Area Study.* New York: The Free Press.

Rogers, C.R. (1957) The necessary and sufficient conditions of therapeutic personality change. *Journal of Consulting Psychology, 21,* 95–103.

Romijn, C.M., Platt, J.J. & Schippers, G.M. (1990) Family therapy for Dutch drug abusers: Replication of an American study. *International Journal of the Addictions, 25*, 1127–1149.

Ronald, P.J.M, Robertson, J.R. & Roberts, J.J.K. (1992) Risk-taking behaviour on the decline in intravenous drug users. *British Journal of Addiction, 87*, 115–116.

Rosenbaum, M. (1981) *Women on Heroin*. U.S.A.: Rutgers University Press.

Rosenbaum, M. (1985) A matter of style: Variation among methadone clinics in the control of clients. *Contemporary Drug Problems, 12*, 375–400.

Rosenbaum, M. (1991) Staying off methadone. *Journal of Psychoactive Drugs, 23*, 251–260.

Rosenbaum, M. & Murphy, S. (1984) Always a junkie?: The arduous task of getting off methadone maintenance. *Journal of Drug Issues, 14*, 527–552.

Rosenbaum, M., Irwin, J. & Murphy, S. (1988) De facto destabilisation as policy: The impact of short-term methadone maintenance. *Contemporary Drug Problems, 15*, 491–517.

Rosenblum, A., Magura, S. & Joseph, H. (1991) Ambivalence towards methadone treatment among intravenous drug users. *Journal of Psychoactive Drugs, 23*, 21–27.

Ross, H.E., Glaser, F.B. & Germanson, T. (1988) The prevalence of psychiatric disorders in patients with alcohol and other drug problems. *Archives of General Psychiatry, 45*, 1023–1031.

Ross, M., Gold, J., Wodak, A., & Miller, M.E. (1991) Sexually transmissible diseases in injecting drug users. *Genitourinary Medicine, 67*, 32–36.

Roszell, D.K. & Calsyn, D.A. (1986) Methadone dosage: Patient characteristics and clinical correlates. *International Journal of the Addictions, 21*, 1233–46.

Rounsaville, B.J. & Kleber, H.D. (1985a) Untreated opiate addicts: How do they differ from those seeking treatment? *Archives of General Psychiatry, 42*, 1072–1077.

Rounsaville, B.J. & Kleber, H.D. (1985b) Psychotherapy/Counseling for opiate addicts: Strategies for use in different treatment settings. *International Journal of the Addictions, 20*, 869–896.

Rounsaville, B.J., Glazer, W., Wilber, C.H., Weissman, M.M. & Kleber, H.D. (1983) Short-term interpersonal psychotherapy in methadone-maintained opiate addicts. *Archives of General Psychiatry, 40*, 629–636.

Rounsaville, B.J., Kosten, T.R., Weissman, M.M. & Kleber, H.D. (1986b) A 2.5-year follow-up of short-term interpersonal psychotherapy in methadone-maintained opiate addicts. *Comprehensive Psychiatry, 27*, 201–210.

Rounsaville, B.J., Kosten, T.R., Weissman, M.M. & Kleber, H.D. (1986b) Prognostic significance of psychopathology in treated opiate addicts: A 2.5-year follow-up study. *Archives of General Psychiatry, 43*, 739–745.

Rounsaville, B.J., Kosten, T.R., Williams, J.B.W., & Spitzer, R.L. (1987) A field trial of DSM-III-R psychoactive substance dependence disorders. *American Journal of Psychiatry, 144*, 351–355.

Rounsaville, B.J., Spitzer, R.L. & Williams, J.B.W., (1986) Proposed changes in DSM-III substance use disorders: Description and rationale. *American Journal of Psychiatry, 143*, 463–468.

Rounsaville, B.J., Weissman, M.M., Kleber, H. & Wilber, C. (1982) Heterogeneity of psychiatric diagnosis in treated opiate addicts. *Archives of General Psychiatry, 39*, 161–166.

San, L., Camí, J., Peri, J.M., Mata, R. & Porta, M. (1990) Efficacy of clonidine, guanifacine and methadone in the rapid detoxification of heroin addicts: A controlled clinical trial. *British Journal of Addiction, 85*, 141–147.

Sanchez-Ramos, J.R. & Senay, E.C. (1987) Ophthalmic naloxone elicits abstinence in opioid-dependent subjects. *British Journal of Addiction, 82*, 313–315.

Saunders, B. & Wilkinson, C. (1990) Motivation and addiction behaviour: A psychological perspective. *Drug and Alcohol Review, 9*, 133–142.

Saunders, B., Wilkinson, C. & Allsop, S. (1991) Motivational intervention with heroin users attending a methadone clinic. In W.R. Miller & S. Rollnick (Eds),

Motivational Interviewing: Preparing People to Change Addictive Behavior. J.S.A.: Guilford.

Säwe, J. (1986) High-dose morphine and methadone in cancer patients: Clinical pharmacokinetic considerations of oral treatment. *Clinical Pharmacokinetics, 11*, 87–106.

Schlesselman, J.J. (1978) Assessing effects of confounding variables. *American Journal of Epidemiology, 108*, 3–8.

Schoenbaum, E.E., Hartel, D., Selwyn, P.A., Klein, R.S., Davenny, K., Rogers, M., Feiner, C., & Friedland, G. (1989) Risk factors for human immunodeficiency virus infection in intravenous drug users. *New England Journal of Medicine, 321*, 874–879.

Schuster, C.R. (1989) Methadone maintenance: An adequate dose is vital in checking the spread of AIDS. *NIDA Notes, 4* (2), pp. 3, 33.

Schut, J., Wohlmuth, T.W., & File, K. (1973) Low dosage maintenance: A re-examination. *International Journal of Clinical Pharmacology and Toxicology, 7*, 48–53.

Schwartz, B., Lauderdale, R.M., Montgomery, M.L., Burch, E.A. & Gallant, D.M. (1987) Immediate versus delayed feedback on urinalyses reports for methadone maintenance patients. *Addictive Behaviors, 12*, 293–295.

Selwyn, P.A. (1991) Injection drug use, mortality, and the AIDS epidemic. *American Journal of Public Health, 81*, 1247–1249.

Selwyn, P.A., Feiner, C., Cox, C.P. Lipshutz, C., & Cohen, R.L. (1987) Knowledge about AIDS and high-risk behavior among intravenous drug users in New York City. *AIDS, 1*, 247–254.

Selwyn, P.A., Hartel, D., Wasserman, W., & Drucker, E. (1989b) Impact of the AIDS epidemic on morbidity and mortality among intravenous drug users in a New York City methadone maintenance program. *American Journal of Public Health, 79*, 1358–62.

Selwyn, P.A., Schoenbaum, E.E., Davenny, K., Robertson, V.J., Feingold, A.R., Shulman, J.F., Mayers, M.M., Klein, R.S., Friedland, G.H. & Rogers, M.F. (1989a) Prospective study of human immunodeficiency virus infection and pregnancy outcomes in intravenous drug users. *Journal of the American Medical Association, 261*, 1289–1294.

Senay, E.C., Dorus, W., Goldberg, F. & Thornton, W. (1977) Withdrawal from methadone maintenance: Rate of withdrawal and expectation. *Archives of General Psychiatry, 34*, 361–367.

Seow, S.S.W., Swensen, G., Willis, D., Hartfield, M. & Chapman, C. (1980) Extraneous drug use in methadone-supported patients. *Medical Journal of Australia, 1*, 269–271.

Siassi, I., Angle, B.P. & Alston, D.C. (1977a) Comparison of the effect of high and low doses of methadone on treatment outcome. *International Journal of the Addictions, 12*, 993–1005.

Siassi, I., Angle, B.P. & Alston, D.C. (1977b) Who should be counselors in methadone maintenance programs: Ex-addicts or nonaddicts? *Community Mental Health Journal, 13*, 125–132.

Siegal, H.A., Carlson, R.G., Falck, R., Li, L., Forney, M.A., Rapp, R.C., Baumgartner, K., Myers, W. & Nelson, M. (1991) HIV infection and risk behaviors among intravenous drug users in low seroprevalence areas in the midwest. *American Journal of Public Health, 81*, 1642–1644.

Simpson, D.D. (1979) The relation of time spent in drug abuse treatment to posttreatment outcome. *American Journal of Psychiatry, 136*, 1449–1453.

Simpson, D.D. (1981) Treatment for drug abuse: Follow-up outcomes and length of time spent. *Archives of General Psychiatry, 38*, 875–880.

Simpson, D.D., & Sells, S.B. (1982) Effectiveness of treatment for drug abuse: An overview of the DARP research program. *Advances in Alcohol and Substance Abuse, 2* (1), 7–29.

Simpson, D.D., Joe, G.W. & Bracy, S.A. (1982) Six-year follow-up of opioid addicts after admission to treatment. *Archives of General Psychiatry, 39*, 1318–1323.

Simpson, D.D., Joe, G.W., Lehman, W.E.K. & Sells, S.B. (1986) Addiction careers: Etiology, treatment, and 12-year follow-up outcomes. *Journal of Drug Issues, 16*, 107–121.

Sisk, J E., Hatziandreu, E.J. & Hughes, R. (1990) *The Effectiveness of Drug Abuse Treatment: Implications for Controlling AIDS/HIV Infection*. U.S.: Congress of the United States, Office of Technology Assessment.

Skinner, J.A. & Goldberg, A.E. (1986) Evidence for a drug dependence syndrome among narcotic users. *British Journal of Addiction, 81*, 479–484.

Snowden, L.R. (1978) Personality tailored covert sensitization of heroin abuse. *Addictive Behaviors, 3*, 43–49.

Sobel, J.D. (1991) Aquired Immune Deficiency Sydrome in intravenous drug abusers. In D.P. Levine & J.D. Sobel (Eds), *Infections in Intraveous Drug Abusers*. New York: Oxford University Press.

Sontag, S. (1988) *AIDS and Its Metaphors*. New York: Farrar, Straus and Giroux.

Sorensen, J.L., Acampora, A.P. & Deitch, D.A. (1984b) From maintenance to abstinence in a therapeutic community: Preliminary results. *Journal of Psychoactive Drugs, 16*, 73–77.

Sorensen, J.L., Acampora, A.P. & Iscoff, D. (1984a) From maintenance to abstinence in a therapeutic community: Clinical treatment methods. *Journal of Psychoactive Drugs, 16*, 229–239.

Sorensen, J.L., Batki, S.L., Good, P. & Wilkinson, K. (1989a) Methadone maintenance program for AIDS-affected opiate addicts. *Journal of Substance Abuse Treatment, 6*, 87–94.

Sorensen, J.L., Constantini, M.F. & London, J.A. (1989b) Coping with AIDS: Strategies for patients and staff in drug abuse treatment programs. *Journal of Psychoactive Drugs, 21*, 435–440.

Stanton, M.D., Todd, T.C. & Associates (1982) *The Family Therapy of Drug Abuse and Addiction*. New York: Guilford.

Stark, M.J. & Campbell, B.K. (1991) A psychoeducational approach to methadone maintenance treatment: A survey of client reactions. *Journal of Substance Abuse Treatment, 8*, 125–131.

State Coroner of Victoria. (1990) *Records of Investigation into Deaths: Case Nos. 623/89, 3273/89, 4439/88*. Melbourne: State Coroner's Office.

Steer, R.A. & Kotzker, E. (1980) Affective changes in male and female methadone patients. *Drug and Alcohol Dependence, 5*, 115–122.

Stimmel, B., Goldberg, J., Cohen, M. & Rotkopf, E. (1978) Detoxification from methadone maintenance: Risk factors associated with relapse to narcotic use. *Arnals of the New York Academy of Sciences, 311*, 173–180.

Stimmel, B., Goldberg, J., Rotkopf, E. & Cohen, M. (1977) Ability to remain abstinent after methadone detoxification: A six year study. *Journal of the American Medical Association, 237*, 1216–1220.

Stimson, G. & Lart, R. (1991) HIV, drugs, and public health in England: New worlds, old tunes. *International Journal of the Addictions, 26*, 1263–1277.

Stimson, G.V. (1990) AIDS and HIV: The challenge for British drug services. *British Journal of Addiction, 85*, 329–339.

Stimson, G.V. & Oppenheimer, E. (1982) *Heroin Addiction: Treatment and Control in Britain*. London: Tavistock.

Stitzer, M.L., Bickel, W.K., Bigelow, G.E. & Liebson, I.A. (1986) Effect of methadone dose contingencies on urinalysis test results of polydrug-abusing methadone-maintenance patients. *Drug and Alcohol Dependence, 18*, 341–348.

Stitzer, M.L., Bigelow, G.E. & McCaul, M.E. (1985) Behavior therapy in drug abuse treatment: Review and evaluation. In R.J. Ashberry (Ed), *Progress in the development of cost-effective treatment for drug abusers*. NIDA Research Monograph 58. Maryland: National Institute on Drug Abuse.

Strain, E.C., Brooner, R.K. & Bigelow, G.E. (1991a) Clustering of multiple substance use and psychiatric diagnoses in opiate addicts. *Drug and Alcohol Dependence, 27,* 127–134.

Strain, E.C., Stitzer, M.L. & Bigelow, G.E. (1991b) Early treatment time course of depressive symptoms in opiate addicts. *Journal of Nervous and Mental Disease, 179,* 215–221.

Strang, J. & Gossop, M. (1990) Comparison of linear versus inverse exponential methadone reduction curves in the detoxification of opiate addicts. *Addictive Behaviors, 15,* 541–547.

Stripp, A.M., Burgess, P.M., Pattison, P.E., Pead, J. & Holman, P. (1990) An evaluation of the psychoactive substance dependence syndrome in its application to opiate users. *British Journal of Addiction, 85,* 621–627.

Suffet, F. & Brotman, R. (1984) A comprehensive care program for pregnant addicts: Obstetrical, neonatal, and child development outcomes. *International Journal of the Addictions, 19,* 199–219.

Sutherland, G., Edwards, G., Taylor, C., Phillips, G., Gossop, M. & Brady, R. (1986) The measurement of opiate dependence. *British Journal of Addiction, 81,* 485–494.

Sutherland, G., Edwards, G., Taylor, C., Phillips, G.T. & Gossop, M.R. (1988) The opiate dependence syndrome: Replication study using the SODQ in a New York clinic. *British Journal of Addiction, 83,* 755–760.

Sutton, L.R. & Hinderliter, S.A. (1990) Diazepam abuse in pregnant women on methadone maintenance: Implications for the neonate. *Clinical Pediatrics, 29,* 108–111.

Swensen, G. (1989) The cost of the Western Australian methadone program. *Australian Drug and Alcohol Review, 8,* 35-37.

Swift, W., Williams, G., Neill, O. & Grenyer, B. (1990) The prevalence of minor psychopathology in opioid users seeking treatment. *British Journal of Addiction, 85,* 629–634.

Szapocznik, J. & Ladner, R. (1977) Factors related to successful retention in methadone maintenance: A review. *International Journal of the Addictions, 12,* 1067–1085.

Task Force on DSM-IV. (1991) *DSM-IV Options Book: Work in Progress 9/1/91.* U.S.A.: American Psychiatric Association.

Tennant, F.S. (1987) Inadequate plasma concentrations in some high-dose methadone maintenance patients. *American Journal of Psychiatry, 144,* 1349–1350.

Tennant, F.S. Jr., Rawson, R.A., Cohen, A., Tarver, A., & Clabough, D. (1984) Methadone plasma levels and persistent drug abuse in high dose maintenance patients. *NIDA Research Monograph, 49,* 262–8.

Thakur, N., Kaltenbach, K., Peacock, J., Weiner, S. & Finnegan, L. (1990) The relationship between maternal methadone dose during pregnancy and infant outcome. *Pediatric Research, 27,* 227a.

Thorley, A. (1980) Longitudinal studies of drug dependence. In G. Edwards and C. Rush (Eds), *Drug Problems in Britain: A Review of Ten Years.* London: Academic Press.

Thornton, L., Clune, M., Maguire, R., Griffin, E. & O'Connor, J. (1990) Narcotic addiction: The expectant mother and her baby. *Irish Medical Journal, 83,* 139–142.

Todd, T.C. (1984) A contingency analysis of family treatment and drug abuse. In J. Grabowski, M.L. Stitzer & J.E. Henningfield (Eds), *Behavioural Intervention Techniques in Drug Abuse Treatment.* NIDA Research Monograph 46. U.S.A.: National Institute on Drug Abuse.

Torrens, M., San, L., Peri, J.M. & Olle, J.M. (1991) Cocaine abuse among heroin addicts in Spain. *Drug and Alcohol Dependence, 27,* 29–34.

Trapido, E.J., Lewis, N., & Comerford, M. (1990) HIV-1-related and nonrelated diseases among IV drug users and sexual partners. *Journal of Drug Issues, 20,* 245–266.

Treece, C. & Nicholson, B. (1980) DSM-III personality type and dose levels in methadone maintenance patients. *The Journal of Nervous and Mental Disease, 168*, 621–8.

Trellis, E.S., Smith, F.F., Alston, D.C. & Siassi, I. (1975) The pitfalls of urine surveillance: The role research in evaluation and remedy. *Addictive Behaviors, 1*, 83–88.

Turner, C. F., Miller, H.G., & Moses, L.E. (Eds), (1989) *AIDS: Sexual behavior and intravenous drug use*. National Academy Press: Washington.

Uchtenhagen, A. (1990a) Impact of AIDS epidemiology on methadone policy. In A. Arif & J. Westermeyer (Edsa. *Methadone Maintenance in the Management of Opioid Dependence: An International Review*. New York: Praeger.

Uchtenhagen, A. (1990b) Policy and practice of methadone maintenance: An analysis of worldwide experience. In A. Arif & J. Westermeyer (Eds), *Methadone Maintenance in the Management of Opioid Dependence: An International Review*. New York: Praeger.

Vaillant, G.E. (1973) A 20 year follow-up of New York narcotic addicts. *Archives of General Psychiatry, 29*, 237–241.

Vaillant, G.E. (1966) A twelve-year follow-up of New York narcotic addicts: I. The relation of treatment to outcome. *American Journal of Psychiatry, 122*, 727–737.

van den Hoek, J.A.R., van Haastrecht, H.J.A., & Coutinho, R.A. (1990) Heterosexual behaviour of intravenous drug users in Amsterdam: Implications for the AIDS epidemic. *AIDS, 4*, 449–453.

van den Hoek, J.A.R., van Haastrecht, H.J.A., Scheeringa-Troost, B., Goudsmit, J., & Coutinho, R.A. (1989) HIV infection and STD in drug addicted prostitutes in Amsterdam: Potential for heterosexual HIV transmission. *Genitourinary Medicine, 65*, 146–50.

Vanichseni, S., Wongsuwan, B., Staff of the BMA Narcotics Clinic No. 6, Choopanya, K. & Wongpanich, K. (1991) A controlled trial of methadone maintenance in a population of intravenous drug users in Bangkok: Implications for prevention of HIV. *International Journal of the Addictions, 26*, 1313–1320.

Verebely, K.V., Volavka, J., Mulé, S., & Resnick, R. (1975) Methadone in man: Pharmacokinetic and excretion studies in acute and chronic treatment. *Clinical Pharmacology and Therapeutics, 18*, 180–190.

Verebey, K. (Ed), (1982) Opioids in mental illness: Theories, Clinical observations, and treatment possibilities. *Annals of the New York Academy of Sciences, 398*.

Volavka, J., Verebely, K., Resnick, R., & Mulé, S. (1978) Methadone dose, plasma level, and cross-tolerance to heroin in man. *Journal of Nervous and Mental Disease, 166*, 104–109.

Walcby, C. (1988) *Mothering and Addiction: Women with Children in Methadone Programs*. National Campaign Against Drug Abuse Monograph Series 4. Canberra: Australian Government Publishing Service.

Walton, R.G., Thornton, T.L., & Wahl, G.F. (1978) Serum methadone as an aid in managing methadone maintenance patients. *International Journal of the Addictions, 13*, 689–694.

Warg, R.I.H., Kochar, C., Hasegawa, A.T. & Roh, B.L. (1982) Initial methadone dose in treating opiate addiction. *International Journal of the Addictions, 17*, 357–363.

Warg, R.I.H., Wiesen, R.L., Lamid, S. & Roh, B.L. (1974) Rating the presence and severity of opiate dependence. *Clinical Pharmacology and Therapeutics, 16*, 653–658.

Ward, J., Darke, S., Hall, W. & Mattick, R. (1992) Methadone maintenance and the human immunodeficiency virus: Current issues in treatment and research. *British Journal of Addiction, 87*, 447–453.

Waters, N., Gaha, T.J., & Reynolds, I. (1975) Random urine analyses from drug addicts in a methadone treatment programme. *Medical Journal of Australia, 2*, 170–172.

Weber, R., Lederberger, B., Opravil, M., Siegenthaler, W. & Lüthy, R. (1990)

Progression of HIV infection in misusers of injected drugs who stop injecting or follow a programme of maintenance treatment with methadone. *British Medical Journal, 301,* 1362–1365.

Weddington, W.W. (1990–91) Towards a rehabilitation of methadone maintenance: Integration of relapse prevention and aftercare. *International Journal of the Addictions, 25,* 1201–1224.

Weiss, R.D., Mirin, S.M., & Griffin, M.L. (1992) Methodological considerations in the diagnosis of coexisting psychiatric disorders in substance abusers. *British Journal of Addiction, 87,* 179–187.

Weissman, M.M., Slobetz, F., Prusoff, B., Mezritz, M. & Howard, P. (1976) Clinical depression among narcotic addicts maintained on methadone in the community. *American Journal of Psychiatry, 133,* 1434–1438.

Wells, R. & McKay, B. (1989) *Review of Funding of Methadone Programs in Australia.* Report to Department of Community Services and Health.

Wermuth, L., Brummett, S. & Sorensen, J.L. (1987) Bridges and barriers to recovery: Clinical observations from an opiate recovery project. *Journal of Substance Abuse Treatment, 4,* 189–196.

Whitehead, C.C. (1974) Methadone pseudowithdrawal syndrome: Paradigm for a psychopharmacological model of opiate addiction. *Psychosomatic Medicine, 36,* 189–198.

Wiesen, R.L., Rich, C.R., Wang, R.I.H. & Stockdale, S.L. (1977) The safety and value of naloxone as a therapeutic aid. *Drug and Alcohol Dependence, 2,* 123–130.

Willet, E.A. (1973) Group therapy in a methadone treatment program: An evaluation of changes in interpersonal behaviour. *International Journal of the Addictions, 8,* 33–39.

Williams, H.R. (1971) Low and high methadone maintenance in the out-patient treatment of the hard core heroin addict. In S.Einstein (Ed), *Methadone maintenance.* New York: Marcel Dekker.

Wilson, G.S. (1989) Clinical studies of infants and children exposed prenatally to heroin. *Annals of the New York Academy of Sciences, 562,* 183–194.

Wittmann, B.K. & Segal, S. (1991) A comparison of the effects of single- and split-dose methadone administration on the fetus: Ultrasound evaluation. *International Journal of the Addictions, 26,* 213–218.

Wodak, A. (1985) The treatment of heroin dependence — an overview. *Proceedings of the Institute of Criminology, 65,* 27–44.

Wodak, A., Dolan, K., Imrie, A.A., Gold, J., Wolk, J., Whyte, B.M., & Cooper, D.A. (1987) Antibodies to the human immunodeficiency virus in needles and syringes used by intravenous drug abusers. *Medical Journal of Australia, 147,* 275–276.

Wolff, K., Hay, A. & Raistrick, D. (1991a) High-dose methadone and the need for drug measurements in plasma. *Clinical Chemistry, 37,* 1651–1654.

Wolff, K., Sanderson, M., Hay, A.W.M. & Raistrick, D. (1991b) Methadone concentrations in plasma and their relationship to drug dosage. *Clinical Chemistry, 37,* 205–209.

Wolk. J., Wodak, A., Guinan, J.J., Macaskill, P., & Simpson, J.M. (1990b) The effect of a needle and syringe exchange on a methadone maintenance unit. *British Journal of Addiction, 85,* 1445–1450.

Wolk, J., Wodak, A., Morlet, A., Guinan, J.J., & Gold, J. (1990a) HIV-related risk-taking behaviour, knowledge and serostatus of intravenous drug users in Sydney. *Medical Journal of Australia, 152,* 453–458.

Wolk, J., Wodak, A., Morlet, A., Guinan, J.J., Wilson, E., Gold, J., & Cooper, D.A. (1988) Syringe HIV seroprevalence and behavioural and demographic characteristics of intravenous drug users in Sydney, Australia, 1987. *AIDS, 2,* 373–377.

Woody, G., O'Hare, K., Mintz, J. & O'Brien, C. (1975) Rapid intake: A method for increasing retention rate of heroin addicts seeking methadone treatment. *Comprehensive Psychiatry, 16,* 165–169.

Woody, G.E., Luborsky, L., McLellan, A.T. & O'Brien, C.P. (1986) Psychotherapy as an adjunct to methadone treatment. In R.E. Meyer (Ed), *Psychopathology and Addictive Disorders*. U.S.A.: Guilford Press.

Woody, G.E., Luborsky, L., McLellan, A.T., O'Brien, C.P., Beck, A.T., Blaine, J., Herman, I. & Hole, A. (1983) Psychotherapy for opiate addicts. Does it help? *Archives of General Psychiatry, 40*, 639–645.

Woody, G.E., McLellan, A.T., Luborsky, L., & O'Brien, C.P. (1985b) Sociopathy and psychotherapy outcome. *Archives of General Psychiatry, 42*, 1081–1086.

Woody, G.E., McLellan, A.T., Luborsky, L. & O'Brien, C.P. (1990) Psychotherapy and counseling for methadone-maintained opiate addicts: Results of research studies. In L.S. Onken & J.D. Blaine (Eds), *Psychotherapy and Counseling in the Treatment of Drug Abuse*. NIDA Research Monograph 104. Maryland: National Institute on Drug Abuse.

Woody, G.E., McLellan, A.T., Luborsky, L., & O'Brien, C.P. (1987) Twelve-month follow-up of psychotherapy for opiate dependence. *American Journal of Psychiatry, 144*, 590–596.

Woody, G.E., McLellan, A.T., Luborsky, L., O'Brien, C.P., Blaine, J., Fox, S., Herman, I. & Beck, A.T. (1984) Severity of psychiatric symptoms as a predictor of benefits from psychotherapy: The Veterans Administration–Penn study. *American Journal of Psychiatry, 141*, 1172–1177.

World Health Organization. (1990) *Guidelines for Counselling About HIV Infection and Disease*. Geneva: WHO.

Wu, C.H. & Henry, J.A. (1990) Deaths of heroin addicts starting on methadone maintenance. *Lancet, 335*, 424.

Yancovitz, S.R., Des Jarlais, D.C., Peyser, N.P., Drew, E., Freidmann, P., Trigg, H.L. & Robinson, J.W. (1991) A randomized trial of an interim methadone maintenance clinic. *American Journal of Public Health, 81*, 1185–1191.

Zilm, D.H. & Sellers, E.M. (1978) The quantitative assessment of physical dependence on opiates. *Drug and Alcohol Dependence, 3*, 419–428.

Zweben, J.E. (1986) Recovery oriented psychotherapy. *Journal of Substance Abuse Treatment, 3*, 255–262.

Zweben, J.E. (1991) Counseling issues in methadone maintenance treatment. *Journal of Psychoactive Drugs, 23*, 177–190.

INDEX

INDEX

Ball J.C. (see Three Cities Study)
blockade (see narcotic blockade)
breastfeeding: hepatitis B and, 249;
  hepatitis C and, 249; HIV and, 248;
  methadone maintenance and, 253

clonidine, 205–208
cocaine: effectiveness of methadone
  maintenance and, 57–58; use
  associated with HIV seropositivity, 47
contingency management, 127–131
counselling, 138–147, 163–169, 154–156,
  223–228: as practised in methadone
  clinics, 139–143; characteristics of
  effective counsellors, 163–166;
  cognitive behavioural therapy,
  149–153, 154, 155–156, 163, 199;
  during withdrawal from methadone,
  208–209; enforcing clinic rules and,
  223–224; group therapy, 155–156; HIV
  and 223–225, 226–228; motivational
  interviewing/counselling, 81–83,
  154–155, 165–166, 228; necessity of,
  143–146; role in methadone
  maintenance treatment, 139; training
  and effectiveness, 146–147; unsafe
  sexual behaviour and, 224–225

detoxification fear, 199–201
Dole and Nyswander model of methadone
  maintenance, 1, 2, 37, 40, 67, 90–91,
  139, 170–171, 195, 222, 272, 273, 275,
  279, 283, 285, 286
dosage (methadone), 86–115: during
  pregnancy, 239–241; flexibility in
  setting, 111–112; high dose (see high
  dose methadone maintenance); initial
  dosing, 86–87, 88–90; low dose (see
  low dose methadone maintenance);
  patient characteristics and, 109–111,
  112; patient self-regulation of, 112–114;
  prior opioid use and initial dosing, 88
Drug Abuse Reporting Program (DARP),
  28–29, 174–175
DSM-III-R: criteria for opioid
  dependence, 75–76; criteria for
  antisocial personality disorder,
  262–263
duration of treatment, 170–195:
  characteristics of methadone programs
  and, 185–187; models of treatment
  and, 188–193; patient characteristics
  and, 183–185; reason for leaving
  treatment and, 179–180; time-limited
  methadone maintenance and, 180–182;
  treatment outcome and, 171–182

effectiveness of methadone maintenance:
  cocaine, 57–58; HIV, 53–61;
  observational studies, 22–40; overall
  appraisal of, 281–286; randomised
  controlled trials, 12–21

family therapy, 156–161

hair analysis, 134–135
Hargreaves, W.A., 92–97, 99, 100, 102,
  103, 109, 113, 114, 171–172, 173, 175,
  179, 189
harm reduction: abstinence as goal of
  treatment and, 45–46, 220–222,
  233–234; assessment of harm, 77–79;
  HIV and, 219–221; iatrogenic
  methadone dependence and, 82;
  methadone maintenance and, 220, 222,
  224;
hepatitis (B and C), 41–42: deaths due to
  methadone overdose and, 88;
  pregnancy, 249–250; prevalence
  among injecting drug users, 47, 54
high dose methadone maintenance;
  effectiveness of, 103–104; heroin use
  and, 99–102; rationale for, 90–91;
  retention rates and, 96–99
HIV (see also AIDS), 41–61, 219–234:
  Australian injecting drug users and, 45;
  breastfeeding, 248; changes in
  treatment for drug dependence, 221;
  clinic staff, 232–233; counselling and,
  223–225, 226–228; education to
  change behaviour and, 225–226; effect
  of pregnancy on HIV-disease status,
  246–247; epidemiology of, 43–46;
  groups to change behaviour, 226–227;
  harm reduction and, 220–221;
  homosexual and bisexual male
  injectors and, 52; injecting drug use
  and, 43–53; management of
  seropositive patients, 231–232;
  methadone maintenance and, 53–57;
  methadone treatment dropouts and,
  58–59; needle sharing and, 47–50;
  perinatal transmission, 245–246;
  pregnancy and indeterminate antibody
  test results, 248; reducing risk
  behaviours, 229; risk factors associated
  with infection, 47–48, 50; sex and,
  50–53; termination of pregnancy and,
  247; testing for HIV antibodies in
  methadone programs, 229–231; unsafe
  sexual behaviour and, 52–53

injecting drug users (see also HIV, needle